LORRAINE PASCALE'S

A Lighter Way to Bake

LORRAINE PASCALE'S

A Lighter Way to Bake

Harper
Collins

Photography by Myles New

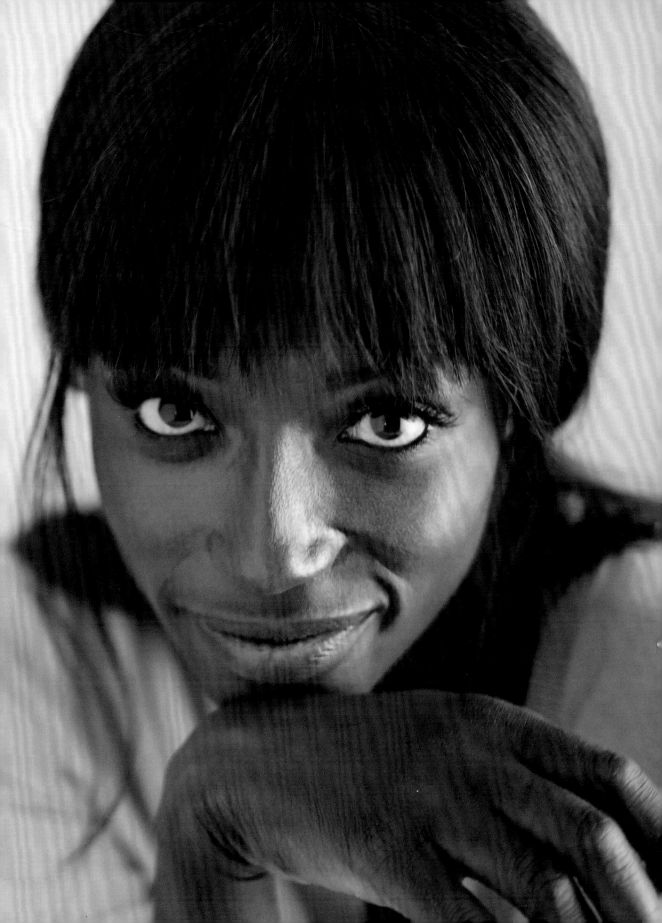

HarperCollins*Publishers*
77-85 Fulham Palace Road
London
W6 8JB
www.harpercollins.co.uk

First published by HarperCollins*Publishers* 2013
10 9 8 7 6 5 4 3 2 1
Text © Lorraine Pascale 2013
Photography © Myles New 2013
Lorraine Pascale asserts her moral right to be identified as the author of this work.
A catalogue record of this book is available from the British Library.

Food styling: Katie Giovanni and Beatrice Ferrante
Props styling: Tony Hutchinson
Art direction and design: Martin Topping
Consultant dieticians: Fiona Hinton BSc, M Nut Diet, Registered Dietician and
Elsa Robson BSc (Hons), Registered Dietician

HB ISBN: 978-0-00-753833-1
Ebook ISBN: 978-0-00-753834-8

Printed and bound in the UK by Butler, Tanner and Dennis Ltd, Frome, Somerset

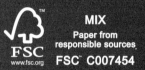

MIX
Paper from
responsible sources
FSC™ C007454

FSC™ is a non-profit international organisation established to promote the
responsible management of the world's forests. Products carrying the FSC
label are independently certified to assure consumers that they come from
forests that are managed to meet the social, economic and ecological needs
of present and future generations, and other controlled sources.

Find out more about HarperCollins and the environment at
www.harpercollins.co.uk/green

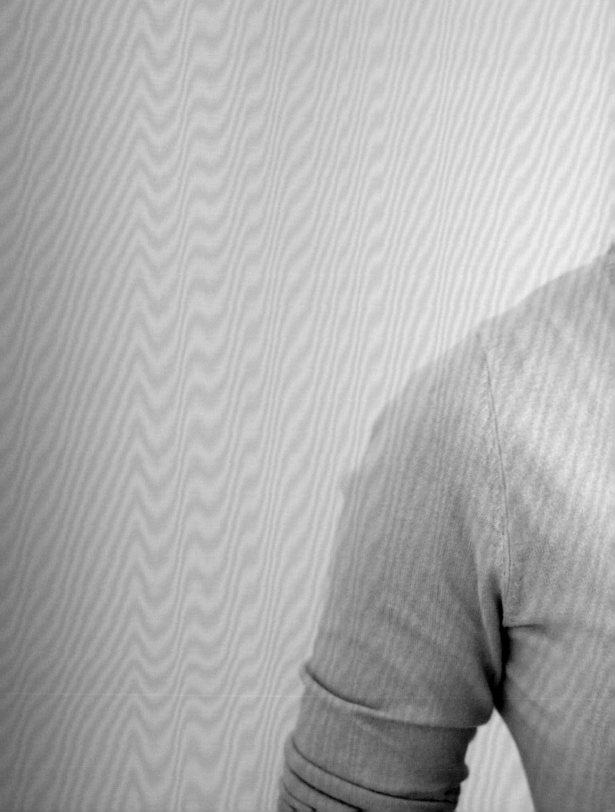

INTRODUCTION

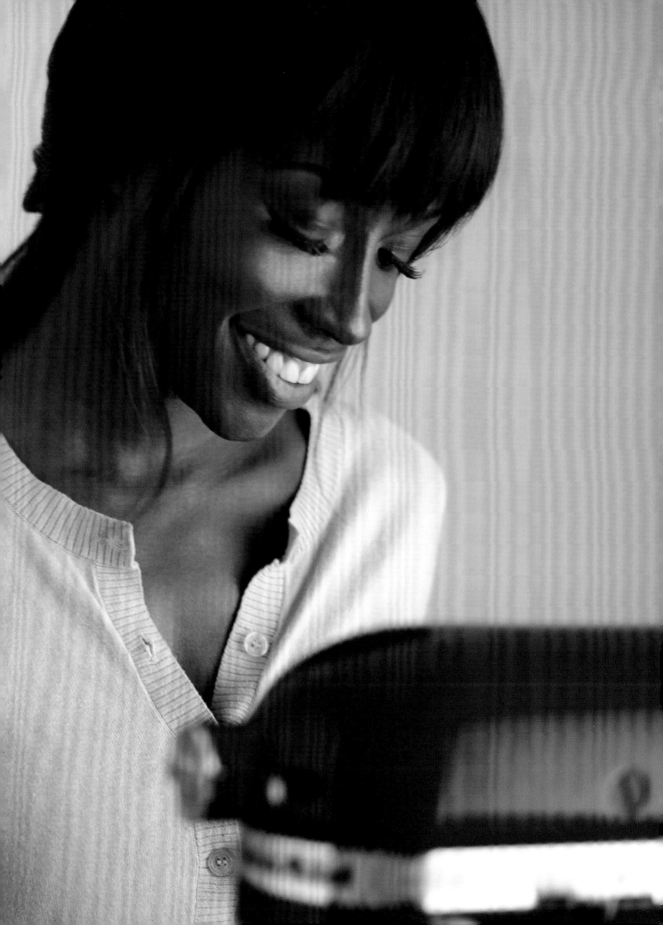

I am sitting alone one Sunday morning doing nothing in particular. Then an idea hits me from nowhere (I am full of thoughts when I am at my most relaxed, like all of us I suppose!) – what if I could create a book of recipes that were lighter in fat, sugar and calories but that tasted just as good as naughty ones? Sounds easy, I think to myself! I phone a friend who, after hearing my latest new idea, responds with, 'Why would anyone not want that... but can you really do it?' At the time I didn't know what a mammoth task I had set myself.

My first challenge was to make a lighter sponge – a lighter Victoria sponge. A doddle, I thought, but 11 attempts later and with a pile of quasi-sponge sandwiches covering my kitchen table, I thought it had beaten me. I genuinely felt despondent and a little bit stupid. But I was encouraged by my loyal publishers and a close circle of friends to keep going, which I did, thankfully. I hadn't realized that as I approached the eleventh attempt of the sponge, I had been getting close to the magic formula. The twelfth came out of the oven exactly like I'd envisaged it would. Eureka! I had cracked it, and my journey to lighter baking began in earnest.

I own an unashamedly indulgent cupcake shop in Covent Garden, and have done so for a good few years. It could therefore perhaps seem strange for me to be writing a book on how to lighten your baking. However, in the shop we do our best to reduce the fat and sugar in the cakes, constantly tweaking them to make them more healthy while retaining the flavours people know and love. These cakes were sources of much inspiration as I embarked on developing lighter bakes.

Writing the recipes for this book was totally counterintuitive. When developing 'normal' recipes, the way to guarantee they'll taste great is by loading them with lots of full-fat butter and sugar. So how on earth was I going to create 'lighter' indulgences that still had you going back for more? I started to do lots of research, scouring magazines, books, the web, and reports by associations such as the British Nutrition Foundation, the NHS and the British Heart Foundation, to see their recommendations on nutritious sweet treats. Funnily enough there is not much information out there (yet I believe there will be) so it was going to be a journey of trial and error. Many a trial and many an error!

I went to the supermarket and bought a stack of dairy products (cream cheese, crème fraîche, cottage cheese, etc. – low-, full- and no-fat versions) and began decreasing the butter, substituting it with other dairy. Some cakes came out flat, some thin, but eventually I found a rhythm which enabled the bakes to work.

A team of dietitians and nutritional specialists helped me too (I say helped, they pretty much did all of the nutritional calculations!), figuring out the nutritional breakdown of each recipe as we sought to achieve the optimum mix. We then scoured other recipes out there to find a comparative full-fat, plenty-of-sugar reference point. I thought it would be good to share these comparisons with you so you can see exactly what you are getting and exactly how the recipes compare to their less-healthy comparisons per same-size serving. It's not an exact science, and is not intended to be so, but hopefully it offers a clear indication of what the difference is. I struggled to reduce the sugar and fat in significant enough quantities in some of the recipes, so some are pretty much the same as the recipe I compare them to, but I have taken the liberty of leaving the analyses in and, wherever possible, added wholemeal flour to make them a healthier bite at the very least.

Some cheeky books wax lyrical about how low fat or low sugar a cake is, but when I read the recipe carefully it says that a cake that would usually serve 8 people, serves 16 people. Therefore each meagre slice looks really low in calories, sugar and fat however the cake itself is not. I have tried really hard not to do that. If I feel the slices are a little on the small side, I say just that: 'makes 16 skinny slices'. Transparency is the best policy , I find!

On the next page are my 'lighter' baking tips, the essence of what makes a successful light bake, for those wanting to eat healthier baked foods, those wanting to cut calories, and those wanting to eat slightly fewer or healthier carbs.

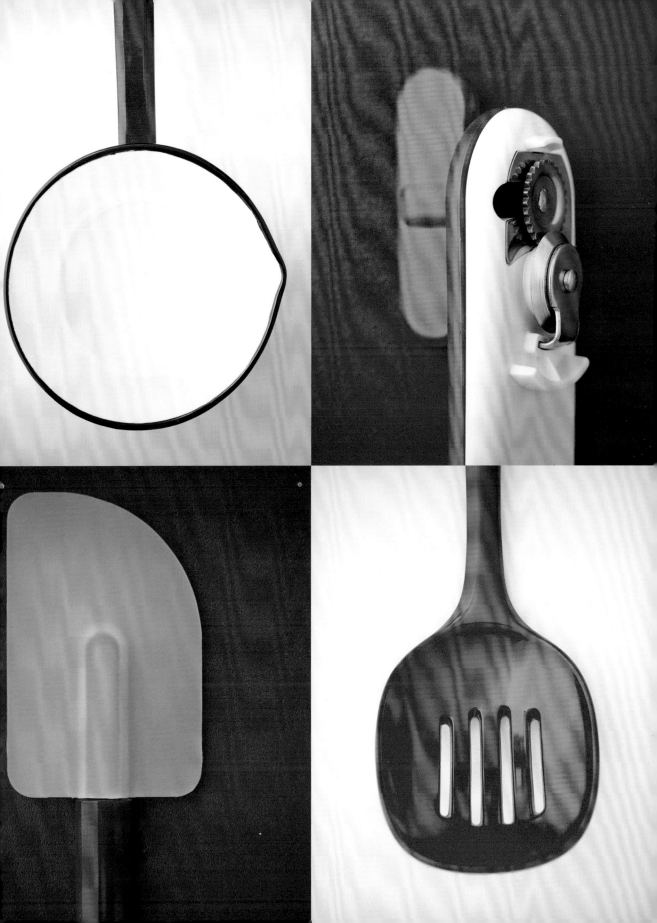

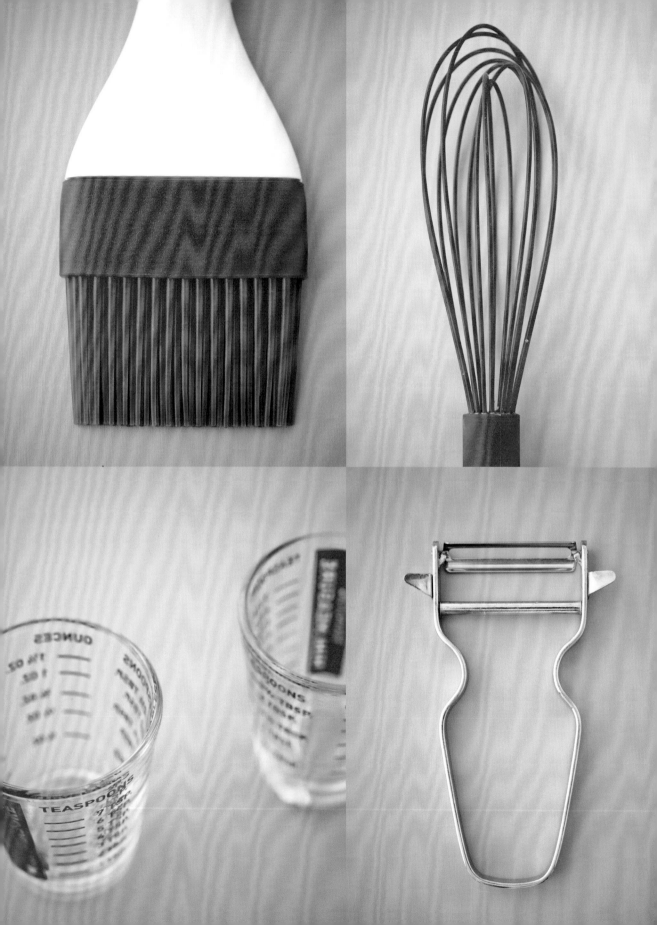

INGREDIENTS

– I tried and tested many different ways of making the cakes lighter but still keeping the naughty flavour. So beware of freestyling with the ingredients – you may not get the results you are after.

– I've substituted butter in some recipes with less naughty products like yogurt, so the texture may not be quite what you are used to; still delightful, but a little different. Cakes with lower fat and sugar content can sometimes have a firmer outside (crust) – but inside it will be like a fluffy cloud.

– All eggs are medium unless otherwise stated.

– Wholemeal flour makes an appearance in many of my recipes. It offers added fibre and a wonderfully nutty flavour, and apparently the carbohydrate is more slowly absorbed by the body than white flour.

– Truvia, Stevia, fructose, xylitol (and the list goes on) are all sugar derivatives or substitutes available in shops and online. I had a good play with them all and, to be fair, I rather liked some of them but after much research and soul searching I decided to leave them out. They are often expensive, not always available and some have received mixed reports from scientists and dietitians.

– I also decided not to use low sodium salt: nutritional experts advise it's far better to get accustomed to the taste of food with little or no salt, than replace it with a substitute, and I agree.

– Ground almonds are a good substitute for flour, if you want to head down the low-carb route. If I was brave I would have used almond flour or coconut flour instead of wheat flour – I believe this is the future in eating, as people start realizing that perhaps fat does not make you fat, it's the sugar and carbs which cause the problem. But I acknowledge that lots of people have cut fat and sugar from their diets with favourable results, and I wanted to write a book which would suit as many people as possible.

– Dried fruit is laden with sugar. I do love dried fruit, and it makes an appearance in some recipes, but I have replaced dried fruit with fresh fruit in many recipes because fresh fruit contains less concentrated sugar.

– Rapeseed oil is my oil of choice, as it is very low in saturated fat compared with other oils.

– Use the best vanilla you can afford. You can get the pods online much cheaper than in the supermarkets, or you can get vanilla bean paste or vanilla extract which are almost black in colour and smell great. Sadly vanilla essence (which comes in a tiny bottle and is the colour of dodgy beer) really is no good for flavour.

METHODS & RESULTS

– Before baking, check your oven with an oven thermometer. Because of the lower butter and sugar content of the cookies, it is really important that they are not over-cooked. If you think your bake is almost ready, that would be a good time to pull it out so it stays nice and moist.

– Lighter cakes are often lighter in colour than you might be used to. They will still taste yumsters but you can feel a lot less guilty about your tum.

– Due to their lower fat content, some of the cookies will be softer than usual, but still very tasty.

SERVING & STORING

– Keep an eye on serving sizes: indulgence needn't mean a doorstop of cake – a modest slice will hit all your sweet-tooth buttons without leaving an indelible impression on your waist.

– Cakes that are made lighter keep for a shorter length of time than other cakes. With that in mind, ideally bake them on the morning that you need them, rather than the night before. If you need to keep them overnight, put them in a tin and wrap the tin a couple of times with cling film to make it airtight. Or pop them in the fridge to keep fresh.

I sincerely hope you enjoy this book. Obviously full-fat, full-sugar bakes have their place in our hearts, but when you are thinking about wanting to enjoy your food and cooking and yet still watch your tum, this baking book is most definitely the one to reach for as a source of little guilt but oodles of pleasure.

BREAKFAST & BRUNCH

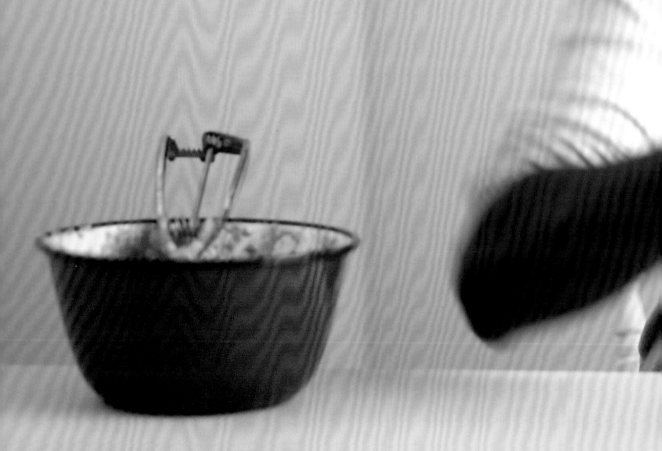

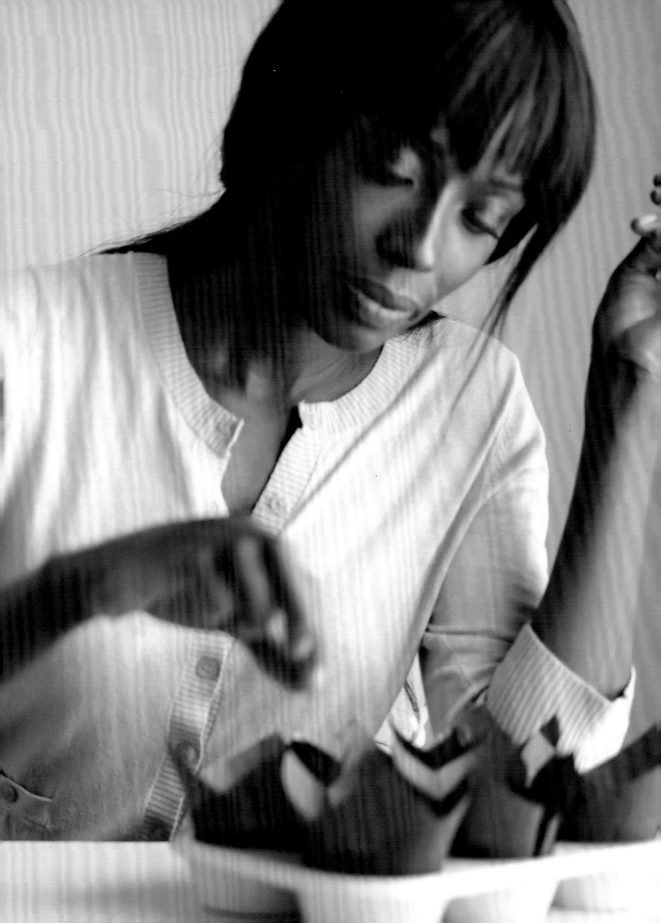

RASPBERRY & BANANA NO-KNEAD BREAKFAST LOAF

As with the Extra-Bananery Banana Loaf (see page 21), if your bananas are too hard, put them (unpeeled) on a baking tray lined with baking parchment and bake in a preheated 180°C, (Fan 160°C), 350°F, Gas Mark 4 oven for about 20 minutes. The skins will blister and go brown, but the bananas will caramelize and become sweeter and tastier.

Makes
1 loaf with 10 slices

Equipment
22 x 10cm loaf tin

50g unsalted butter
50g soft light brown sugar
2 eggs, lightly beaten
100g wholemeal flour
125g plain flour
2 tsp baking powder
2 ripe bananas, roughly mashed
125g raspberries
Handful of rolled oats

Preheat the oven to 180°C, (Fan 160°C), 350°F, Gas Mark 4 and line a 22 x 10cm loaf tin with baking parchment. I make sure that the paper overlaps a little bit, which makes it much easier to remove the loaf from the tin once it is cooked.

Cream the butter and sugar together in a large bowl until it is nicely combined. Add the eggs in two batches, beating well between each addition. The mixture won't quite look its best, but it will soon come good! Add the wholemeal flour, plain flour and baking powder and stir through until nicely mixed in. Then stir the bananas in, followed by a gentle fold in of the raspberries.

Pour the mixture into the loaf tin, smooth out a bit with the back of a spoon, and then sprinkle the oats evenly over the top. Bake in the oven for 50–55 minutes or until a skewer comes out clean when pierced in the centre.

Leave to cool in the tin for a few minutes before lifting out and leaving to cool completely on a wire rack. The loaf will stay at its best for 1 to 2 days when stored in an airtight container.

(PER SLICE)	ENERGY	FAT	SAT FAT	SUGAR	PROTEIN	SALT
LORRAINE'S RECIPE	180 Kcal	6.1g	3g	10.2g	4.7g	0.29g
COMPARISON RECIPE	225 Kcal	10.4g	6.1g	17.8g	3.3g	0.47g

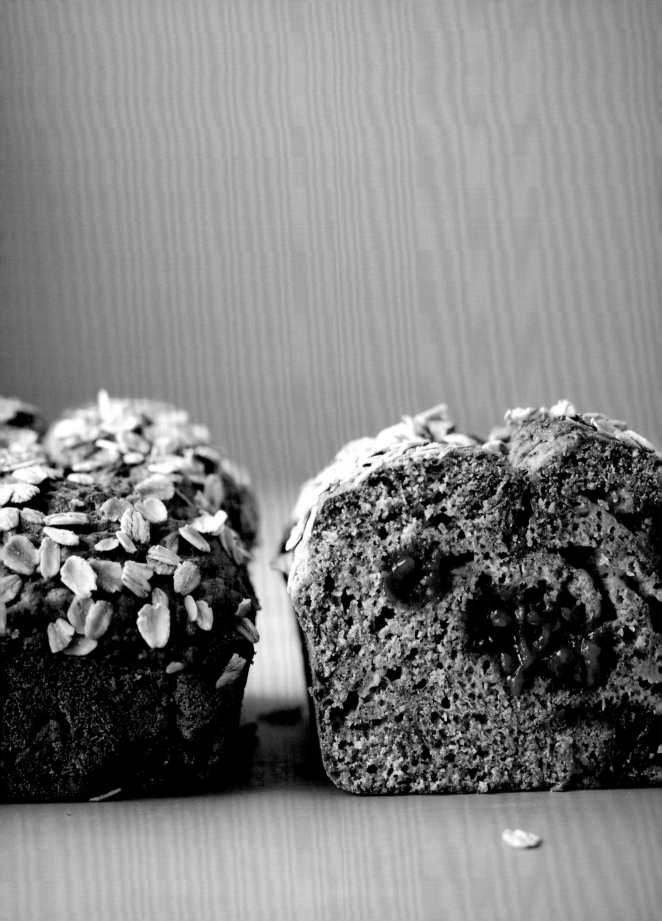

BEAUTIFUL BOILED THEN BAKED BREAKFAST BAGELS

I have been shoving wholemeal flour into everything in this book. It is a little better for you than white flour, has less calories and more fibre and iron, and I find it imparts a nutty flavour to baked goods. However, if you are really not a fan, then just substitute the 200g strong wholemeal flour for 200g strong white bread flour, so you use 500g white flour altogether. As ever, I like to keep some bagels in the freezer (sliced horizontally in half), so that when anyone wants one, I can just pop it into the toaster to heat through.

Makes

8 bagels

Equipment

Large bowl or freestanding electric mixer set with the dough hook

200g strong wholemeal bread flour

300g strong white bread flour, plus extra for dusting

7g sachet of fast-action dried yeast

1 heaped tsp salt

325ml warm water (from the tap)

Spray oil

3 tbsp honey (optional)

1 egg, lightly beaten

2 tbsp toppings in total (eg sesame seeds, poppy seeds and the reserved bran in the recipe)

Sieve the wholemeal flour (unprecedented I know, as I am not a fan of the sieving flour thing, but there is a method to my madness) into a large bowl (or food mixer bowl fitted with a dough hook). Put three-quarters of the bran that remains in the sieve back into the flour and save the remainder for later. Add the white flour (no need to sieve this one!) and then add the yeast and salt. Toss everything together and make a well in the centre. Pour in the warm water and mix together to form a soft, but not sticky dough.

Knead the dough for 10 minutes if doing by hand or 5 minutes if by machine. To test if the dough is kneaded enough, form it into a ball with a nice taut top. Put some flour onto your finger and prod the top of the bread, making an indent of about ½cm. The dough should spring back all the way if it is kneaded and be stretchy. If necessary, knead it a bit more.

Weigh the dough and divide the weight of the dough by eight, then separate the dough into eight equal-size portions weighing the amount you came up with. Place seven of the pieces under a tea towel so they don't dry out. Take one piece and roll it into a ball with a nice taut top, then dip your index finger in a little flour to coat and push it through the centre of the dough ball until it touches the work surface. With your finger still in the hole, pick it up and spin it around to make the hole bigger — about 4cm wide is ideal as the hole will close up quite a bit as the dough rises. Place the bagel onto a baking sheet lined with baking parchment and repeat with the rest of the dough balls. Space the bagels quite far apart on the baking sheet as they will expand quite a bit.

Spray the bagels with some oil and then cover them with cling film. The cling film should be loose enough for the bagels to increase in size, but still airtight.

Leave the bagels in a warm place to rise for about 40 minutes or until they have increased in size by about a third. To test if they are ready, put some flour on your finger and prod the side of the bagel, making an indent of about 5mm. The indent should spring back about halfway.

When they are ready, cover them back up and preheat the oven to 200°C, (Fan 180°C), 400°F, Gas Mark 6.

Pour 2 litres of water into a wide pan and bring to the boil (popping a lid on will help do this more quickly). Once boiling, stir the honey through. This will add shine and flavour to the finished bagels. Working in batches of two at a time, drop the bagels into the boiling water. They will be a bit squidgy to pick up, so the trick is to do so without misshaping them too much. Leave to boil for 15 seconds per side. Remove them from the water with a slotted spoon and place them back on the baking sheet as you go.

Once they have all been boiled, brush the bagels really well with the beaten egg so they are nicely covered. Then, scatter over your choice of toppings. Each bagel will take about ¾ of a teaspoon of topping in total, whether individual or mixed. I like to go for a selection with some coated in just sesame seeds, some just poppy seeds and then a mixture of the two. This is where the reserved bran from the flour comes in also. It is best scattered on the bagel with the seeds rather than on its own.

Finally, bake the bagels in the oven for 25–30 minutes or until they are golden brown and sound hollow when tapped underneath.

(PER BAGEL)	ENERGY	FAT	SAT FAT	SUGAR	PROTEIN	SALT
LORRAINE'S RECIPE	229 Kcal	3.2g	0.5g	1g	9.4g	1.02g
COMPARISON RECIPE	244 Kcal	3g	0.4g	5.1g	8.1g	1.34g

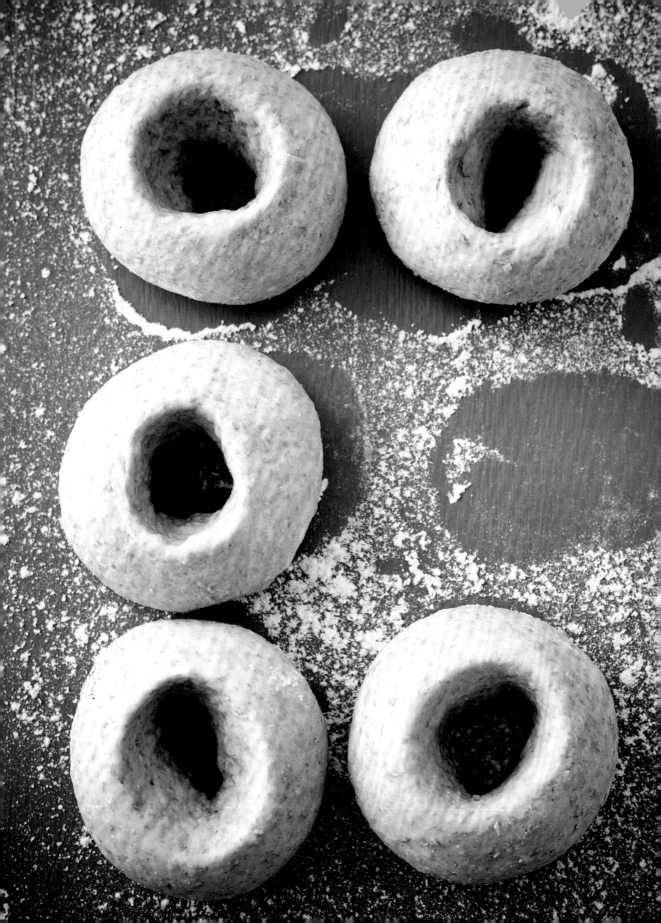

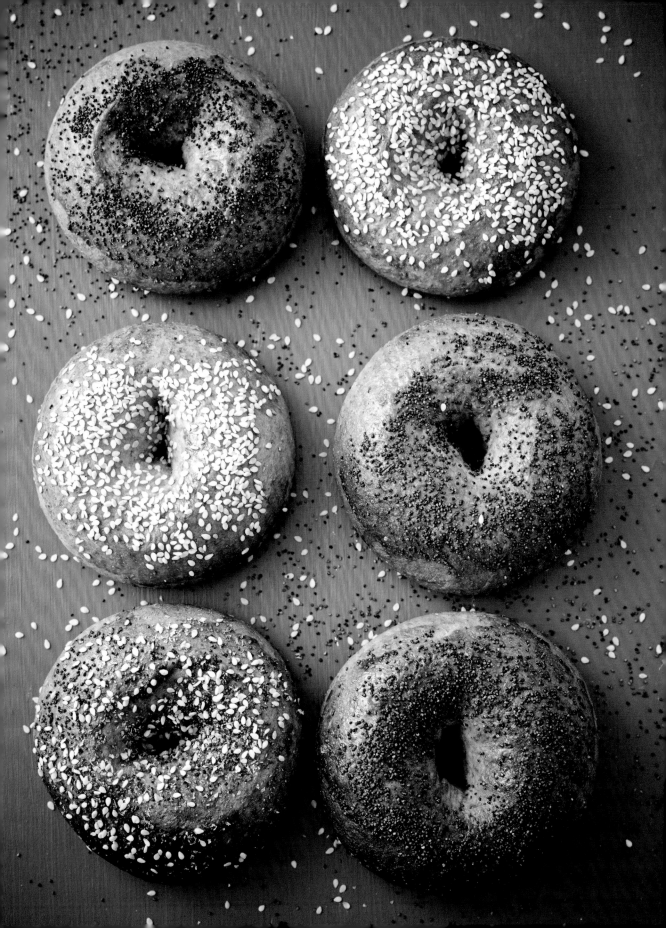

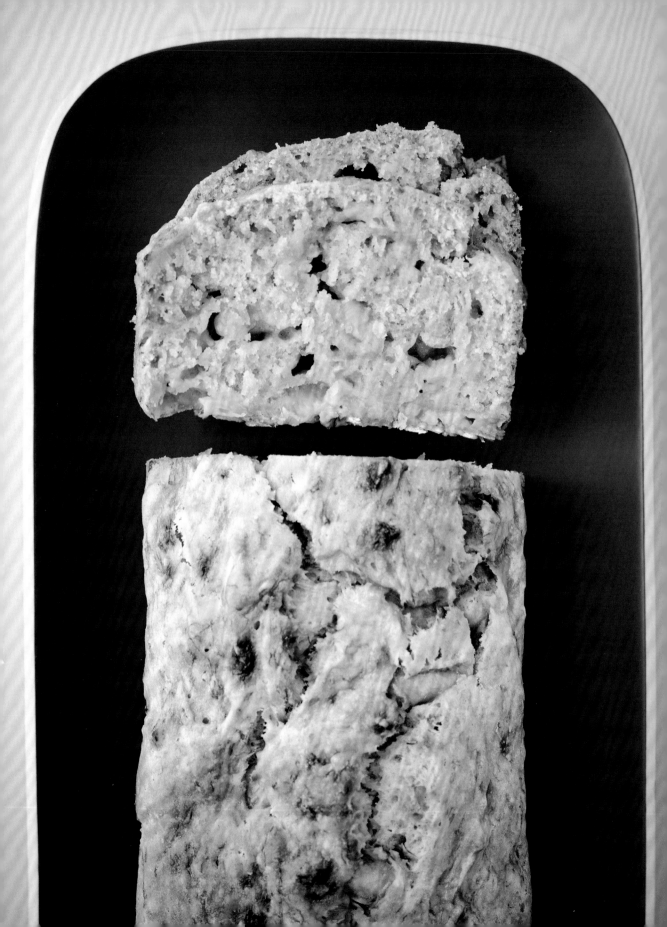

EXTRA-BANANERY BANANA LOAF

I did my online supermarket shop the other day and was waiting patiently, as I do every morning when recipe testing, for my shopping to arrive. The delivery driver, who is fast becoming my new BFF, dutifully carried the bags up the stairs, handed me the receipt and, after a brief chat, went on his way. I tore through the noisy plastic bags looking for the canary-coloured Caribbean fruit only to find, to my dismay, that the bananas were a lighter shade of lime. Unable to wait for them to mature, I turned the oven on to 200°C, (Fan 180°C), 400°F, Gas Mark 6, shoved them in and baked them for about 20 minutes until their skins turned black. After cooling, the bananas were peeled to reveal their expedited overripe mushiness, just perfect for this dish.

Makes
1 loaf with 10 skinny slices

Equipment
22 x 10cm loaf tin

25g rolled oats
4 just overripe bananas
  (or see recipe intro)
200g self-raising flour
50ml maple syrup
25g unsalted butter, melted
50ml olive oil
Pinch of salt

Preheat the oven to 180°C, (Fan 160°C), 350°F, Gas Mark 4 and line a 22 x 10cm loaf tin with baking parchment. I make sure that the paper overlaps a little bit, which makes it easier to remove the baked loaf from the tin.

Scatter about a third of the oats in the bottom of the loaf tin. Cut one banana up into ½cm-thick rounds and lay them out in an even layer on top of the oats.

Peel and roughly mash the remaining bananas in a large bowl. Add the flour, maple syrup, butter, olive oil, salt and remaining oats and stir everything together until well mixed to a soft dropping consistency. Carefully pour the mixture into the loaf tin on top of the bananas. Spread out evenly with the back of a spoon and bake in the oven for 45 minutes.

Once cooked, remove from the oven and allow to cool a little in the tin before lifting out and leaving to cool a little more. This loaf is delicious served warm or cold and stays at its best for 1 to 2 days in an airtight container.

(PER SLICE)	ENERGY	FAT	SAT FAT	SUGAR	PROTEIN	SALT
LORRAINE'S RECIPE	191 Kcal	7.2g	2.1g	12.7g	2.7g	0.21g
COMPARISON RECIPE	202 Kcal	7.1g	4g	19.8g	3.1g	0.46g

APPLE & APRICOT SPICED HOT-CROSS MUFFINSKIS

Sometimes I come up with a name for a recipe that I like the ring to and then spend time coming up with a recipe to suit. This is one of those very recipes. The muffinskis are really just hot-cross buns shoved in baking parchment, but they still look a bit different to the buns baked in a tin. The cross on the buns is not ultra-bright Simon Cowell teeth white due to the addition of the cinnamon. So if you want your buns to have a bit more of the X Factor, then just leave the cinnamon out.

Makes

12 muffinskis

Equipment

12-hole muffin tin, large bowl or freestanding electric mixer set with the dough hook, disposable piping bag

Buns

300g strong white bread flour, plus extra for dusting
200g wholemeal flour
3 tsp mixed spice
2 tsp ground cinnamon
1½ tsp fast-action dried yeast
Good pinch of salt
325ml warm water (from the tap)
1 small apple, peeled, cored and very finely diced
50g dried apricots, finely chopped
Finely grated zest of 1 orange
Spray oil
1 tbsp maple syrup

Cross

2 tbsp strong white bread flour
1 tsp ground cinnamon
2 tbsp water

Cut out 12 squares of baking parchment and set them aside along with a 12-hole muffin tin.

Toss the flours, mixed spice, cinnamon, yeast and salt in a large bowl (or food mixer bowl). Make a well in the centre and pour in the warm water. Mix everything together well (by hand or in the machine set with a dough hook) to give a smooth, soft dough ball.

If doing by machine, continue to knead for 5 minutes. Otherwise, put the dough onto a clean work surface sprinkled with a little flour and knead for about 10 minutes. To test if the dough has been kneaded enough, form the dough into a ball with a nice taut smooth top and then put some flour on your finger. Make an indent on the side of the dough about 5mm deep. The dent should spring back completely, showing that the dough is ready for the next stage. If it does not spring back, then keep kneading for a little longer.

Roll the dough out on a lightly floured surface into about a 25-cm wide circle. Toss the apple, apricots and orange zest together in a small bowl and pile the mixture into the centre of the dough. Then fold the edges of the dough up and over the filling to enclose, turn it over and roll out again to about the same size circle. Once again gather the edges up and over, but then knead the dough by hand to incorporate the filling ingredients evenly throughout. You may need to dust with a little more flour as you go if the apples make things a little damp.

Preheat the oven to 200°C, (Fan 180°C), 400°F, Gas Mark 6.

Divide the dough into 12 equal-sized pieces and shape each one into a ball with a smooth, taut top. Push a baking parchment square into a hole in the muffin tin and sit a dough ball, seam side down, into it. Repeat with the remaining dough balls.

Spray a little oil on top of the buns and then cover them loosely with cling film so they are airtight, but leaving room for them to rise. Leave the buns to rise for about 30 minutes in a warm place (I leave them to rise on a chair about a metre from the preheating oven) or until they have doubled in size.

About 5 minutes before the end of the dough rising time, prepare the cross mixture. Put the flour and cinnamon into a small bowl and gradually add the water, stirring all the time, to make a smooth, thick paste. Pour this into the piping bag, seal it closed and snip a 3mm piece off the end.

Once the dough balls have risen, remove the cling film and slowly and carefully pipe a cross on each one. Bake in the oven for 10–15 minutes or until the buns are well risen and crusty on top. Once they are cooked, remove them from the oven, brush with the maple syrup and leave to cool in the tin. Serve warm or cold.

(PER MUFFINSKI)	ENERGY	FAT	SAT FAT	SUGAR	PROTEIN	SALT
LORRAINE'S RECIPE	160 Kcal	1g	0.1g	2.7g	5.8g	0.1g
COMPARISON RECIPE	243 Kcal	8.4g	4.8g	10.2g	5.5g	0.36g

SWEET POTATO, BUTTERNUT SQUASH, APPLE & SAGE MUFFINS

This muffin started out as a soup. In my laziness, I bought a few packets of prepared butternut squash and sweet potato, an apple, some sage and some good liquid stock. A boil and a blend later, I was left with an autumnal soup with a divinely delicious difference. Left with an abundance of fruit and veg, I then tossed the remainder into my muffin batter. As a side note, much like the other muffin recipes, this will not give you a huge muffin top when you pull the muffins hot from the oven.

Makes
12 muffins

Equipment
12-hole muffin tin, muffin cases

200g ready-prepared sweet potato and butternut squash mix, chopped further until quite fine
300g wholemeal flour
1 tsp baking powder
½ tsp bicarbonate of soda
1 egg
2 egg whites
250ml semi-skimmed milk
100g low-fat natural yogurt
50ml sunflower oil
1 tbsp maple syrup
3 tsp finely chopped fresh sage leaves
Pinch of salt
1 eating apple, peeled, cored and roughly grated

Preheat the oven to 200°C, (Fan 180°C), 400°F, Gas Mark 6 with the middle shelf at the ready. Line a muffin tin with 12 paper muffin cases.

Bring a steamer pan of water to the boil and steam the sweet potato and butternut squash for 5 minutes until just tender.

Meanwhile, toss the flour, baking powder and bicarbonate of soda together in a large bowl. Beat the egg and egg whites briefly in a large jug, and then beat in the milk, yogurt, oil and maple syrup until smooth and well combined. Mix the wet mixture into the dry ingredients with as few stirs as possible to give a wet, sloppy mixture. Add the now cooked sweet potato and butternut squash along with the sage and salt and gently fold in.

Pouring the mixture into a jug or using two spoons (or I like to use a mechanical ice-cream scoop), divide the mixture among the 12 cases. Scatter the grated apple evenly over the top of each one, then pop into the oven to bake for 20–25 minutes or until a skewer inserted into one of the muffins comes out clean. The centre may be a little damp from the moisture of the vegetables, but the cakey part shouldn't look raw.

Leave to cool for a few minutes in the tin before removing. Then tuck in!

(PER MUFFIN)	ENERGY	FAT	SAT FAT	SUGAR	PROTEIN	SALT
LORRAINE'S RECIPE	155 Kcal	5.3g	1g	4.9g	5.7g	0.34g
COMPARISON RECIPE	282 Kcal	13.3g	2.1g	23.5g	4.6g	0.99g

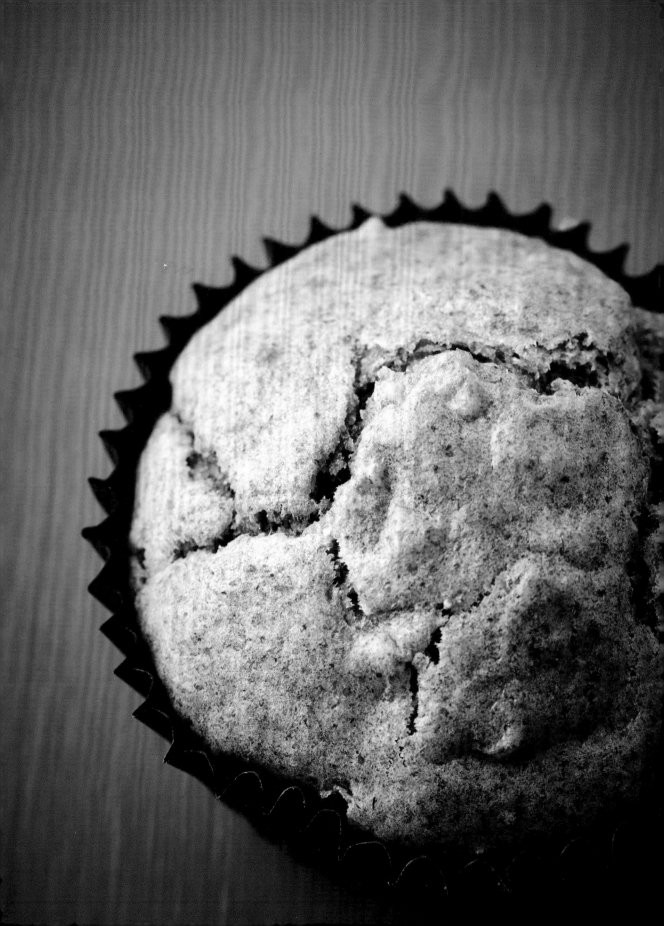

BANANA & HONEY MUFFINS

During my modelling days in New York, when I was not working I loved the Manhattan luxury of being able to order breakfast in bed. The choice would oscillate between a toasted poppy seed bagel with salmon (hold the cream cheese, I just don't like it with salmon) OR a double chocolate muffin with double chocolate chips. Now, a New York muffin is a behemoth, and don't get me wrong there is a time and a place for great big muffins, but just not in this particular book! So, these almost guilt-free muffinskis are made with yogurt, wholemeal flour, egg whites and sweetened with honey and bananas. If you look really closely, you may even see a little halo hovering above them when you pull them hot from the oven.

Makes

12 muffins

Equipment

12-hole muffin tin, muffin cases

300g wholemeal flour
1 tsp baking powder
½ tsp bicarbonate of soda
1 egg
2 egg whites
200ml semi-skimmed milk
100g low-fat natural yogurt
50ml sunflower oil
2 tbsp honey
1 tsp vanilla extract
4 overripe bananas

Preheat the oven to 200°C, (Fan 180°C), 400°F, Gas Mark 6 with the middle shelf at the ready. Line a muffin tin with 12 paper muffin cases.

Toss the flour, baking powder and bicarbonate of soda together in a large bowl. Beat the egg and egg whites briefly in a large jug, and then beat in the milk, yogurt, oil, honey and vanilla extract until smooth and well combined. Mix the wet mixture into the dry ingredients with as few stirs as possible to give a wet, sloppy mixture. Finally, roughly mash three of the bananas in a small bowl and then gently fold them into the mixture.

Pouring the mixture into a jug or using two spoons (or I like to use a mechanical ice-cream scoop), divide the mixture among the 12 cases. Peel and cut the remaining banana into 12 slices about ½cm thick and arrange one slice on top of each muffin. Then pop them into the oven to bake for 20 minutes or until a skewer inserted into one of the muffins comes out clean.

Leave to cool for a few minutes and then tuck in! Once completely cool, I like to freeze them and get one out each night so that it defrosts in time for the morning. Lovely cold and also scrumptious reheated and eaten warm.

(PER MUFFIN)	ENERGY	FAT	SAT FAT	SUGAR	PROTEIN	SALT
LORRAINE'S RECIPE	179 Kcal	5.4g	1g	12g	5.8g	0.3g
COMPARISON RECIPE	253 Kcal	7.9g	1.1g	16.3g	6.6g	0.44g

DOUBLE-CHOCOLATE CHIP 'CUPCAKE' MUFFINS

I struggled with this one, I mean really struggled. When tasting recipes, I am usually really good and will just wrap up one muffin and nibble at it throughout the day. Well, let me tell you dear reader/ budding chef, I could not get enough of these. I had a bite and put it down. Then had another bite, then put it down. Then popped them all in a tin, paced up and down the kitchen trying hard to focus on the next recipe, went back into the cupboard, unwrapped the muffin and polished it off in two bites. But that was not enough... in a blink of an eye all that was left of a second muffin was its chocolaty paper case scrumpled up into a ball.

Makes
12 muffins

Equipment
12-hole muffin tin, muffin cases

200g wholemeal flour
75g plain flour
50g dark chocolate chips
25g cocoa powder
1 tsp baking powder
½ tsp bicarbonate of soda
1 egg
2 egg whites
200 semi-skimmed milk
100g low-fat natural yogurt
50ml maple syrup
50ml sunflower oil

Preheat the oven to 200°C, (Fan 180°C), 400°F, Gas Mark 6, with the middle shelf at the ready. Line a muffin tin with 12 paper muffin cases.

Place the flours, chocolate chips, cocoa powder, baking powder and bicarbonate of soda in a large bowl and make a well in the centre. Beat the egg and egg whites briefly in a large jug, and then beat in the milk, yogurt, maple syrup and oil until smooth and well combined. Mix this wet mixture into the dry ingredients with as few stirs as possible to give a wet, sloppy mixture.

Pouring the mixture into a jug or using two spoons (or I like to use a mechanical ice-cream scoop), divide the mixture among the 12 cases. Pop the muffins in the oven to cook for about 20 minutes or until a skewer inserted into the middle comes out clean and the cupcakes feel spongy to the touch.

Remove from the oven and once cool enough to handle, transfer them out onto a wire rack to cool completely (although these are most delicious eaten warm).

(PER MUFFIN)	ENERGY	FAT	SAT FAT	SUGAR	PROTEIN	SALT
LORRAINE'S RECIPE	173 Kcal	6.8g	1.9g	7.6g	5.7g	0.36g
COMPARISON RECIPE	258 Kcal	13g	7.9g	14.6g	5g	0.62g

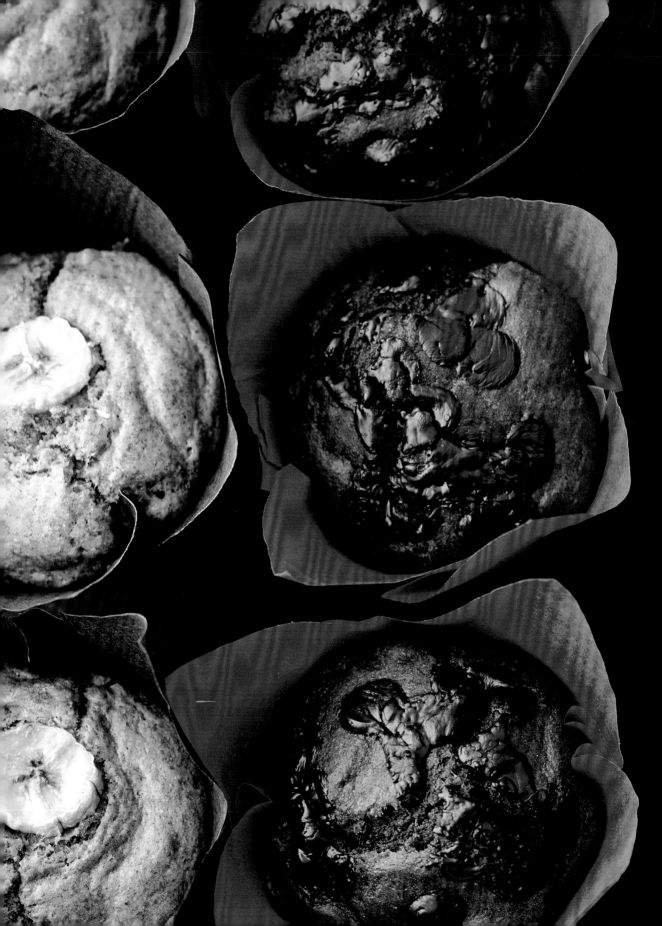

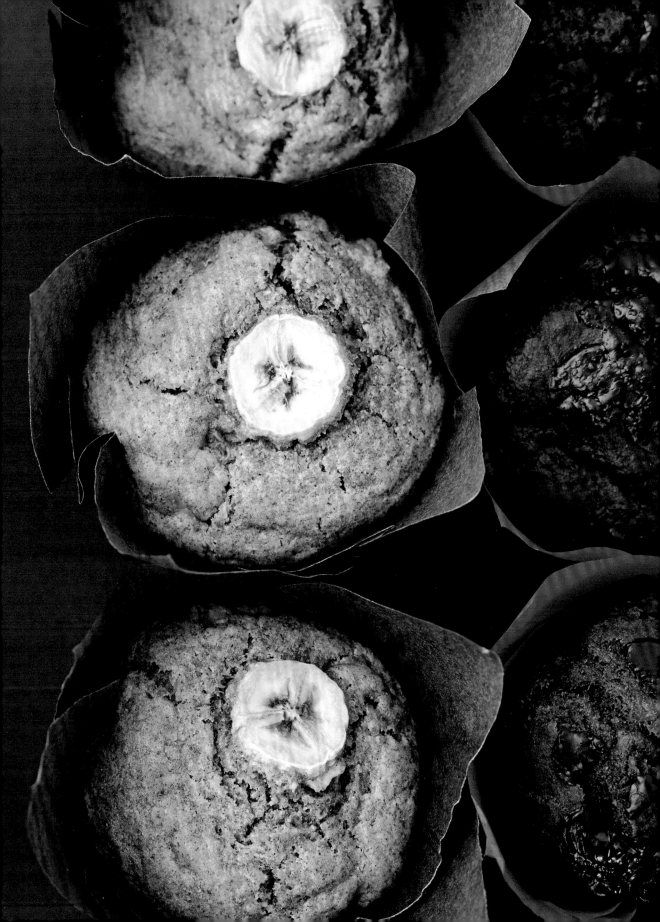

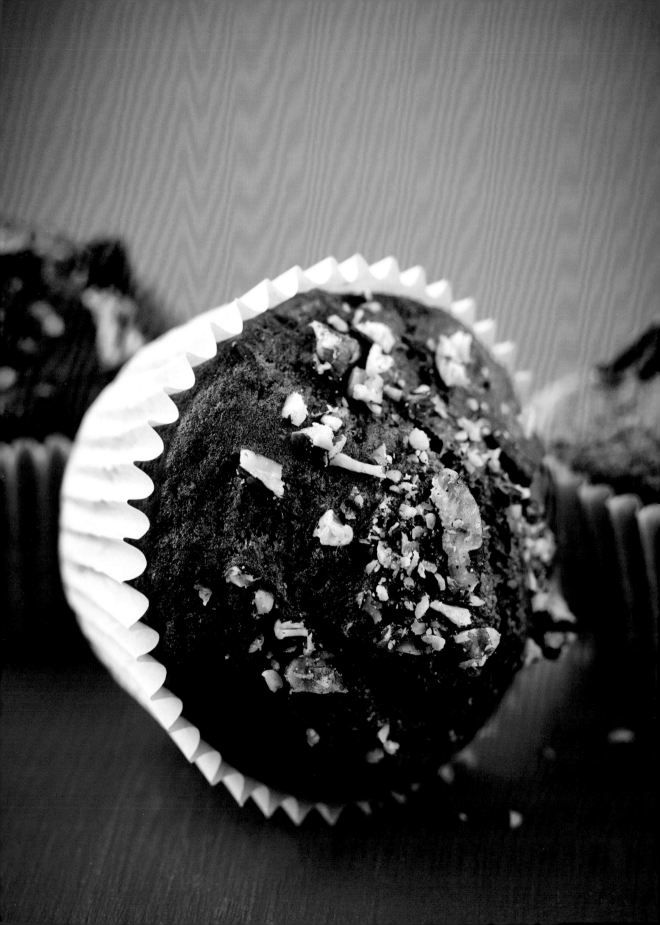

CAPPUCCINO, CINNAMON PECAN MUFFINS

I'm not a huge fan of coffee in a cup, but love the taste in cookies, muffins and cakes. These are less weighty than your average coffee-shop muffin, but are still stuffed with loads of flavour. I trawled my local supermarket looking for Camp Coffee essence, which is a brilliant thing to have, but could not find it, so used coffee granules in hot water to give these cappuccino muffins just the flavour they need.

Makes

12 muffins

Equipment

12-hole muffin tin, muffin cases, food processor

75g pecans, roughly chopped
100g soft light brown sugar
4 tbsp instant coffee granules
150g wholemeal flour
150g plain flour
1 tsp ground cinnamon
1 tsp baking powder
½ tsp bicarbonate of soda
1 egg
2 egg whites
175ml semi-skimmed milk
100g low-fat natural yogurt
50ml sunflower oil

Preheat the oven to 200°C, (Fan 180°C), 400°F, Gas Mark 6, with the middle shelf at the ready. Line a muffin tin with 12 paper muffin cases.

Toast the pecan nuts in a dry frying pan for 3–4 minutes. Tip two thirds of them into a large bowl and reserve the rest for later. Blitz the sugar and coffee in a food processor for a few seconds to give a finely chopped mixture and add to the bowl. Then, toss the flours, cinnamon, baking powder and bicarb through and make a well in the centre.

Beat the egg and egg whites briefly in a large jug and then beat in the milk, yogurt and oil to combine. Mix the wet mixture into the dry ingredients with as few stirs as possible to give a wet, sloppy consistency.

Pouring the mixture into a jug or using two spoons (or I like to use a mechanical ice-cream scoop), divide it among the 12 cases. Sprinkle the reserved pecans evenly over the tops and then pop the tin into the preheated oven to bake for 15 minutes or until a skewer inserted into one of the muffins comes out clean.

Leave to cool for a few minutes and then enjoy! They are lovely served cool, but also scrumptious reheated and eaten warm.

(PER MUFFIN)	ENERGY	FAT	SAT FAT	SUGAR	PROTEIN	SALT
LORRAINE'S RECIPE	211 Kcal	9.5g	1.2g	10.5g	5.6g	0.3g
COMPARISON RECIPE	241 Kcal	10.7g	3.3g	15.6g	4.4g	0.24g

MIXED BERRY & CINNAMON MUFFINS

I like to freeze these and get one out at night so that it defrosts in time for the morning. They taste lovely cold, but are also scrumptious reheated and eaten warm. They are also packed full of high-fibre wholemeal flour, so are perfect for powering you through to lunch.

Makes
12 muffins

Equipment
12-hole muffin tin, muffin cases

300g wholemeal flour
1 tsp baking powder
½ tsp bicarbonate of soda
1 tsp ground cinnamon
1 egg
2 egg whites
200ml semi-skimmed milk
100g low-fat natural yogurt
50ml sunflower oil
4 tbsp maple syrup
200g frozen summer berry or fruits
  of the forest berry mix

Preheat the oven to 200°C, (Fan 180°C), 400°F, Gas Mark 6, with the middle shelf of the oven at the ready. Line a muffin tin with 12 paper muffin cases.

Place the flour, baking powder, bicarbonate of soda and cinnamon in a large bowl and quickly toss together. Beat the egg and egg whites in a large jug briefly and then beat in the milk, yogurt, oil and maple syrup until smooth and well combined. Mix this wet mixture into the dry ingredients to give a wet, sloppy consistency. Finally, gently fold in two-thirds of the frozen berry mix.

Pouring the mixture into a jug or using two spoons (or I like to use a mechanical ice-cream scoop), divide it among the 12 cases. Scatter the remaining frozen berries evenly over the tops and press them in lightly. Pop into the oven to bake for 20 minutes or until a skewer inserted into one of the muffins comes out clean.

Remove from the oven and leave to cool for a few minutes in the tin. Then tuck in!

(PER MUFFIN)	ENERGY	FAT	SAT FAT	SUGAR	PROTEIN	SALT
LORRAINE'S RECIPE	155 Kcal	5.2g	0.9g	7g	5.5g	0.3g
COMPARISON RECIPE	208 Kcal	8.5g	4.8g	12.4g	4.3g	0.65g

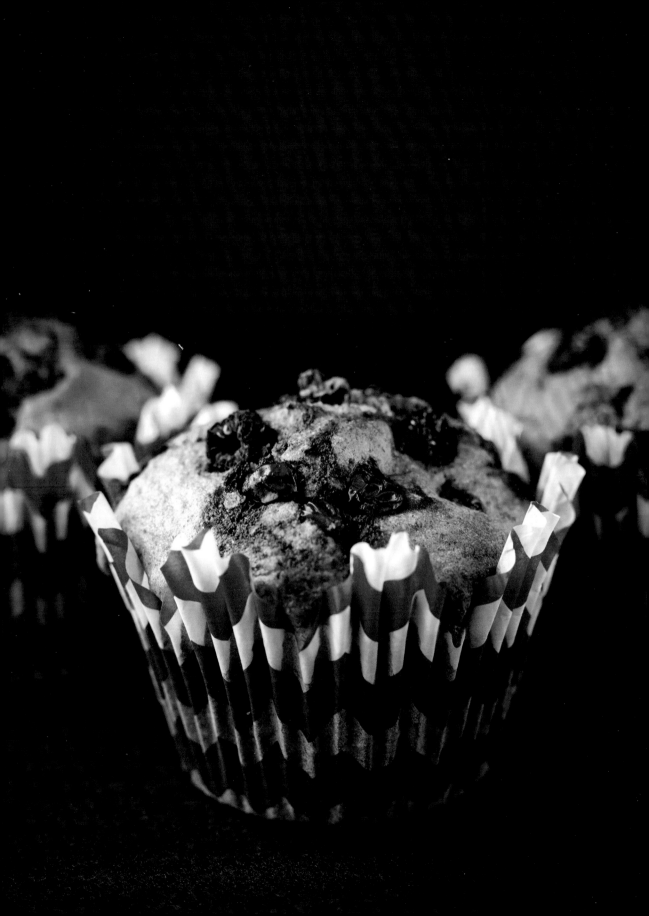

WHEN YOU REACH THE END OF YOUR ROPE,
TIE A KNOT IN IT AND HANG ON.
THOMAS JEFFERSON

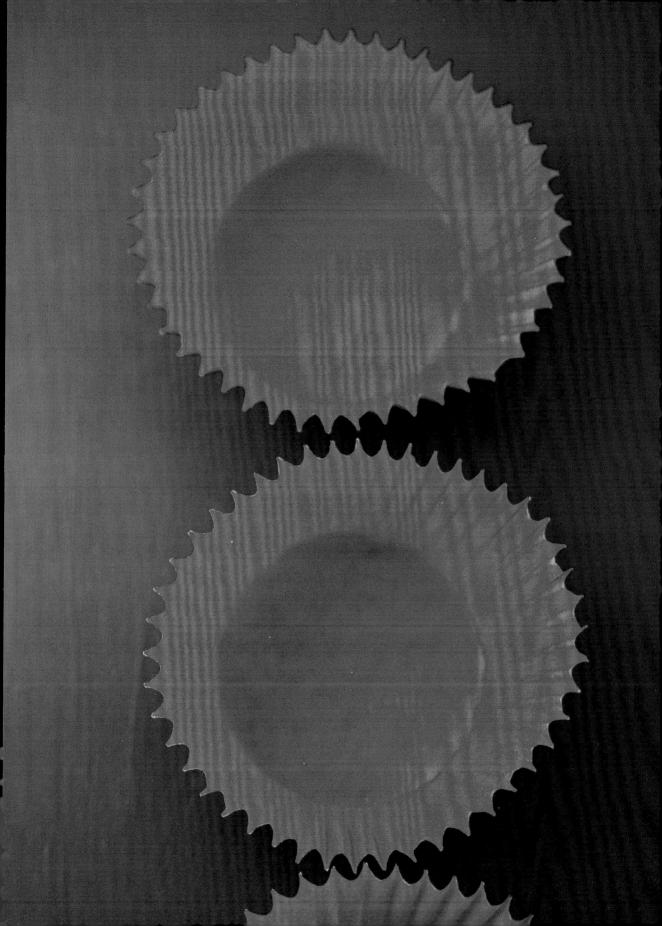

BREAD

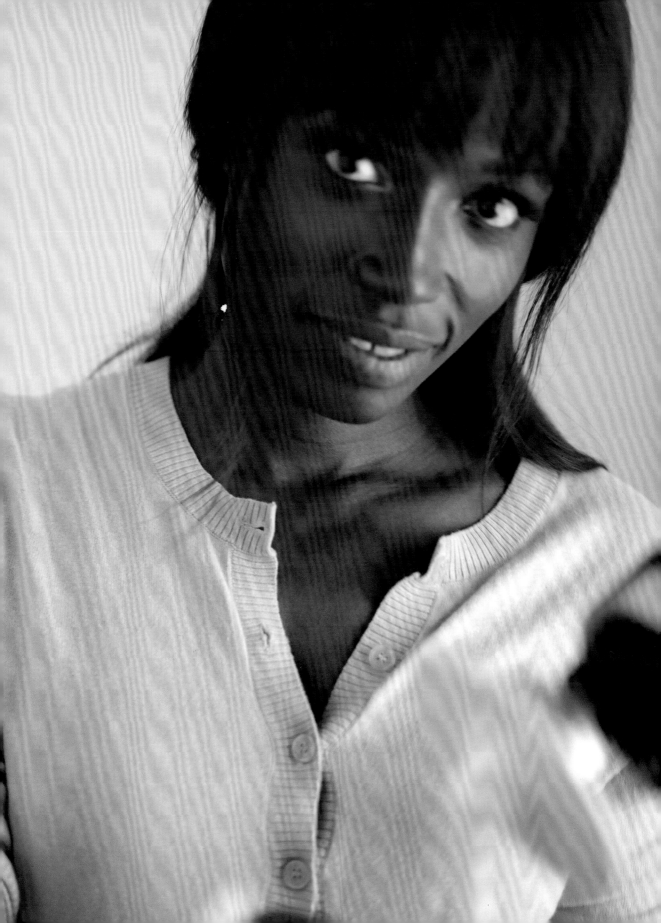

HONEY & OAT BREAD

This loaf is relatively traditional in its making method, but the amount of flour is slightly reduced and oats are added for extra fibre, with gratifyingly flavoursome results. If a whole loaf is too much to eat in one go, then once the bread is cool, cut it into slices and lay them out on a tray that will fit into your freezer. Freeze for 20 minutes to firm up and then put them all in a bag and back in the freezer (this way they will be easier to separate when you need them). Pull out and toast as and when you fancy a honey and oat bread bite.

Makes
1 loaf with 12 skinny slices

Equipment
1½ lb loaf tin
Large bowl or freestanding electric mixer set with the dough hook,

Spray oil
200g strong white bread flour, plus extra for dusting
125g strong wholemeal bread flour
50g rolled oats, plus 3 tsp extra for sprinkling
1½ tsp fast-action dried yeast
1 tsp salt
225ml warm water
2 tbsp honey
1 egg, lightly beaten

Preheat the oven to 180°C, (Fan 160°C), 350°F, Gas Mark 4. If you choose to make this by machine, then set the food mixer with a dough hook. Spritz the inside of 1½lb loaf tin with the oil.

Put the flours, 50g of oats, yeast and salt in a large bowl (or the food mixer bowl). Make a well in the centre and pour in the water and honey. Mix everything together well (by hand or machine) to give a smooth, soft dough ball.

If doing by machine, continue to knead for 4 minutes. Otherwise, put the dough onto a clean work surface sprinkled with a little flour and knead for about 8 minutes.

Shape the dough into a rugby ball shape with a nice smooth and taut top and place in the loaf tin. Spray the top of the loaf with a little oil and then cover it with cling film so that it is airtight, but loose enough to allow room for the loaf to grow. Leave the dough to rise in a warm place (I sit mine on a chair by the oven) for about 45 minutes or until the loaf has doubled in size.

Once the bread has risen, remove the cling film, brush with the egg and sprinkle over the extra oats. Bake in the oven for 35–40 minutes until golden brown on top and sounding hollow when tapped underneath. Loosen the loaf from the tin and leave it to cool completely on a wire rack before serving.

(PER SLICE)	ENERGY	FAT	SAT FAT	SUGAR	PROTEIN	SALT
LORRAINE'S RECIPE	132 Kcal	1.5g	0.2g	3g	4.8g	0.44g
COMPARISON RECIPE	167 Kcal	5.9g	3.3g	4.2g	3.3g	0.62g

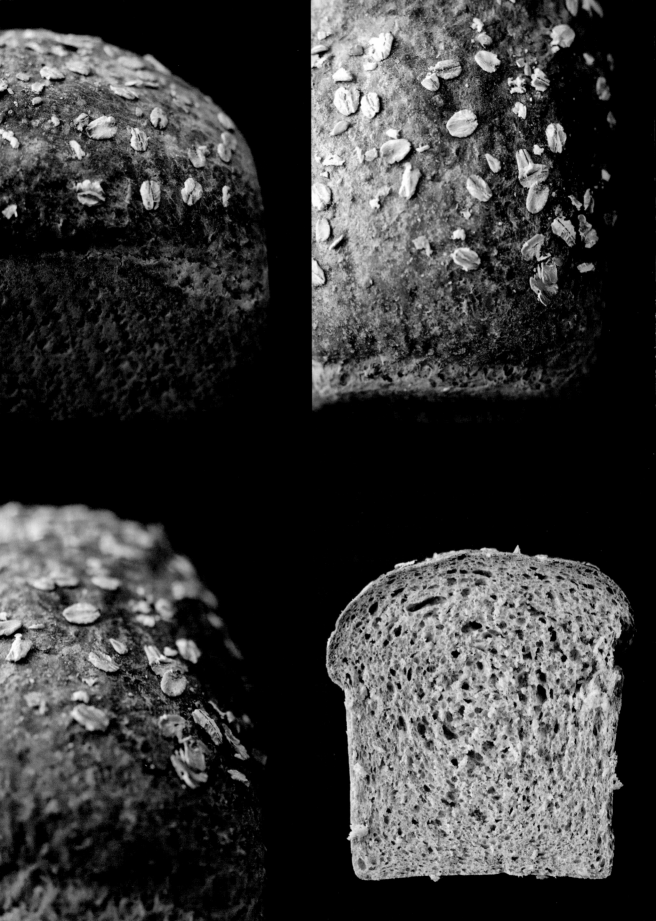

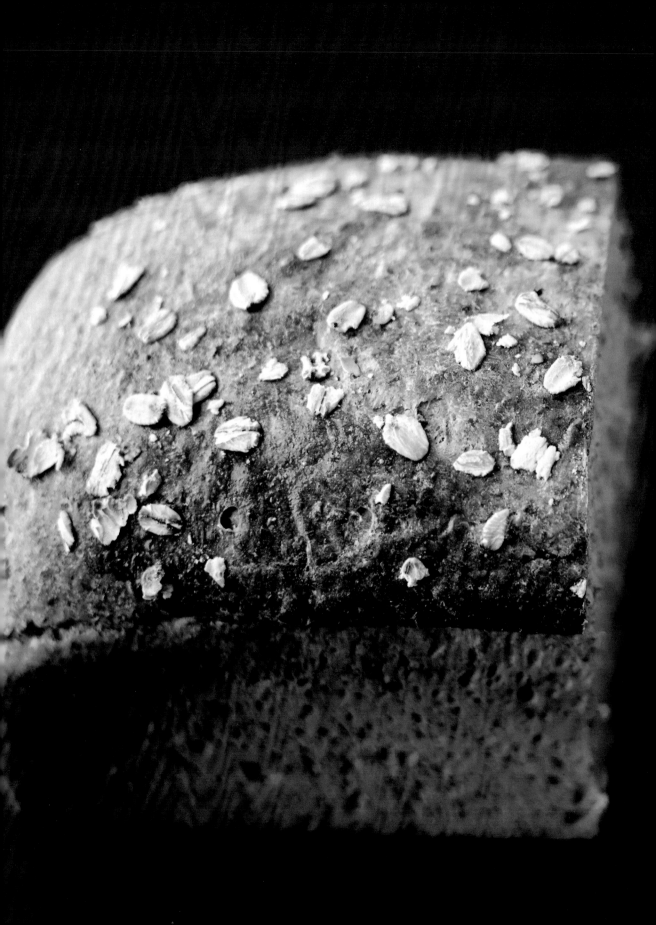

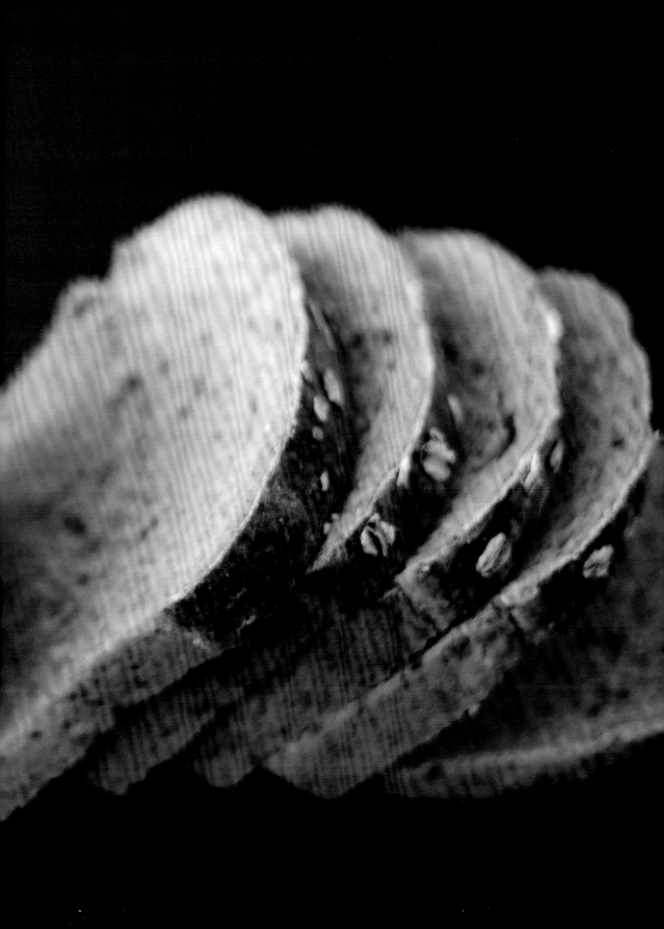

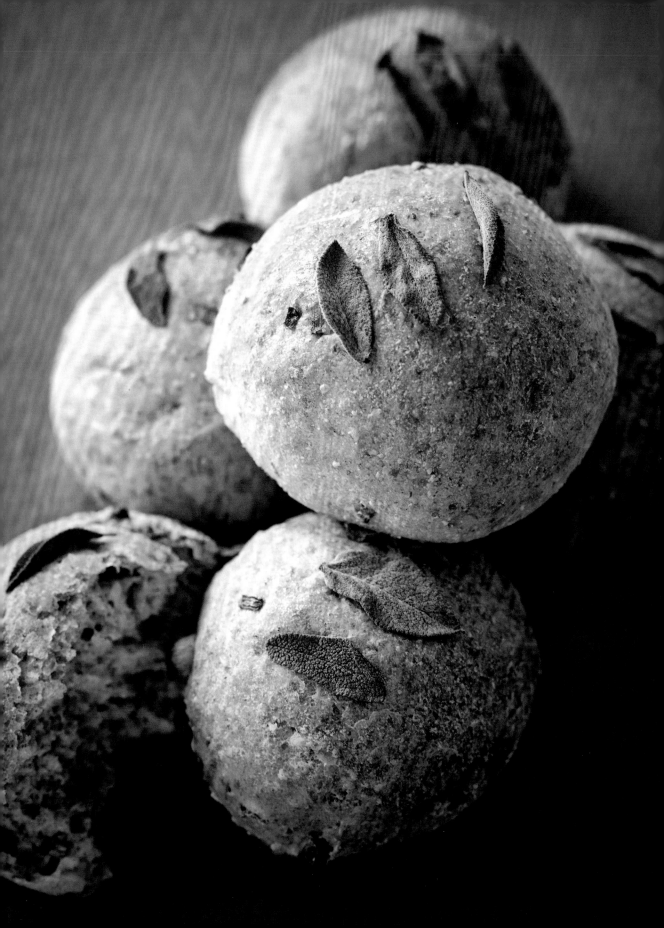

SPRING ONION, THYME & SAGE ROLLS

Bread is essentially just flour, yeast, salt and water, so reducing the fat and sugar is really not the challenge. For me, it is about making the bread more healthy. Some breads fare well with just wholemeal flour, but others, such as these rolls, become a little tough and heavy like a rounders ball. So the trick is to mix white and wholemeal flours together to get the benefits of wholemeal flour, with its higher volume of nutrients and slower energy release, and white flour, which keeps the bread from being too stodgy. If you can get organic flour (I know it is a bit more costly), then this will give an even better end product.

Makes
10 rolls

Equipment
Large bowl or freestanding electric mixer set with the dough hook

300g strong white bread flour, plus extra for dusting
200g strong wholemeal bread flour
7g sachet of fast-action dried yeast
1½ tsp salt
375ml warm water (from the tap)
6 spring onions, finely sliced
Leaves from 5 sprigs of fresh thyme, finely chopped
Spray oil
1 egg, lightly beaten
30 fresh sage leaves

Put the flours, yeast and salt into a large bowl (or food mixer bowl). Make a well in the centre and pour in the water. Mix everything together well (by hand with a wooden spoon or if by machine, then set with a dough hook) to give a smooth, soft dough ball. If doing by machine, continue to knead for 5 minutes. Otherwise, put the dough onto a clean work surface sprinkled with a little flour and knead for about 10 minutes.

To test to see if it has been kneaded enough, form the dough into a ball with a nice taut top. Put some flour on your finger and then prod the dough to make an indent about 5mm deep. If the dent springs back all the way, this means the dough is kneaded enough. If not, then knead it a little bit more.

Put the dough down on the work surface (sprinkled with a little flour if you haven't already done so) and then flatten it out to about a 20cm round, 2–3cm thick, with a rolling pin. Put the spring onions and thyme in a pile in the centre and then bring the sides of the dough up over the filling to enclose. Flip it over so the seam side is down and roll it out to the same size again. Once again, gather the edges up and over, but then knead the dough by hand to incorporate the filling ingredients evenly throughout. You may need to dust with a little more flour as you go if the spring onions make things a little damp.

Divide the dough into 10 equal-sized pieces and knead each one into a ball with a nice taut top. Put each roll, seam side down and spaced apart, on a large non-stick baking sheet. Spray the rolls with a light spritz of oil and then cover with cling film so that it is airtight, but not too tight as the bread needs to grow.

Preheat the oven to 200°C, (Fan 180°C), 400°F, Gas Mark 6 and then leave the bread on a chair about a metre away from the oven for 45 minutes or until the bread has almost doubled in size. To test that the rolls are ready, remove the cling film, put some flour on your finger and prod the side of the dough to make a 5mm dent. The dent should spring back about halfway. When it does it is ready. If necessary, leave it to rise for a bit longer.

Once ready, brush the dough balls with the beaten egg and lay three sage leaves in whatever decorative fashion you like on top of each one. Bake in the oven for 20 minutes or until the rolls are golden brown and sound hollow when tapped underneath. Once ready, remove from the oven and serve warm or cold.

(PER ROLL)	ENERGY	FAT	SAT FAT	SUGAR	PROTEIN	SALT
LORRAINE'S RECIPE	186 Kcal	1.2g	0.2g	0.9g	6.7g	0.75g
COMPARISON RECIPE	237 Kcal	4.6g	0.7g	4.8g	6.3g	0.93g

ALL-GRAIN, NUTTY, SEEDY SODA BREAD LOAF

Here I am wheeling out the old soda bread again. This time in loaf form, making it easier to slice, and with added nuts and seeds for extra texture and, of course, fibre. Due to the loaf being all packed up, unlike regular soda bread that spreads out, this tasty delight will require a little more cooking time than usual. Bread's low fat content means there really is not a whole lot that can be reduced by way of making it lighter, so this loaf is enriched with wholemeal flour and seeds, while full-fat buttermilk is replaced by semi-skimmed milk.

Makes
1 loaf with 14 skinny slices

Equipment
22 x 10cm loaf tin

375g wholemeal flour
100g self-raising flour
5 tbsp seeds and finely chopped
  mixed nuts (like pumpkin,
  sunflower or linseeds and
  hazelnuts, walnuts or almonds)
1 tsp bicarbonate of soda
1 tsp salt
450ml semi-skimmed milk
1 tbsp rolled oats

Preheat the oven to 200°C, (Fan 180°C), 400°F, Gas Mark 6. Line a 22 x 10cm loaf tin with baking parchment. I just cut a long strip of paper to cover the bottom and come up either side of the tin with the excess hanging over a little. This makes it easier to lift the baked loaf out of the tin.

Toss the flours, seeds and nuts, bicarb and salt together in a large bowl and make a hole in the centre. Pour in the milk and mix again until everything starts to come together to a soft, dropping consistency (you want the dough to be soft, but not sticky).

Spoon the mixture into the loaf tin, spreading the top down evenly with the back of a spoon. Sprinkle the oats evenly over and bake in the oven for 35–40 minutes or until the bread is a nice golden brown colour and sounds hollow when tapped underneath.

Once cooked, remove from the oven and allow to cool for a few moments in the tin before lifting it out. If you find that the loaf gets stuck, then just run a knife around the edge to loosen it a bit. Peel off the paper and allow to cool on a wire rack. This bread is best served just a little warm and eaten on the day that it is cooked.

(PER SLICE)	ENERGY	FAT	SAT FAT	SUGAR	PROTEIN	SALT
LORRAINE'S RECIPE	151 Kcal	3.6g	0.7g	2.2g	6g	0.65g
COMPARISON RECIPE	164 Kcal	5.2g	0.8g	2g	6.5g	0.72g

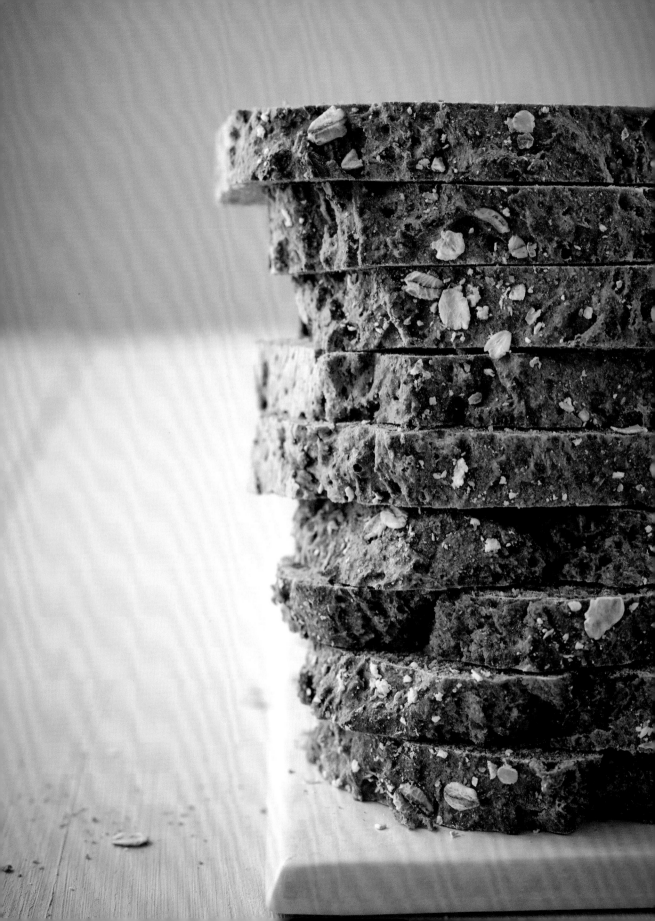

ANCHOVY, OLIVE, ONION & ROSEMARY FOCACCIA

I often make a focaccia full of salt and sprigs of rosemary, a reminder of the first focaccia I ate as a 'side' dish in Italy sometime way back in the eighties. And as gorgeous as that was, by adding some more flavour to it, this springy Italian bread almost becomes a meal in itself. Although the habit is often to dip it into some oil and balsamic vinegar, due to the added anchovies, olives and onion in this bread it's good to go, just as it is.

Makes
1 focaccia with 9 slices

Equipment
Large bowl or freestanding electric mixer set with the dough hook

300g strong white bread flour, plus extra for dusting
100g strong wholemeal bread flour
7g sachet of fast-action dried yeast
1 tsp salt
1 tbsp extra virgin olive oil
250ml warm water (from the tap)
Spray oil
1 large red onion, halved and thinly sliced
125g pitted black olives (or 150g if stone in and needs to be removed), halved
2 stalks of fresh rosemary, broken into smaller sprigs
25g anchovies, drained

Line a large baking sheet with baking parchment and set aside.

Toss the flours, yeast and salt together in a large bowl (or food mixer). Make a well in the centre and add the oil and warm water. Mix everything together well with a wooden spoon if doing by hand or in a mixer set with the dough hook, to give a smooth, soft dough ball. If doing by machine, continue to knead for 5 minutes. Otherwise, put the ball onto a clean work surface sprinkled with a little flour and knead for about 10 minutes.

To test if the dough is kneaded enough and that the gluten (protein) in the flour is nice and stretchy, form the dough into a ball with a nice taut top, and then put a little flour on your finger. Prod the dough to make a dent about 5mm deep. If the dough has been kneaded enough, the dent will spring back and disappear. If it requires more kneading, then the dent will remain.

Place the kneaded dough on the baking sheet and roll it into a 25cm circle. Spray the top with some oil and cover with cling film, loose enough to allow the dough space to rise, but all enclosed so it is airtight. Leave the dough to rise in a warm place for about 45 minutes or until it has almost doubled in volume. I like to leave mine on a chair close to a hot oven. Set the oven to preheat to 200°C, (Fan 180°C), 400°F, Gas Mark 6.

Meanwhile, spritz a little oil into a large frying pan set over a low to medium heat. Add the onion and gently fry for 15 minutes, stirring regularly, until soft and just beginning to turn golden. Remove from the heat and set aside.

Once the dough has had its rising time, test to see if it has risen enough. Put some flour on your finger and prod the side of the dough to make an indent about 5mm deep. The dough should spring back halfway. Once the dough is ready, prod your fingers all over it to make those dents traditional to focaccia. Then stick an olive half and rosemary sprig out of each hole. Spread the onions evenly all over, scatter with the remaining olives and lay the anchovies on top. Bake for 20–25 minutes or until the dough is firm and sounds hollow when tapped underneath.

Once cooked, remove the focaccia from the oven. Leave until cool enough to handle before cutting into wedges or bite-sized squares. This can be served warm or cold.

(PER SLICE)	ENERGY	FAT	SAT FAT	SUGAR	PROTEIN	SALT
LORRAINE'S RECIPE	195 Kcal	3.9g	0.6g	2.2g	6.8g	1.61g
COMPARISON RECIPE	236 Kcal	6.5g	0.9g	1.7g	5.5g	1.94g

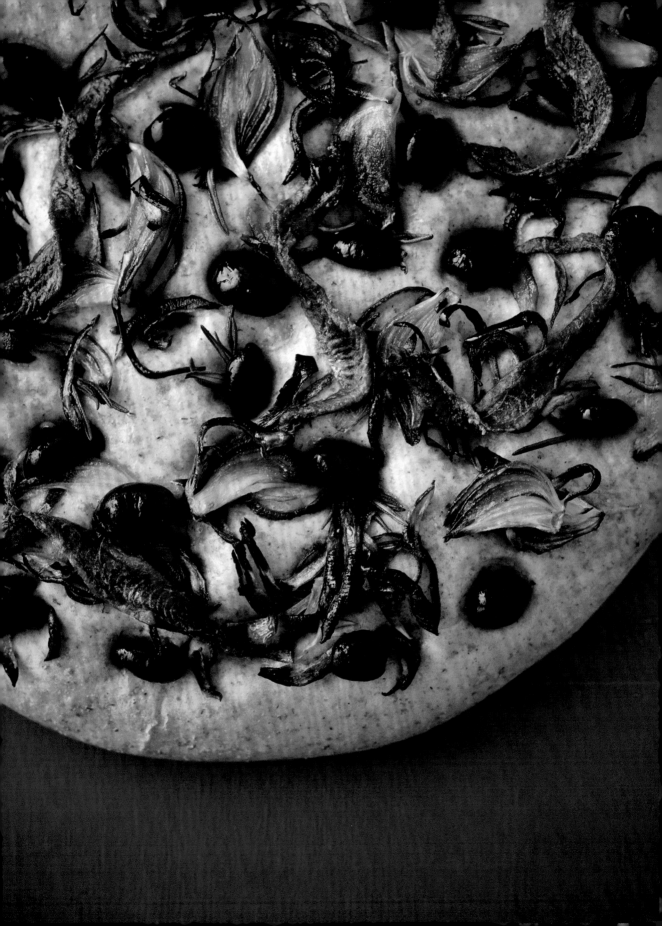

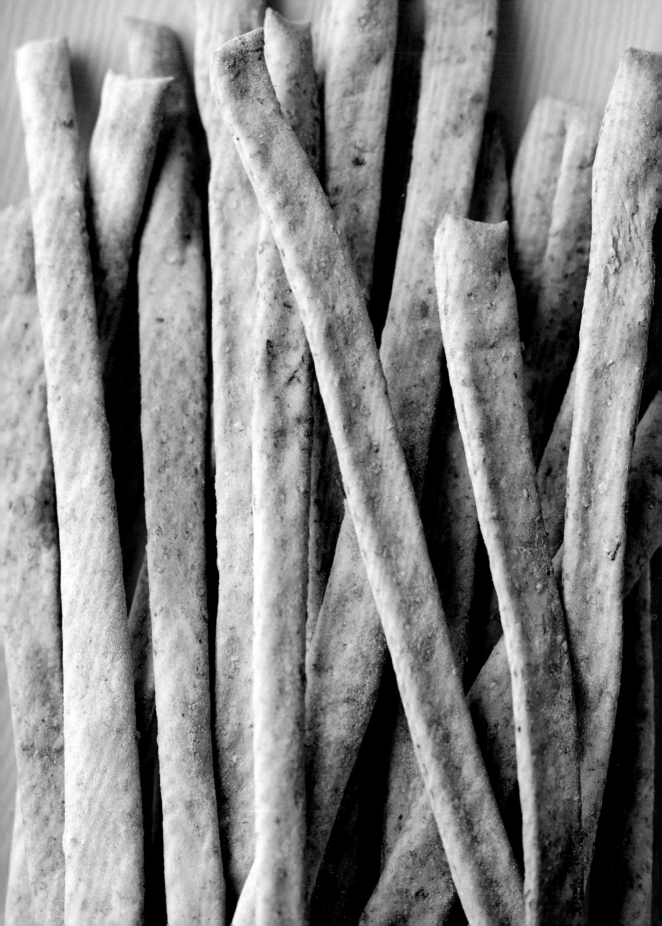

OREGANO & THYME GRISSINI

There is a little Italian restaurant down where I live in London and when they sit you down, you get a teeny bowl of olive and anchovy paste (sounds not quite right, but tastes very right) and a little packet of long, skinny breadsticks or grissini. *Baking Made Easy* had a tasty recipe for salt and pepper breadsticks, which were big and fat, but these slim and slender alternatives mean you can have a whole one with a little less guilt. Great with dips and/or olive oil.

Makes
About 36 grissini

Equipment
Large bowl or freestanding electric mixer set with the dough hook

Spray oil
200g strong white bread flour, plus extra for dusting
100g strong wholemeal bread flour
1 tsp fast-action dried yeast
3 tbsp fresh thyme leaves
1 tbsp dried oregano
1 tsp salt
225ml warm water (from the tap)

Preheat the oven to 200°C, (Fan 180°C), 400°F, Gas Mark 6. Spritz 2 large baking trays with a little oil and set aside.

Toss the flours, yeast, thyme, oregano and salt together in a large bowl (or food mixer bowl). Make a well in the centre and pour in the warm water. Mix everything together well (by hand with a wooden spoon or by the machine fitted with a dough hook) to give a smooth, soft dough ball. If doing by machine, continue to knead for 5 minutes. Otherwise, put the dough onto a clean work surface sprinkled with a little flour and knead for about 10 minutes.

Once you have kneaded the dough for the allocated time, cut it in half and cover one half with cling film. Then, working on a large chopping board well dusted with flour, roll the other half of the dough into a rectangle about 30 x 22cm in size and about 3mm in thickness. Using a long, sharp knife (or a pizza cutter also makes an excellent tool for cutting these), cut out about 18 strips, each one about 1½cm wide along the width, rather than the length. Carefully transfer each one to a baking sheet. They may stretch a bit as you lift them, but that is fine – these can come in all lengths! Repeat with the remaining dough half.

Bake the grissini in the oven for about 15–18 minutes or until they are slightly puffed up and crisp. The ends may catch quickly near the end of cooking time, so keep a good eye on them, especially those bits that may be a bit thinner than others.

Once cooked, remove from the oven and leave to cool a little before serving warm or cold. These will keep in an airtight container for up to a week.

(PER GRISSINI)	ENERGY	FAT	SAT FAT	SUGAR	PROTEIN	SALT
LORRAINE'S RECIPE	30 Kcal	0.2g	0.01g	0.1g	1.1g	0.14g
COMPARISON RECIPE	38 Kcal	1.1g	0.2g	0.3g	1.2g	0.26g

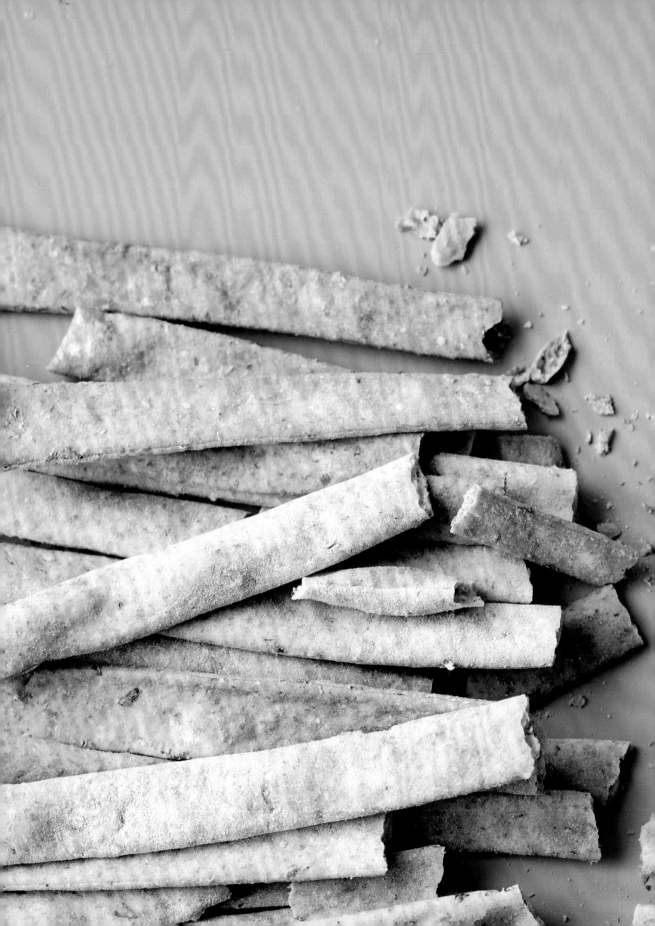

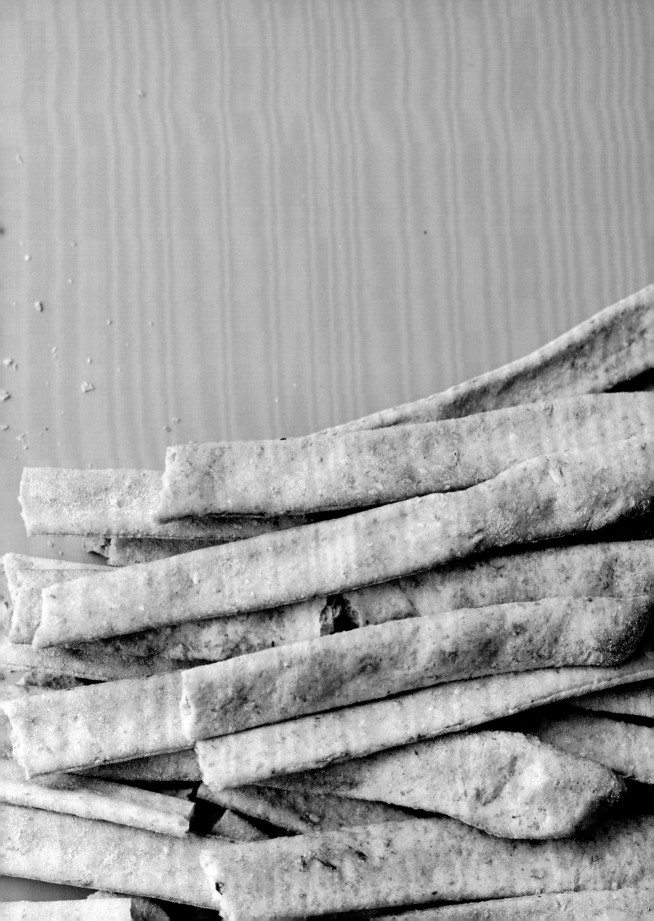

SESAME PRETZEL BUNS

I cannot pretend that pretzels are an all-encompassing part of the UK eating psyche, but with a little recipe experimentation, failure, followed by tears and then some progress, I genuinely believe that these are quite literally some of the tastiest buns I have ever made. Despite being only fractionally lower in fat and sugar than similar recipes out there, they get their nutritional brownie points from a boost of high-fibre wholemeal flour. They're really easy on the eye too.

Makes

12 buns

Equipment

Large bowl or freestanding electric mixer set with the dough hook

200g strong wholemeal bread flour
175g strong white bread flour
125g plain flour, plus extra for dusting
1½ tsp fast-action dried yeast
1 tsp salt
325ml warm water (from the tap)
Spray oil
125g bicarbonate of soda
1 egg, lightly beaten
1½ tsp sesame seeds

Put the flours, yeast and salt together in a large bowl (or food mixer bowl). Make a well in the centre and pour in the warm water. Mix everything together well (by hand with a wooden spoon or in a machine fitted with a dough hook) to give a smooth, soft dough ball. Knead the dough for 10 minutes on a lightly floured surface if doing by hand or for 5 minutes if using a food mixer.

To test to see if it has been kneaded enough, form the dough into a ball with a nice taut top. Put some flour on your finger and then prod the dough to make an indent about 5mm deep. If the dent springs back all the way, this means the dough is kneaded enough. If not, then knead it a little bit more.

Divide the dough into 12 equal-sized pieces. I like to find out the weight of the dough and divide it by 12 to get the exact weight each one should be — that way they all look nice and uniform. Knead each piece into a ball with a nice taut top and place them seam side down and spaced apart on a large baking sheet.

Spray the dough balls with a little oil and cover them well with cling film. The cling film should be airtight so that it provides a nice cosy atmosphere for the bread, but not too tight as it needs some room to grow. Leave the dough in a nice warm, but not too hot, place for about 45 minutes, until it grows by about a quarter. It will not grow that much due to the types of flours used in it (the wholemeal flour makes it much heavier and the plain flour is not as stretchy as strong flour, but the buns will still be great).

About 15 minutes before the end of the rising time, preheat the oven to 200°C, (Fan 180°C), 400°F, Gas Mark 6.

Bring about 2 litres of water to the boil in a large, wide pan. Once it is boiling, add the bicarbonate of soda and allow it to fizzle up and then calm down a little. Remove the cling film from the buns and, using a slotted spoon, drop three of the buns into the boiling (and slightly fizzing) water. Leave to boil for about 30 seconds, constantly turning them around so all sides are immersed in the water. Remove the buns and place back on the baking tray, again seam side down. Repeat with the rest of the buns. This part of the process will give the buns a very deliciously distinct flavour and it will also make the tops take on a characteristic dark brown 'pretzel' look.

Brush the tops of the buns with the beaten egg and sprinkle the sesame seeds evenly over. Use a sharp knife to slash the tops of the buns. I like to either use three small slashes that are fairly deep or put a little cross in the centre. Bake in the oven for 20–25 minutes or until the buns sound hollow when tapped underneath and the tops have gone a medium to dark brown.

(PER BUN)	ENERGY	FAT	SAT FAT	SUGAR	PROTEIN	SALT
LORRAINE'S RECIPE	147 Kcal	1.3g	0.2g	0.7g	5.4g	0.43g
COMPARISON RECIPE	150 Kcal	1.5g	0.3g	0.8g	5.1g	0.69g

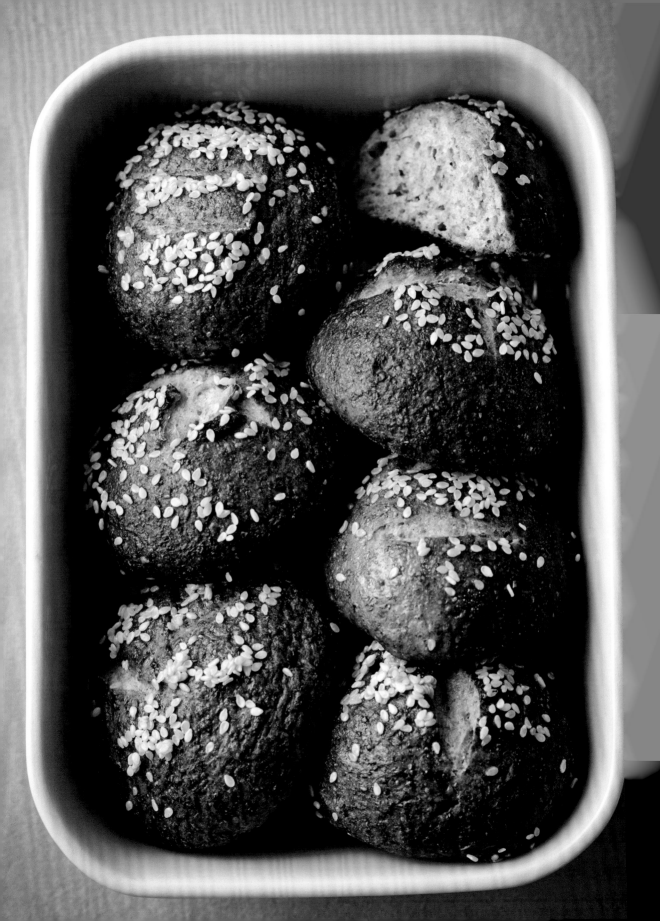

THE BEST THING ABOUT THE FUTURE
IS THAT IT COMES ONE DAY AT A TIME.
ABRAHAM LINCOLN

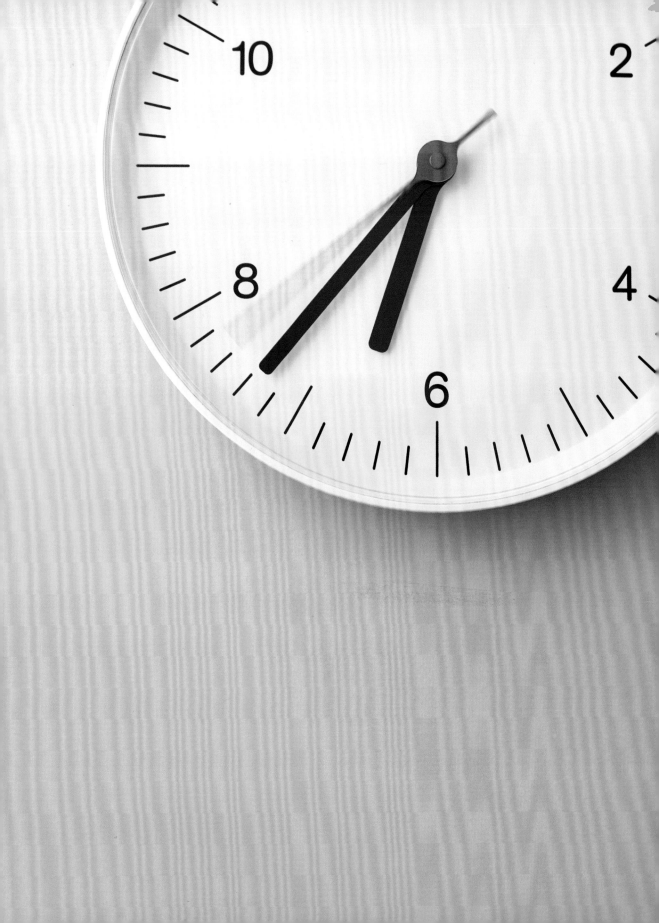

SAVOURY
BAKES

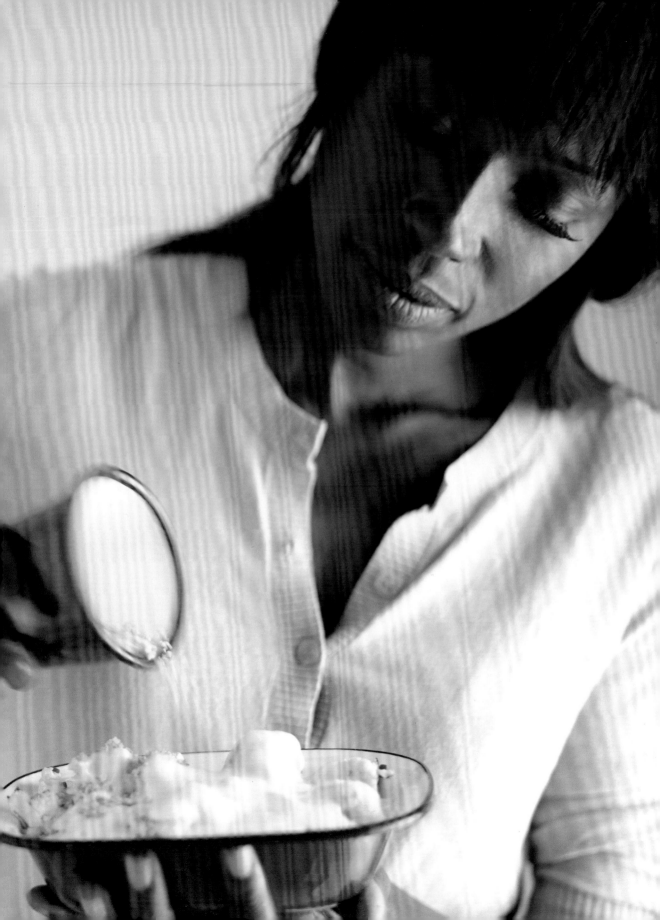

MOROCCAN CHICKEN POT PIES WITH CUMIN & CORIANDER & A CRISP FILO TOP

Traditionally pot pies are not from North Africa, nor are they made with the lighter-than-light filo pastry, but as we are baking a lighter way I hope you can forgive me for all that. The usual way I make them is with chicken, peas and carrots but without the benefit of buttery flaky pastry, these little pies were missing some oompfh. So I turned to the tastes of the Casbah for a flamboyant flavour boost. Spiced chicken on the inside, sweetened with apricots (hence the slightly higher natural sugar content), and a crispy crunchy filo topping scattered with rich nutty almonds. Delish.

Serves
6

Equipment
6 ramekins or hot pot dishes about 10cm wide, 6cm high and 450ml in volume

Filling
Spray oil
2 large onions, finely sliced
1 garlic clove, finely chopped
3cm piece of fresh ginger, peeled and finely chopped
2 tsp ground cinnamon
2 tsp ground cumin
1 tsp paprika
4 large chicken breasts, cut into 3cm chunks
3 tbsp cornflour
600ml good chicken stock
2 carrots, peeled and sliced into ½cm slices
100g frozen peas
50g dried apricots, roughly chopped
Leaves from a small bunch of fresh coriander or flat leaf parsley, roughly chopped
Salt and freshly ground black pepper

Topping
3 sheets of filo pastry
25g flaked almonds

To serve
Crisp green salad

Preheat the oven to 180°C, (Fan 160°C), 350°F, Gas Mark 4.

Spray a little oil into a large pan over a medium heat. Add the onion and cook gently for about 5 minutes, stirring from time to time, until softened. Add the garlic and ginger and cook for a further minute before adding the cinnamon, cumin and paprika. Then, allow them to toast for a minute.

In the meantime, toss the chicken pieces in the cornflour and a little salt and pepper until evenly coated. Stir these into the onion mixture and cook for 1 minute. Gradually add the stock, stirring all the time to blend in the cornflour without any lumps. Turn up the heat and add the carrots, peas, apricots and seasoning. Allow to come to the boil, then pop a lid on and reduce to simmer gently for 5 minutes until the chicken is cooked through and the sauce thickened.

Meanwhile, prepare the topping. Lay the filo sheets out in one pile and cut them into 1cm wide strips across the width (rather than down the length). I use a pastry cutter for this, but a sharp knife or even scissors or a pizza wheel will do the trick. Keep covered with a lightly dampened tea towel until ready to use to stop it from drying out.

Once ready, divide the pie filling among six ramekins or hot pot dishes about 10cm wide, 6cm high and 450ml in volume. Scatter the coriander or parsley over each one, then divide the filo strips into six even-sized bunches (they may have stuck together a bit, so just separate the layers). Pick up the bunches and lay one messily on top of each pie. The more bits that are sticking up and messy, the more likely the filo is to crisp up. Scatter the almonds evenly over, then spray each pie with two squirts of the spray oil. Bake in the oven for 15 minutes or until the chicken is cooked through and piping hot, the filo is crisp and golden brown and the sauce bubbling.

Once cooked, remove from the oven and serve at once with a crisp green salad.

(PER SERVING)	ENERGY	FAT	SAT FAT	SUGAR	PROTEIN	SALT
LORRAINE'S RECIPE	320 Kcal	5.4g	0.9g	12.9g	27g	1.08g
COMPARISON RECIPE	358 Kcal	9.4g	2.7g	9.3g	32g	0.81g

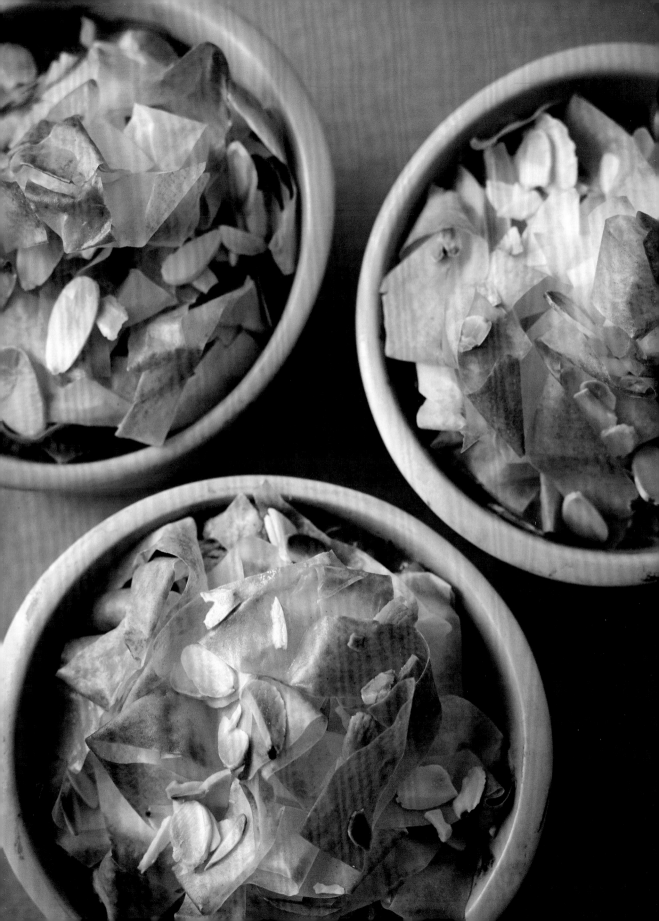

LOVELY, LIGHTER HERBED LASAGNE WITH COURGETTE 'PASTA'

If you are not a fan of courgettes, carrots can be used in their place. This makes the recipe nice and low-carb. However, if you fancy getting your teeth stuck into some carbs, then wholemeal pasta has a great nutty flavour. I really tried hard to make a roux which was super tasty using reduced flour and butter, but I just could not come up with a satisfactory product. The best way I found was to make a faux white sauce with flavourings, olive oil, milk, cheese and flour – still bags of flavour, but a lot better for you. I experimented with low-fat cheeses, but I found that the reduced and half-fat cheese was full of stuff we may not like to be eating, and was very, very stringy and stretchy and did not really melt. So I opted for a reduced quantity of regular cheese.

Serves

6

Equipment

2½ litre baking dish measuring
   25.5cm square and 6cm deep

White sauce

475ml semi-skimmed milk
1 sprig of rosemary, bashed a bit
   to release the flavours
1 bay leaf
5 black peppercorns
¼ tsp freshly grated nutmeg
25g plain flour
25ml olive oil
50g mature Cheddar cheese,
   roughly grated

Ragù

2 tbsp olive oil
2 onions, finely chopped
3 carrots, finely diced
2 tsp finely chopped rosemary
2 tsp thyme leaves
2 tsp dried oregano
2 garlic cloves, finely chopped
600g lean beef mince
2 tbsp cornflour
1 tbsp smoked paprika (optional)
2 x 400g tins chopped tomatoes
400ml Marsala or a good red wine
   or a good liquid beef stock
3 tbsp Worcestershire sauce
3 tbsp tomato purée
1–1½ tsp caster sugar (optional)
Salt and freshly ground black pepper

Courgette 'pasta'

4 courgettes, trimmed and cut
   lengthways into 0.5cm-thick slices
   (use wholemeal or regular pasta if
   courgettes are not your thing)

Topping

A little freshly grated nutmeg
25g mature Cheddar cheese,
   roughly grated
8 basil leaves

To serve

Crisp green salad

Preheat the oven to 180°C, (Fan 160°C), 350°F, Gas Mark 4. Sit a 2½ litre baking dish measuring 25.5cm square and 6cm deep on a baking sheet, and set aside.

First, flavour up the milk for the white sauce. Pour the milk into a medium pan over a medium heat and add the rosemary, bay leaf, peppercorns and nutmeg. Once the milk is just beginning to steam, take it off the heat and leave to one side for the flavours to infuse.

Next, make the ragù. Heat 1 tablespoon of the oil in a large, wide pan over a low heat. Add the onions and cook for about 6 minutes, stirring from time to time so they don't catch. Once softened, add the carrots, rosemary, thyme and oregano and cook these gently for 5 minutes, adding the garlic for the final minute. Tip this mixture out into a bowl and set aside for a moment.

Heat the remaining tablespoon of oil in the pan on a high heat and add half of the mince. It may need to be broken up a bit with a wooden spoon. Cook for 4–5 minutes, stirring regularly until this turns from pink to brown. Using a slotted spoon, scoop the meat out (leaving the oil behind) and add to the onion mixture. Repeat with the remaining meat, leaving it in the pan once browned. Then, return the onion and beef mix to the pan and stir in the cornflour, paprika (if using) and seasoning and cook for a further minute. Then stir in the tomatoes, Marsala, Worcestershire sauce and tomato purée. Taste and add some sugar if you feel it is necessary (there may be some bitterness from the tomatoes). Turn up the heat and bring to the boil before reducing to simmer for a good 45 minutes for the sauce to thicken and the flavours to intensify.

About 5 minutes before the ragù is cooked, continue to make the white sauce. Strain the infused milk through a sieve into a large jug and discard the flavourings. Return the empty pan to a low heat and put in the flour and oil. Stir together to combine and cook for about 30 seconds before removing from the heat. Gradually add the infused milk, stirring all the time so no lumps form. Then, once all the milk is added, return the pan to a medium heat and bring to a simmer. Allow it to bubble away for a couple of minutes until it thickens, stirring from time to time so it does not stick on the bottom. Then, add the Cheddar cheese (for the sauce, not topping), stirring until melted. Season to taste, remove from the heat and set aside.

Now, time to assemble everything in the baking dish. Arrange a third of the courgette slices in a just-overlapping single layer in the bottom of the dish. Spoon in half of the ragù and spread it out evenly, followed by a layer using half of the white sauce. Then, add another layer of courgette slices, again using a third of them, followed by the remaining ragù, the remaining courgette slices, and then finish with the remaining white sauce. Finally grate over a little nutmeg and scatter the cheese on top.

Bake in the oven for 40–45 minutes until piping hot, golden on top and the courgettes feel just tender when pierced with a knife. Remove from the oven, scatter over ripped basil leaves and serve with a crisp green salad.

(PER SERVING)	ENERGY	FAT	SAT FAT	SUGAR	PROTEIN	SALT
LORRAINE'S RECIPE	457 Kcal	24.4g	9.1g	14.3g	32.5g	1.31g
COMPARISON RECIPE	803 Kcal	54.2g	26g	14g	48.6g	1.83g

HERBED-BAKED CHICKEN STRIPS WITH HONEY & MUSTARD DIPPING SAUCE

Herbed-baked chicken strips or 'goujons' to the catering cognoscenti. Nice and easy to do this one, much like the other recipes in the book. If you want chicken strips without the spice, then you can substitute the harissa for two egg whites. Simply beat them lightly and then dip the chicken in to coat before tossing in the crumbs.

Makes
16 strips (serves 4 as a main)

Equipment
Food processor

Chicken strips
2 slices of wholemeal bread
2 tsp finely chopped fresh
   rosemary
3 tsp dried oregano
3 tbsp rolled oats
4 large skinless, boneless chicken
   breasts, trimmed of any fat
2–4 tbsp harissa paste (depending
   on how hot you like it)
Salt and freshly ground black
   pepper

Dipping sauce
200g low-fat crème fraîche
2 tbsp honey
3 tbsp Dijon mustard (or to taste)
Salt and freshly ground black
   pepper

To serve
1 lemon, cut into quarters

Preheat the oven to 200°C, (Fan 180°C), 400°F, Gas Mark 6. Line a roasting tray with baking parchment and set aside.

Lightly toast the bread in a toaster or under the grill and then blitz in a food processor to give fine, dry breadcrumbs. Tip them into a wide, shallow bowl and toss in the rosemary and oregano, then season with salt and pepper. Blitz the oats in the processor until roughly ground and toss them through the breadcrumbs.

Cut each chicken breast into four long strips. Season them with salt and a good amount of pepper and then brush them all over with the harissa paste. Working in batches, toss the strips into the breadcrumb mixture to stick and evenly coat and lay in a single layer on the baking sheet as you go. Bake in the oven for 10–12 minutes or until the chicken is cooked through and golden brown on the outside.

Meanwhile, prepare the dipping sauce by simply mixing the ingredients together in a small bowl and seasoning to taste. Spoon into a small serving bowl, cover and leave aside in the fridge until ready to serve.

Check the chicken is cooked by cutting through to the centre of the thickest one. If there is any pinkness return the strips to the oven for a little longer. Arrange the cooked chicken strips on plates with the dipping sauce drizzled over and the lemon wedges nestled beside them and serve. The squeeze of lemon really lifts the flavour of the chicken.

(PER SERVING –4 STRIPS)	ENERGY	FAT	SAT FAT	SUGAR	PROTEIN	SALT
LORRAINE'S RECIPE	374 Kcal	12.6g	5.9g	12g	37.8g	1.9g
COMPARISON RECIPE	545 Kcal	28.8g	7.1g	13.1g	35.4g	2.57g

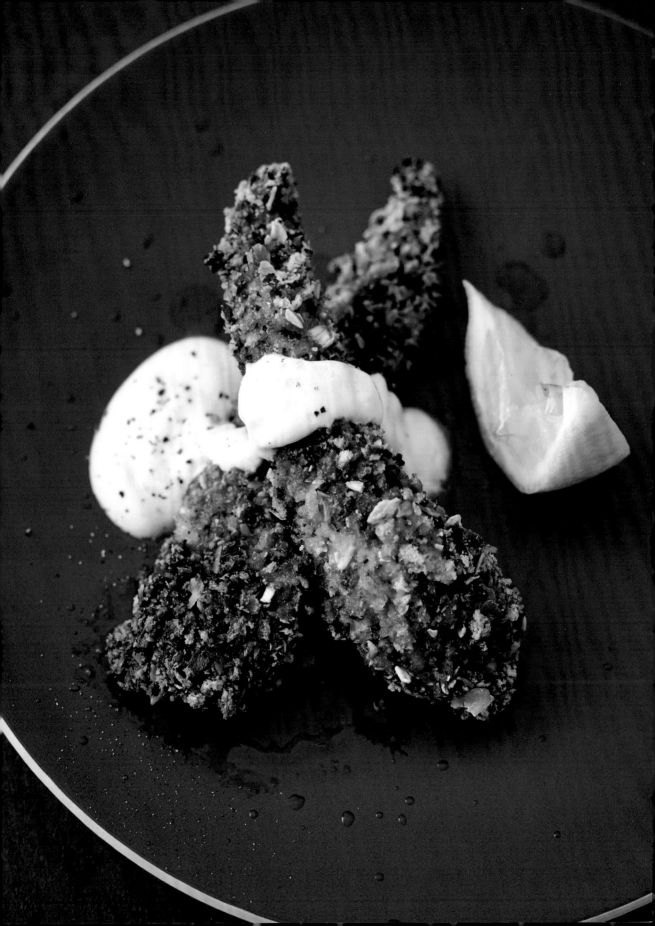

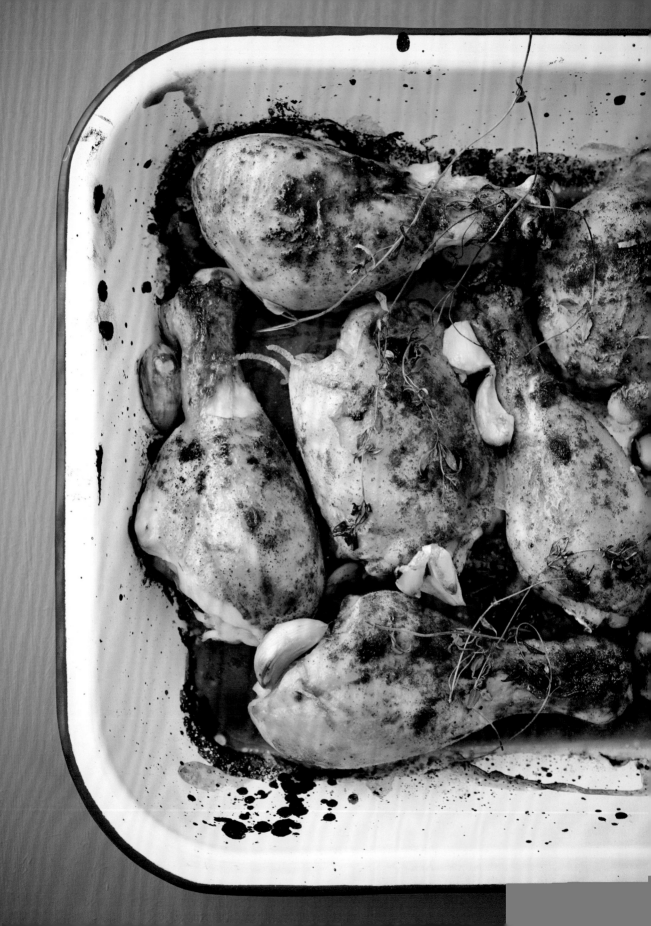

BAKED STORE-CUPBOARD CHICKEN WITH LIME, HONEY & SOY

My mother would get all of our food to eat in the evening ready made and ready to cook. Dinner therefore was a simple affair of sliding off the cardboard sleeve, peeling back the plastic layer, emptying the whole lot into a heatproof dish and shoving it in the oven. Naturally the appeal of this is great, and it is something I am not ashamed to say that I do from time to time. However, it is meals like this one, which can take equally little effort but that is made fresh and from scratch, that the children love to eat – and I as a parent love to make. Fast, fresh, easy and light! There is an increase in sugar due to the addition of honey, but still great savings on calories and fat.

Serves

4

Chicken

8 chicken pieces (either drumsticks or thighs, or a mixture of the two), skin removed
8 garlic cloves, peeled and gently crushed
1 tsp chilli powder
Leaves from 3–4 sprigs of thyme
Juice of 1 lime
Salt and freshly ground black pepper

Glaze

3 tbsp honey
1 tsp English mustard powder
½ tsp soy sauce
½ tsp Worcestershire sauce
Zest of 1 lime

Sauce

300ml chicken stock
2 tsp cornflour

To serve

A small handful of fresh mint leaves
Cauliflower 'couscous' (see page 88), or brown rice with vegetables

Preheat the oven to 220°C, (Fan 200°C), 425°F, Gas Mark 7.

Toss the chicken pieces on a large roasting tray with the garlic, chilli powder, thyme, lime juice and salt and pepper. Lay them out in a single layer and pop them into the oven to bake for 25 minutes.

Meanwhile, mix the honey, mustard powder, soy sauce, Worcestershire sauce and lime zest in a small bowl to give a sticky glaze.

Once the chicken has been cooking for 10 minutes, remove it from the oven and brush over half of the glaze. Then brush over the remaining glaze after another 10 minutes of cooking. Pop it back into the oven for the remaining 5 minutes or until the chicken is piping hot in the centre and cooked through. Remove from the oven, transfer the pieces to a serving plate and cover with foil to keep warm.

Put the roasting tray on a high heat on the hob. Pour in all but about 3 tablespoons of the chicken stock, stirring all the time and scraping up any yumminess from the bottom of the tray. Blend the cornflour with the remaining stock to give a smooth liquid and pour this into the tray, stirring constantly. Let this bubble away for 2–3 minutes or so, stirring occasionally, until reduced and thickened. The sauce may have a few lumps in, which you can just sieve out before serving if you like. Season to taste and remove from the heat.

Serve two pieces of chicken per person with a little sauce poured over and a scattering of mint leaves on top. This is delicious served with my cauliflower 'couscous' (see page 88) or some brown rice with vegetables.

(PER SERVING)	ENERGY	FAT	SAT FAT	SUGAR	PROTEIN	SALT
LORRAINE'S RECIPE	242 Kcal	5.3g	1.5g	11.8g	32.2g	1.38g
COMPARISON RECIPE	499 Kcal	35.8g	9.4g	8g	36.5g	1.47g

CHICKEN, LEEK, BACON & TARRAGON PIE

My first foray into the grown-up world of the herb tarragon, at 15 years old, was not a good one. This relative of the daisy, I now know, is not to be eaten as a snack on its own. But when this faintly aniseedy herb is paired with chicken, the tarragon flavour softens to become something incredibly likeable, and the chicken comes out of its sometimes not-so-flavourful shell to pack a powerful, pungent punch. If you are counting the calories, then feast your eyes on this easy-to-make recipe – with a 40% reduction in calories compared to its full-fat friend. By all means reduce the bacon from four rashers to two, if you are watching your salt intake.

Serves
4

Filling
Spray oil
4 medium chicken breasts, cut into bite-sized chunks
4 rashers of lean back bacon, trimmed of excess fat and cut into strips
2 leeks, finely sliced
2 garlic cloves, finely chopped
1 tbsp fresh thyme leaves
2 tbsp cornflour
150ml chicken stock
200ml white wine
1 tsp Worcestershire sauce
½ bunch of spring onions, cut into 1cm-thick slices
3 tsp Dijon mustard
1 tbsp roughly chopped tarragon
Salt and freshly ground black pepper

Topping
3 sheets of filo pastry, defrosted

To serve
Crisp green salad

Preheat the oven to 180°C, (Fan 160°C), 350°F, Gas Mark 4.

Spritz a few sprays of oil into each of two large non-stick frying pans and set over a medium to high heat. Add half of the chicken to one pan and all of the bacon to the other and fry both for 4–5 minutes until they catch a good golden colour. Tip both into a medium-sized casserole pot and return the frying pans to the heat with another small spritz of oil.

Fry the remaining chicken in the chicken pan and add the leeks to the bacon pan. Again fry them for 4–5 minutes until the chicken turns golden and the leeks soften, stirring occasionally. Add the garlic and thyme to the leeks for the last minute. If the leeks start to look a little dry and stick to the pan, add a tablespoon of water. Tip the chicken and leeks into the casserole pot.

Next, blend the cornflour in about 50ml of the stock until smooth and then stir into the pot, followed by the remaining stock, the wine and the Worcestershire sauce. Bring to the boil on a medium heat, then reduce to a simmer for 5 minutes until thickened and the strong alcohol taste has burned off. Stir in the spring onions, Dijon mustard and tarragon and season to taste.

Finally, rip the filo pastry into pieces, scrunch them up a little and dot them all over the top of the casserole. Pop in the oven and cook for 15–20 minutes or until the chicken is piping hot in the middle and cooked through and the filo is crisp and lightly golden.

Serve hot with a crisp green salad.

(PER SERVING)	ENERGY	FAT	SAT FAT	SUGAR	PROTEIN	SALT
LORRAINE'S RECIPE	378 Kcal	6.3g	1.5g	3.2g	41.8g	2.18g
COMPARISON RECIPE	673 Kcal	54g	27.1g	2.9g	23.5g	1.36g

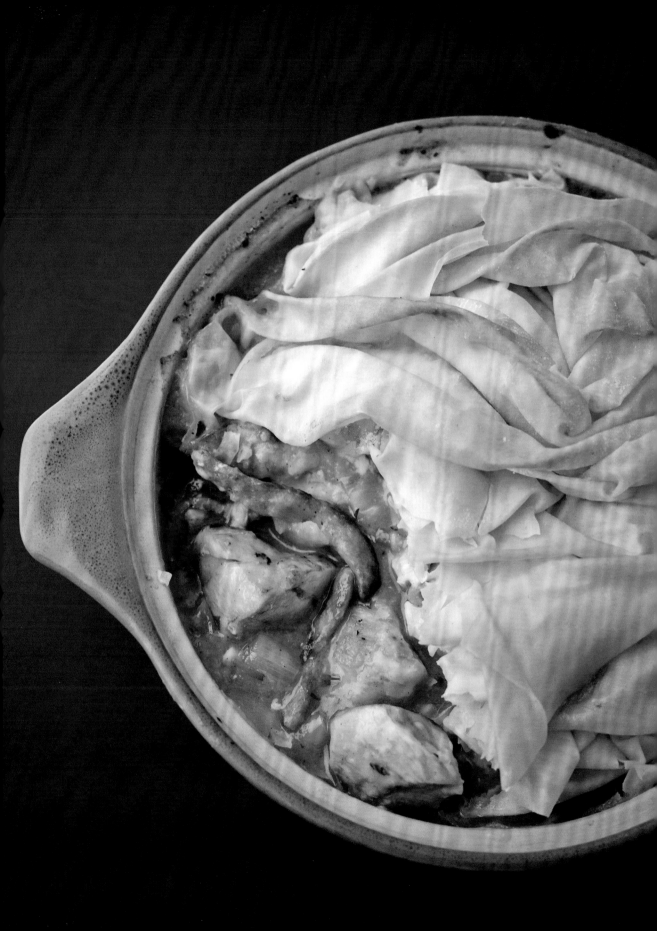

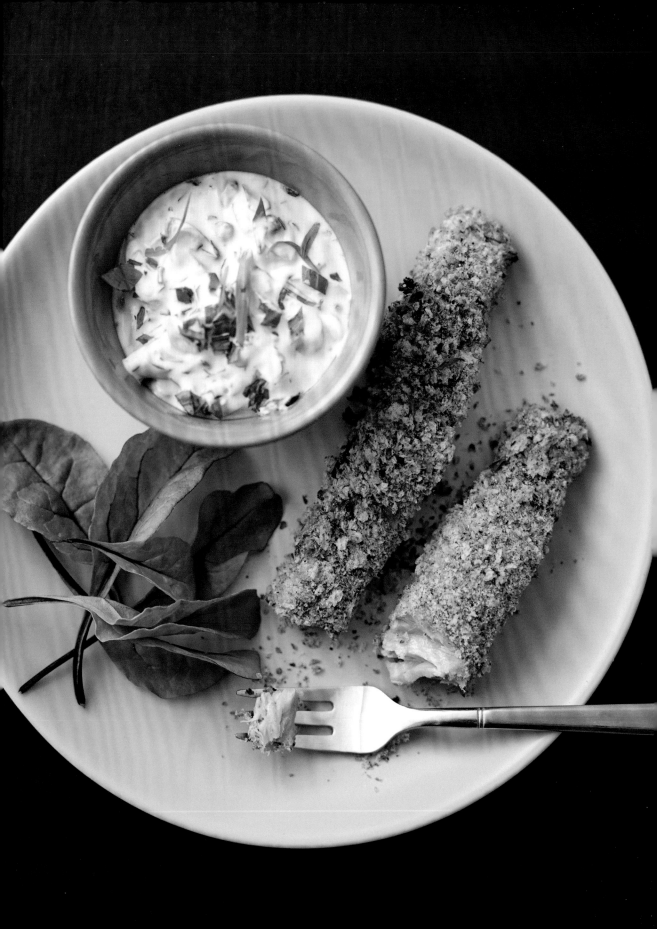

BAKED SALMON & THYME FISH FINGERS & HOME-MADE TARTARE SAUCE

I grew up on fish fingers. Not literally (there were other items of food that came to the table), but fish fingers had their close-up every Friday when my brother and I sat on the purple carpet, staring up at the crackly TV and dipping the bright orange sticks into pools of ketchup whilst mesmerized by Monkey, Pigsey and Tripitaka. These slightly-more-classy-than-I-remember-eating fish fingers were invented to bring me back to the day when fish fingers ruled the Friday roost. I have also tried these out on kiddies, who lap them up and beg for more. Just be doubly sure that there are no bones in the salmon before cooking and cod, haddock and pollock can all be substituted for the salmon too. Don't let the increase in sugar worry you: it is due to the naturally occurring sugars in the yogurt.

Makes
8 fish fingers (serves 4 as a main)

Equipment
Food processor

Fish fingers
4 slices of wholemeal bread
1 tbsp roughly chopped fresh
    thyme leaves
3 egg whites
4 x 125g sustainably caught
    salmon fillets (or 2 x 250g
    chunky cod fillets), skinless

Tartare sauce
150g Greek yogurt (full fat, low
    fat or no fat)
1 tsp English mustard powder or
    2 tsp Dijon mustard
4 tsp capers
3 spring onions, finely chopped
1 tbsp finely chopped fresh flat
    leaf parsley
2 tsp finely chopped fresh tarragon
Juice of ½ lemon
Few drops of Tabasco (optional)
Salt and freshly ground black
    pepper

Preheat the oven to 220°C, (Fan 200°C), 425°F, Gas Mark 7 and line a baking tray with baking parchment.

Lightly toast the bread in a toaster or under the grill and then blitz in a food processor to give fine, dry breadcrumbs. Tip them into a wide, shallow bowl and toss the thyme leaves, a little salt and a good amount of black pepper through. Lightly beat the egg whites in another wide shallow bowl with a bit of seasoning too.

If using salmon, cut each fillet in half along the length or cut each cod fillet down its length into four thick fingers. Either way, this should give you eight fish fingers.

Working in batches, toss the fish fingers firstly through the egg white, followed by the breadcrumbs to stick and coat evenly. Arrange them in a single layer on the baking tray as you go. Bake in the oven for 10–15 minutes.

Meanwhile, prepare the tartare sauce. Simply mix all the ingredients in a medium bowl and season to taste.

To check the fish fingers are cooked, wiggle a knife into the centre of the thickest piece. The fish should be white all through and not opaque. Once cooked, remove from the oven and serve straight away with the tartare sauce.

(PER SERVING – 2 FISH FINGERS AND SAUCE)	ENERGY	FAT	SAT FAT	SUGAR	PROTEIN	SALT
LORRAINE'S RECIPE	370 Kcal	18.8g	5g	2.8g	34.1g	1.31g
COMPARISON RECIPE	761 Kcal	58.7g	9.3g	0.8g	22.7g	1.73g

QUICKISH
THAI FISH PIE

I have a fish pie recipe in my *Baking Made Easy* book – a traditional affair with the ubiquitous eggs, white fish and other usual suspects. Although fish pie is a British favourite, my family simply would not eat it. I love fish, I really do, and I love pie, so I had to come up with something that the whole family could enjoy. Coconut milk and Thai green curry paste lift this subtle-tasting pie into the realms of something rather special. This anglo-Asian dish is not to be sniffed at and has now made it into the top ten dinners on the LP wall of fame – no mean feat with all the demanding mouths around my table! If you want to make it ahead of time, just make the fish filling and pop it in the fridge. Leave the filo off until you are ready to bake it so the pastry retains its crispness. There's a touch more salt in my recipe than the comparison recipe: this comes from the curry paste, but the increase is small and worthwhile for the speed advantage!

Serves
4

Equipment
4 ramekins or hot pot dishes

Filling
500g skinless, boneless sustainably caught fish (I use salmon and haddock) cut into big bite-sized chunks
16 raw, peeled tiger prawns (about 175g)
100g fresh or frozen peas
400ml tin of low-fat coconut milk
4 tbsp Thai green curry paste
2 garlic cloves, finely chopped
2cm piece of ginger, finely chopped
1 red chilli, finely chopped
Juice of ½ lime
A large handful of basil leaves
Salt and freshly ground black pepper

Topping
2 sheets of filo pastry, defrosted

Preheat the oven to 180°C, (Fan 160°C), 350°F, Gas Mark 4.

Toss the fish, prawns, peas and a little salt and pepper together in a medium bowl and then divide the mixture evenly between four ramekins or hot pot dishes. Mine measure about 10cm wide, 6cm high and are 450ml in volume. Arrange them on a baking sheet and set aside.

Put the coconut milk, curry paste, garlic, ginger and chilli into a wide pan. Stir them together well to combine and set over a high heat to bring to the boil. Reduce to simmer for 2–3 minutes, stirring occasionally, until reduced and thickened a little. Stir the lime juice and basil through and season to taste if necessary.

Divide the curry sauce mixture between the four ramekins or dishes. Rip the filo pastry into pieces, lightly scrunch them up and place them on top of the filling to cover. Pop into the oven to bake for 15–20 minutes or until the fish is cooked through and the pastry is crisp and golden brown.

(PER SERVING)	ENERGY	FAT	SAT FAT	SUGAR	PROTEIN	SALT
LORRAINE'S RECIPE	420 Kcal	19.9g	10.8g	3.9g	37.3g	1.14g
COMPARISON RECIPE	526 Kcal	37.6g	24.8g	5.7g	22.3g	0.77g

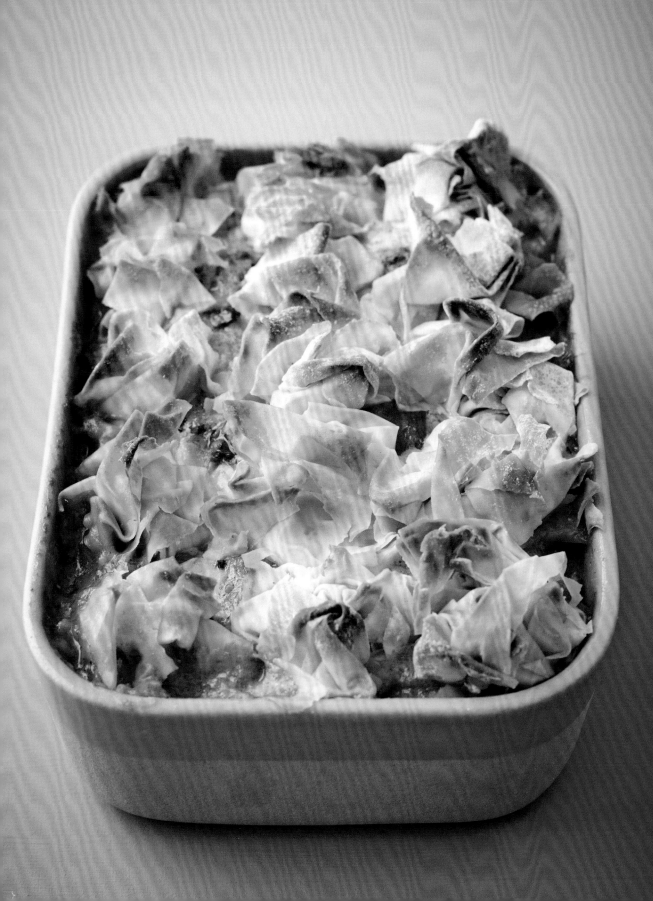

BAKED COCONUT SHRIMP SALAD WITH HONEY DRESSING & SPICY MANGO & CORIANDER SALSA

It may seem a bit odd to bake something as small as the humble curled-up shrimp, but when frying them I found that the shrimps became too rich due to the oil which they soaked up in the pan. If you, like my dear brother, are not a fan of coconut, then forgo our exotic speckled 'fruit' and just use the breadcrumbs instead. 'But surely, Ms Pascale, the shrimp would be even healthier if they did not have any breadcrumbs on at all?' 'Why yes,' I would reply, 'of course, but breaded and baked is of course much better than breaded and fried.' I have served these before as canapés to hand around as my mates arrive. It's hard to get the shrimps with the tails still on, but if you can they look great on the plate as they are passed around to waiting guests!

Serves

4

Prawns

2 egg whites
25g dried breadcrumbs
25g desiccated coconut
¼ tsp dried chilli flakes
20 raw peeled jumbo prawns
   (about 400g), with the tails left
   on if you like

Dressing

2 tbsp honey
2 tbsp balsamic vinegar

Mango salsa

250g prepared mango chunks
   (or 2 medium mangoes), cut into
   1cm cubes
2 red chillies, seeds removed if you
   want less heat, finely chopped
Juice of 2 limes
Leaves from a large handful of
   coriander, roughly chopped

To serve

200g bag of prepared lettuce
Salt and freshly ground black
   pepper

Preheat the oven to 200°C, (Fan 180°C), 400°F, Gas Mark 6. Line a baking sheet with baking parchment and set aside.

Lightly beat the egg whites in a wide, shallow bowl to break them up. Toss the breadcrumbs, coconut, chilli flakes and a little salt and pepper together in another similar-sized bowl.

Working in batches, toss a few of the prawns into the egg whites, making sure they are well coated. Use a slotted spoon to lift them out, allowing the excess egg white to fall back into the bowl. Then, tip the prawns into the coconut crumbs, toss them about and, using another slotted spoon (or you can just pick them up with your hands), transfer them onto the baking sheet in a single layer. Repeat until all are coated and then bake in the oven for 8–10 minutes.

Meanwhile, make the dressing. Simply whisk the honey and vinegar together in a small bowl, season to taste and set aside.

To make the salsa, toss the mango, chilli, lime juice, coriander and a little salt and pepper together and set aside also.

Once cooked, the prawns should have turned from bluish green to pink, be cooked through and the coconut crumbs crisp and lightly golden. Remove from the oven and you are ready to serve.

Divide the salad leaves between four serving bowls. Spoon the salsa over, arrange five prawns on top of each, finish with a drizzle of the dressing and serve.

(PER SERVING – SHRIMP ONLY)	ENERGY	FAT	SAT FAT	SUGAR	PROTEIN	SALT
LORRAINE'S RECIPE	132 Kcal	4.6g	3.5g	0.6g	19.4g	0.66g
COMPARISON RECIPE	271 Kcal	17.7g	6g	0.7g	16.6g	0.51g

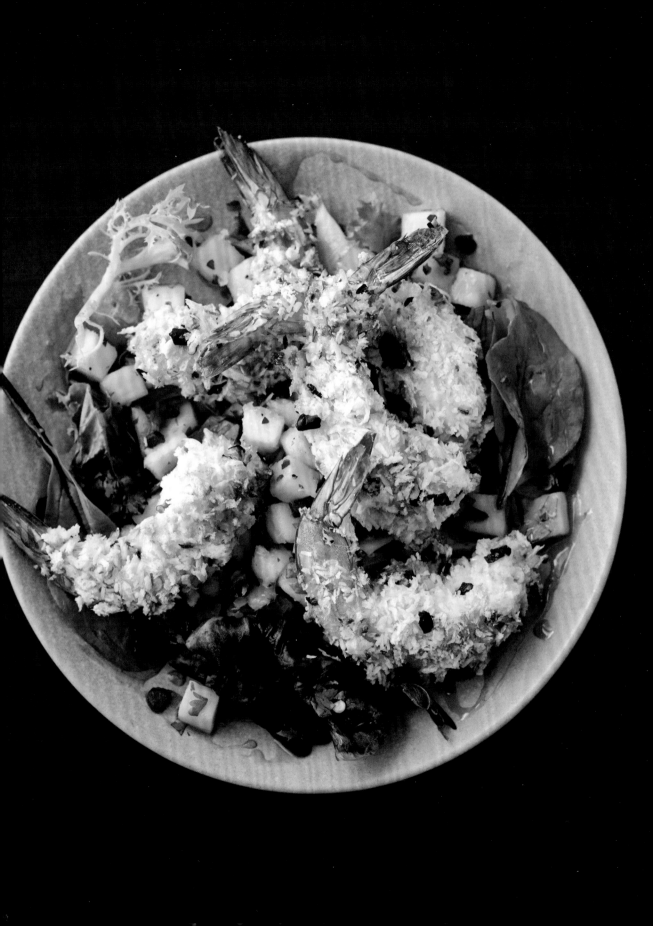

CRÈME FRAÎCHE POTATO DAUPHINOISE WITH THYME & SAGE

This, by its very nature, is a truly indulgent dish. Traditionally made with lashings of double cream, I decided to use a small bit of crème fraîche in its place for flavour which has less fat. Experimenting with low-fat crème fraîche, or even half-fat, meant that the resulting product was watery and tasteless, so I knew that there was definitely a need for something in it to give it a hint of its full-fat decadence. So to make the dish really tasty, I cheated by the use of milk and crème fraîche, plus a little cornflour to thicken the sauce, which gave this French beauty the final lift that it needed.

Serves
4

Equipment
Mandoline or good sharp knife, 2 litre baking dish, measuring 27 x 21cm and 5cm in depth

3 large potatoes (about 1kg)
2 tbsp cornflour
400ml semi-skimmed milk
100g full-fat crème fraîche
200ml vegetable or chicken stock
2 big or 3 small garlic cloves, finely sliced
Leaves from 3 large sprigs of fresh thyme
2 tsp roughly chopped sage leaves
Good pinch of freshly grated nutmeg
50g Gruyère or Parmesan cheese
Salt and freshly ground black pepper

Preheat the oven to 200°C, (Fan 180°C), 400°F, Gas Mark 6.

Peel and slice the potatoes as thinly as possible (preferably to the thickness of half a £1 coin if you can). A mandolin would be ideal for this, but a good sharp knife and a steady hand should do the trick also. Then set aside for a moment while you prepare the sauce.

Put the cornflour into a medium pan off the heat, add a couple of tablespoons of milk and blend to a smooth paste. Then slowly add the remaining milk, whisking all the time until all is added without any lumps. Whisk in the crème fraîche, stock, garlic, thyme, sage and nutmeg. Place on a medium heat and bring slowly to the boil, stirring occasionally.

Reduce to simmer, add the potato slices and season with salt and pepper, to taste. Pop a lid on and let them simmer away for about 12 minutes, stirring it every now and again so nothing catches on the bottom. The potatoes should be partly cooked, but still firm. Remove from the heat and, using a slotted spoon, transfer the potatoes to a 2 litre baking dish, measuring 27 x 21cm and 5cm in depth. Pour over the milky liquid and all the tasty bits in it. Grate the cheese over with a little bit of extra nutmeg also if you like. Cover with foil and pop into the oven for about 30 minutes, removing the foil for the last 10 minutes. The cheese should be bubbling away and the potatoes should be cooked through and soft.

Remove from the oven and serve straight away.

(PER SERVING)	ENERGY	FAT	SAT FAT	SUGAR	PROTEIN	SALT
LORRAINE'S RECIPE	418 Kcal	16.6g	10.6g	7.7g	13.2g	1.08g
COMPARISON RECIPE	767 Kcal	53.5g	32.4g	6.2g	23.4g	1.92g

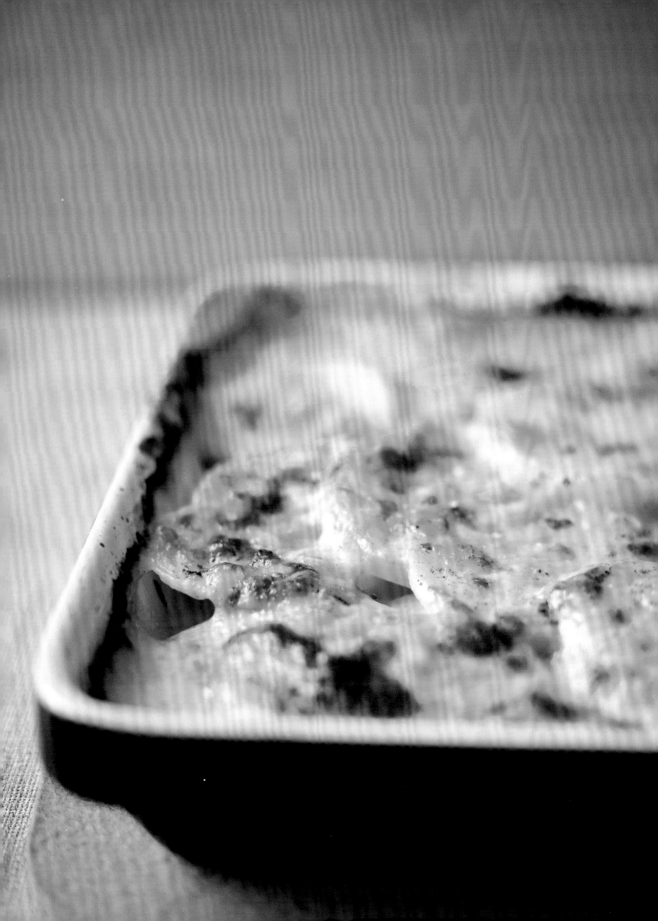

BAKED LENTIL &
BEAN COTTAGE PIE
WITH A POTATO &
PARSNIP MASH TOP

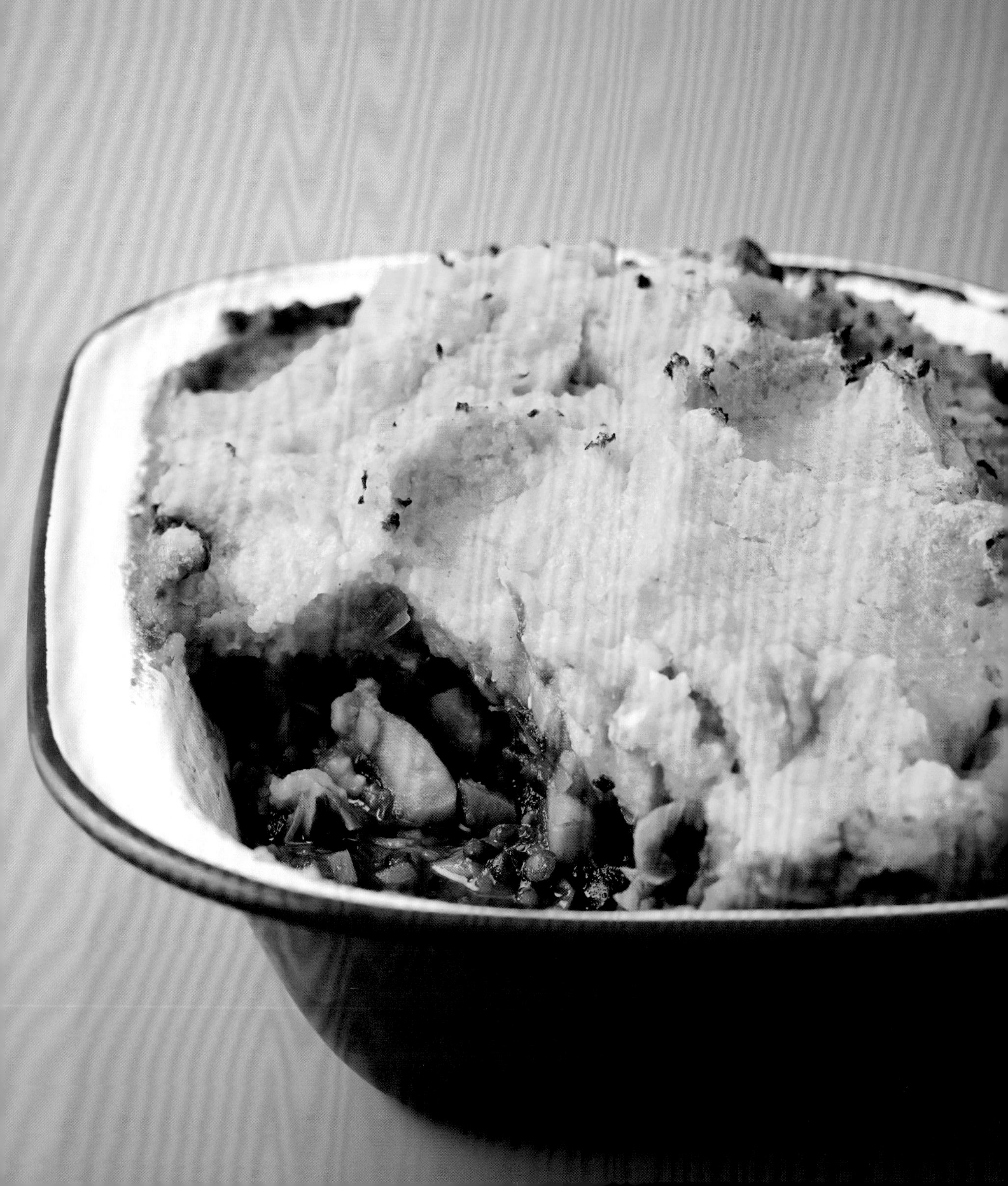

Serves

6

Equipment

2.5 litre baking dish, measuring 25.5cm square and 6cm deep

Filling

Spray oil
2 leeks, finely chopped
2 big garlic cloves, finely chopped
4 carrots, finely chopped
300g chestnut mushrooms, roughly chopped
400g tin of green or Puy lentils, drained
400g tin of kidney beans, drained
400g tin of chopped tomatoes
150ml vegetable stock
1 glass of Marsala, dry sherry or red wine
5 large sage leaves, roughly chopped
Leaves from 3 sprigs of fresh rosemary, finely chopped
1 tsp chilli flakes (optional)
1 tbsp Worcestershire sauce
1 tbsp soy sauce
1 tsp caster sugar (optional)
1 tbsp finely grated Parmesan (optional)
Salt and freshly ground black pepper

Mash top

2 medium sweet potatoes (about 500g), peeled and cut into 2cm chunks
2 medium potatoes (about 500g), peeled and cut into 1cm chunks (save the peelings to make my Baked Potato Crispies on page 87)
1 parsnip, peeled and cut into 1cm chunks
2 tbsp unsalted butter
Salt and freshly ground black pepper

To serve

Crisp green salad

As far as writing a healthier or lighter cookbook is concerned, I always think it is a good idea to include stuff in there that people actually want to bake. I mean, nuts and seeds are great, but if I was given a book of recipes full of stuff that I would never normally cook, then I am not sure I would buy it. Sooo, I was very tempted not to put this recipe in the book and instead place a meaty version in there, but I have it on solemn word from the family that this beany cottage pie really does taste pretty good.

Spray a little oil in a large pan and set over a medium heat. Add the leek and cook gently for 5 minutes until it begins to soften. Then add the garlic and cook for a further minute. Next, add the carrot, mushroom, lentils, kidney beans, tomatoes, stock, Marsala (dry sherry or red wine), sage, rosemary and chilli flakes (if using). Whack up the heat and let it bubble away for 20 minutes while you make the mash.

Preheat the oven to 200°C, (Fan 180°C), 400°F, Gas Mark 6.

Bring a large pan of water to the boil (no need to add salt). Add the sweet potato, potato and parsnip and cook for about 15 minutes or until everything is nice and soft. Then, drain well and return to the pan. Add the butter, season well with salt and pepper, and then mash until smooth and keep warm.

Once the pie filling mixture has had its time, add the Worcestershire sauce, soy sauce and sugar, if using. Let it bubble away for a further minute or two. If the sauce is too thick, add a little water, but if you think the sauce is too thin, then let it bubble away for a little longer. Taste it and adjust the seasoning to your liking.

Once the pie filling is ready, tip it into a 2.5 litre baking dish, measuring 25.5cm square and 6cm deep, and then spoon the mash over the top, spreading it out evenly, fluffing it up in places with a fork so that bits of it crisp up during baking. Sprinkle the Parmesan over, if using, and then bake for 20 minutes or until the mash starts to go a little crispy.

Once baked, remove from the oven and serve straight away with a crisp green salad.

(PER SERVING)	ENERGY	FAT	SAT FAT	SUGAR	PROTEIN	SALT
LORRAINE'S RECIPE	367 Kcal	6g	2.9g	16.2g	15.3g	1.69g
COMPARISON RECIPE	461 Kcal	14.1g	7.3g	22.7g	15.3g	2.39g

SKINNIER MAC & CHEESE WITH THYME

In *Baking Made Easy*, I had a mac and cheese. Boy did I have a mac and cheese. It had all the cheese you could shake a stick at and then some. I received oodles of letters and tweets from people saying how much they had enjoyed it but how they felt they could only make it for a special occasion due to its, er, cheese and cream content. I made this recipe several times, reducing the cheese but still giving you that feeling that you are indeed having a real treat. I served it up to a table of friends, and no one knew that it was the lighter version. So mac and cheese, lighter on the calories, but equally filling and just as tasty on the tongue.

Serves
6

Equipment
2.5 litre baking dish, measuring 25.5cm square, 6cm deep, food processor

400g wholemeal spiralli or macaroni (or you can use regular if you like)
1 slice of wholemeal bread
3 tbsp cornflour
1 tsp English mustard powder
Pinch of cayenne
500ml semi-skimmed milk
200g strong or mature Cheddar cheese, roughly grated
Leaves from 3 sprigs of thyme
Salt and freshly ground black pepper

To serve
Crisp green salad

Turn the grill on to high. Sit a 2.5 litre baking dish measuring 25.5cm square and 6cm deep on a baking sheet and set aside.

Bring a large pan of water to the boil and cook the pasta according to the packet directions.

Meanwhile, lightly toast the bread under the grill and then blitz in a food processor to give fine, dry breadcrumbs and set them aside.

Next, prepare the sauce. Place the cornflour, mustard powder and cayenne in a medium pan with about 4 tablespoons of the milk and blend to give a smooth, lump-free liquid. Continuing to stir, pour the rest of the milk into the pan, season with salt and pepper and set over a high heat. Bring to the boil and then reduce to simmer for 3–4 minutes, stirring from time to time until thickened. Stir in all but 75g of the cheese (reserving that for the top) and allow it to melt before removing from the heat.

Once the pasta is cooked, drain it well and return it to the pan in which it was cooked. Pour the cheese sauce over, add the thyme and mix it all together well. Tip the macaroni cheese into the prepared baking dish. Toss the remaining cheese and breadcrumbs together in a small bowl and scatter them evenly over the top. Then pop it under the grill for a few minutes to get nice and crispy, bubbly and golden brown. Serve with a crisp green salad.

(PER SERVING)	ENERGY	FAT	SAT FAT	SUGAR	PROTEIN	SALT
LORRAINE'S RECIPE	448 Kcal	14.9g	8.4g	6.3g	20.9g	0.77g
COMPARISON RECIPE	471 Kcal	22.3g	13.5g	6.6g	20.7g	1.15g

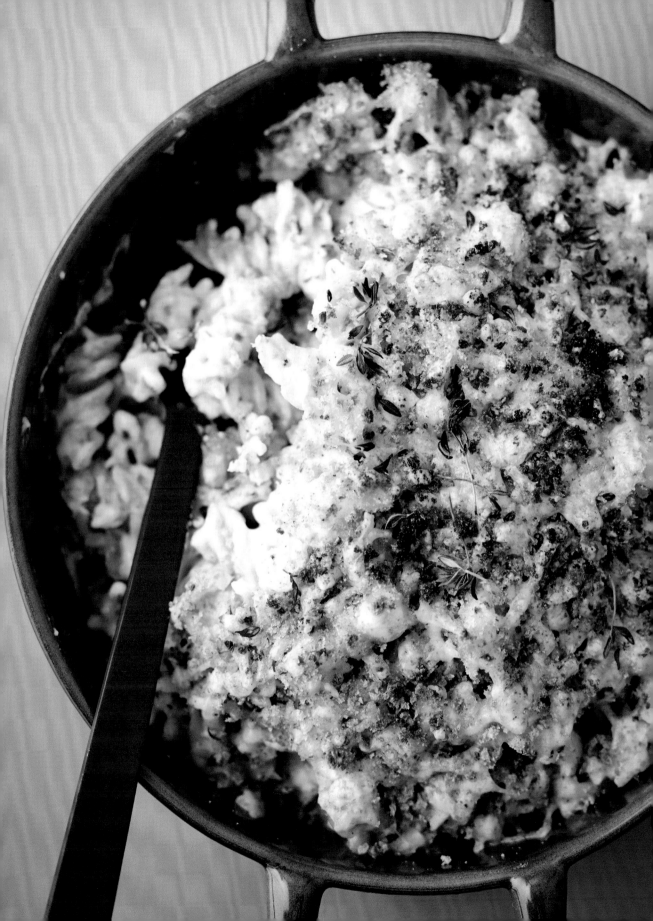

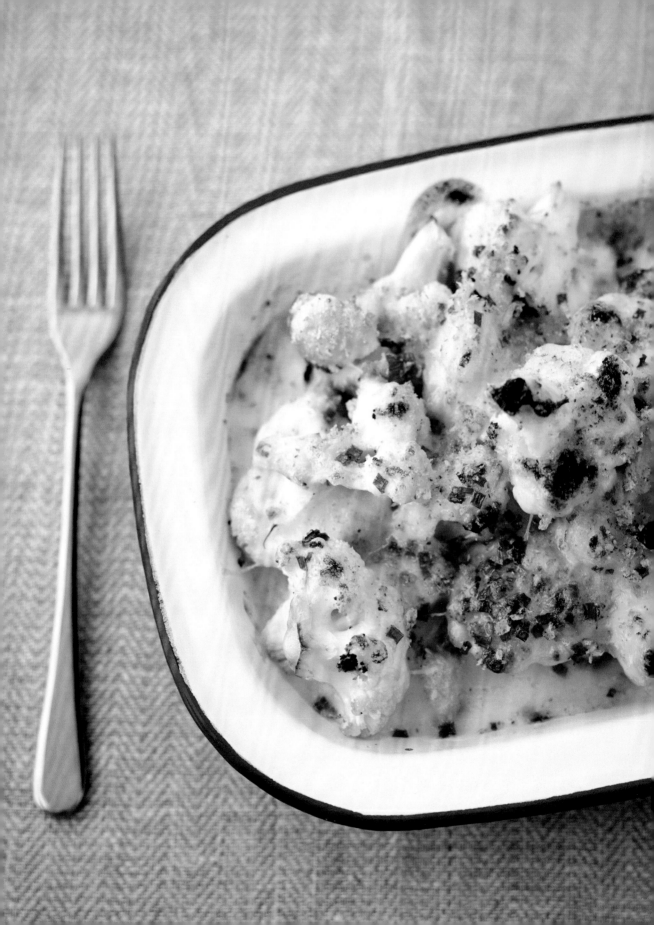

BAKED CAULIFLOWER CHEESE WITH A CREAMY GRATIN SAUCE

Now, I don't know about you, but I am a bit partial to a good cauliflower with way too much cheese. However, in the spirit of the healthier vibe I searched for a way to make cauliflower cheese our friend. In my quest to make it 'lighter', I have come up with a quick white sauce requiring no faffing about with a roux. Add more cheese if you must, but this for me is a great little side number for your veggie friend or as an accompaniment to a meaty roast.

Serves

4 as a side dish

Equipment

25cm square shallow baking dish

1 large cauliflower, trimmed and cut into small bite-sized florets
Spray oil
2 tbsp cornflour
1 tsp English mustard powder
500ml full-fat milk (semi-skimmed milk does not seem to work so well)
2 bay leaves
75g Cheddar cheese, roughly grated
Small handful of fresh chives, finely chopped
3 tbsp wholemeal breadcrumbs (made from about ½ slice of lightly toasted bread, crusts included)
2 tbsp roughly grated Parmesan
Salt and freshly ground black pepper

Preheat the oven to 200°C, (Fan 180°C), 400°F, Gas Mark 6.

Scatter the cauliflower florets into a 25cm square shallow baking dish, season with some salt and pepper and spray a little oil evenly over them. Bake in the oven for 25–30 minutes or until the cauliflower florets have toasty golden brown edges and are just tender when pierced with a fork.

Meanwhile, make the sauce. Put the cornflour and mustard powder into a medium pan and add 2 tablespoons of the milk. Stir them together well until dissolved and smooth, and then gradually stir in the remaining milk. Add the bay leaves and some salt and pepper and place the pan on a medium heat. Bring to the boil and then allow to bubble away, while stirring constantly, for 3–4 minutes until smooth and thickened. Remove from the heat and stir in the Cheddar until melted. Fish the bay leaves out and discard.

Once the cauliflower is ready, remove it from the oven and turn the grill on to high. Scatter the chives over the top of the cauliflower and then pour the sauce evenly over that. Finally, sprinkle the breadcrumbs and the Parmesan cheese over the top. Place under the grill for 3–4 minutes until bubbling and beginning to crisp up. Serve at once.

(PER SERVING)	ENERGY	FAT	SAT FAT	SUGAR	PROTEIN	SALT
LORRAINE'S RECIPE	272 Kcal	14.6g	8.6g	8.9g	15.7g	0.93g
COMPARISON RECIPE	364 Kcal	24.2g	14.7g	8.2g	18.7g	0.91g

BUTTERNUT SQUASH 'NAKED' BEAN BURGER WITH APPLE, MANGO & CHILLI SALSA

Growing up as a teen in Devon, there really was not a lot to do, once you had watched sheep eat grass, observed a few rabbits hopping about the field and been moved on by a farmer telling you to get off his land. The only other thing to do was to head to the very small town centre to sit on the shiny plastic seats down the Wimpy for a catch-up with your mates. They would always go for the full meat burger, but I was one for the bean burger – I just could not get enough of them. I am sure the Wimpy burger did not come with an apple, mango and chilli salsa, but it would have been good if it did! Anyway, Wimpy, I thank you for my introduction to the world that is the beany burger. The sugar content comes mostly from the fruit in the salsa (the added sweetener being just a cheeky squeeze of honey).

Makes
6 burgers

Equipment
Food processor

Bean burger
200g prepared butternut squash, peeled and cut into 1cm pieces
Spray oil
2 red onions, finely chopped
2 garlic cloves, finely chopped
1 red chilli, finely chopped
2 tsp paprika
Small handful of fresh coriander, roughly chopped
400g tin of kidney beans, drained
400g tin of cannellini beans, drained
1 egg white
Finely grated zest of 1 lime
Salt and freshly ground black pepper

Coating
3 slices of wholemeal bread
1 egg white

Salsa
250g prepared mango chunks (or 2 mangoes), cut into 1cm cubes
2 Granny Smith apples, peeled, cored and cut into 1cm cubes
1 red chilli, finely sliced
2 tsp honey
Leaves from a small handful of coriander or flat leaf parsley, roughly chopped

'Bun'
12 iceberg lettuce leaves

Preheat the oven to 200°C, (Fan 180°C), 400°F, Gas Mark 6 and line a baking sheet with baking parchment.

Cook the butternut squash in a pan of boiling, lightly salted, water for 3–4 minutes or until just tender and drain really well. Meanwhile, heat a little spray oil in a medium frying pan over a medium heat and cook the red onion for 8 minutes or so until it goes nice and soft and a little bit brown.

While the onion is cooking, prepare the burger coating. Lightly toast the bread in a toaster or under the grill and then blitz in a food processor to give fine, dry breadcrumbs. Tip them into a wide, shallow bowl and season with a little salt and pepper. Lightly beat the egg white in another shallow bowl until a bit foamy. Set both aside.

Once the onions are cooked, add the garlic, chilli, paprika and coriander, cook for a further minute and remove from the heat.

Tip the kidney and cannellini beans into a large bowl and lightly crush them with a potato masher. Then stir the onion mixture through, followed by the egg white, lime zest and a little salt and pepper. Finally, carefully fold in the cooked butternut squash until well mixed through. Form the mixture into six burger patties about 9cm wide and 1.5cm deep. The mixture is a little sticky, so use dampened hands to shape them.

Next, dip a burger into the prepared egg white, turning it to make sure it is stuck all over. Shake off any excess and dip the burger into the breadcrumbs until evenly coated. Repeat with the remaining burgers, popping them onto the baking sheet as you go. Spray each one with some oil and then bake in the oven for 25 minutes until crisp and golden.

Meanwhile, make the salsa. Simply toss all of the salsa ingredients together in a bowl, season to taste and then cover and set aside in the fridge until needed.

Using a pair of scissors, trim around the edge of the lettuce leaves to make a nice cup shape big enough to hold the burger.

Once the burgers are cooked remove them from the oven. Arrange a lettuce leaf on each serving plate, sit a burger inside and top with a little salsa. Lay the second lettuce-leaf cup just off the burger and serve.

(PER BURGER)	ENERGY	FAT	SAT FAT	SUGAR	PROTEIN	SALT
LORRAINE'S RECIPE	188 Kcal	1.4g	0.2g	18.2g	8.5g	1.06g
COMPARISON RECIPE	494 Kcal	22.4g	10.7g	6.3g	21.4g	3.13g

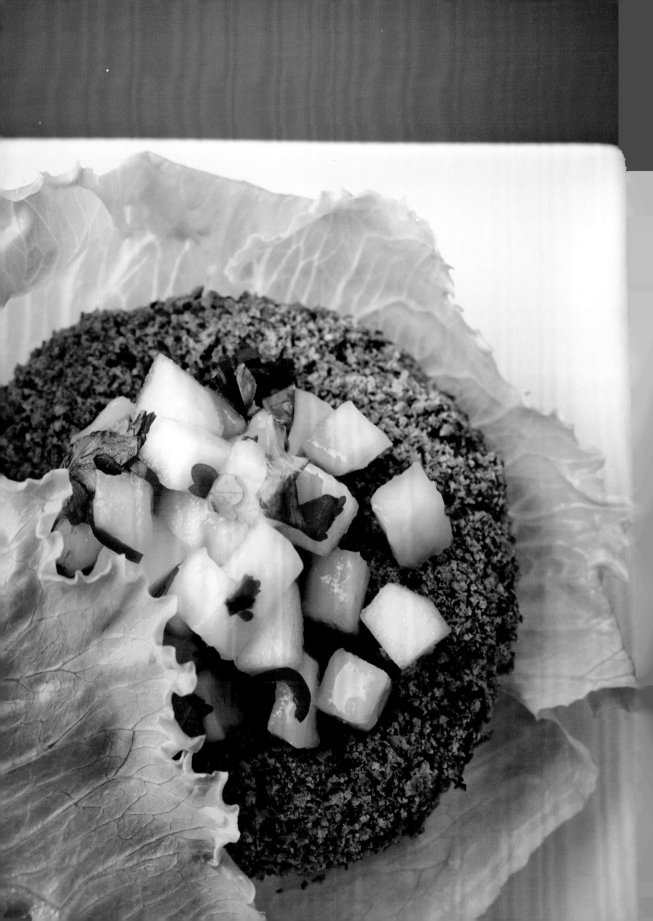

BUTTERNUT SQUASH, BASIL & ONION QUICHE

So the quiche (my namesake!) comes from the Alsace region in eastern France, which has changed hands frequently over the years between the Germans and the French. Now nestled on the French side, the Alsace-Lorraine region's quiche, traditionally has only a little bacon added to the egg custard mix. Being an advocate, wherever possible, of getting as much veg you can get your hands on into your daily diet, I have taken the liberty of adding some other colourful flavourful things to the standard recipe – to help you on your way to getting your five-a-day. Nearly half of the sugar content comes from the onions, and you're saving over 100 calories per portion!

Serves
6

Equipment
20cm round, loose-bottomed, straight-sided flan tin, dried beans or ceramic baking beans

Pastry
A little plain flour for dusting
350g Lower-fat Spread Wholemeal 'Shortcrust' Pastry (see page 263) – or you can use shop-bought light shortcrust pastry

Filling
Spray oil
2 large red onions, finely sliced
220g pack of ready-prepared butternut squash, cut into 1cm cubes
1 garlic clove, finely chopped
2 eggs
1 egg white
100g less than 3% fat crème fraîche
100g semi-skimmed milk
Salt and freshly ground black pepper

To serve
Small handful of basil leaves
50g bag of rocket

Preheat the oven to 180°C, (Fan 160°C), 350°F, Gas Mark 4. Grease a 20cm round, loose-bottomed, straight-sided flan tin.

Lightly dust a clean surface with flour and roll the pastry out into a circle just bigger than the tin and to the thickness of a £1 coin. Lift the pastry up carefully and drape it over the rolling pin to help you lay it into the prepared tin, leaving the excess hanging over. Pinch a little of the spare pastry off, roll it into a ball and then push it down gently into the 'corners' of the tin, so that when the tin is removed after baking the edges are nice and straight. Trim the excess pastry off with a sharp knife. Try not to pull or stretch the pastry too much, otherwise it will just shrink during cooking. If there are any holes in the pastry just patch them up with other bits of pastry, to make sure the filling can't leak out.

The pastry will probably now be a bit soft, so put it in the fridge for about 20 minutes or so or until it is nice and firm. Take a large square of baking parchment, scrunch it up and then open it out to line the pastry – this just makes it a little easier to make it stay where you put it. Then fill the paper-lined pastry with dried beans or ceramic baking beans and bake it for about 20 minutes until just firm to the touch and beginning to turn golden. Lift the paper and beans out and return the pastry case to the oven to bake for 5 more minutes. This should dry the bottom out and make it a bit more evenly golden. Finally, remove from the oven and leave to cool.

While the pastry is cooking, make the filling. Spray a little oil into a medium pan set over a medium heat and fry the onions for 6–8 minutes until they begin to soften and just turn brown. Add the butternut squash and cook for 6–8 minutes, until just tender. Add the garlic for the final minute and then remove from the heat and leave to cool for a few minutes.

Meanwhile, mix the eggs, egg white, crème fraîche and milk together in a large jug and season with a little salt and pepper. Stir the cooled onion and squash mixture into the egg mix and then carefully pour this into the cooked pastry case.

Bake in the oven for 30–35 minutes or until the egg has just set but with the tiniest bit of wobble still in the centre. Once cooked remove from the oven and leave until cool enough to handle. Then carefully remove from the tin, cut into six wedges, scatter the basil and rocket over the quiche and serve.

(PER SERVING)	ENERGY	FAT	SAT FAT	SUGAR	PROTEIN	SALT
LORRAINE'S RECIPE	346 Kcal	15.6g	8g	10.8g	12.7g	0.22g
COMPARISON RECIPE	452 Kcal	30.6g	13.8g	5.2g	15.6g	0.88g

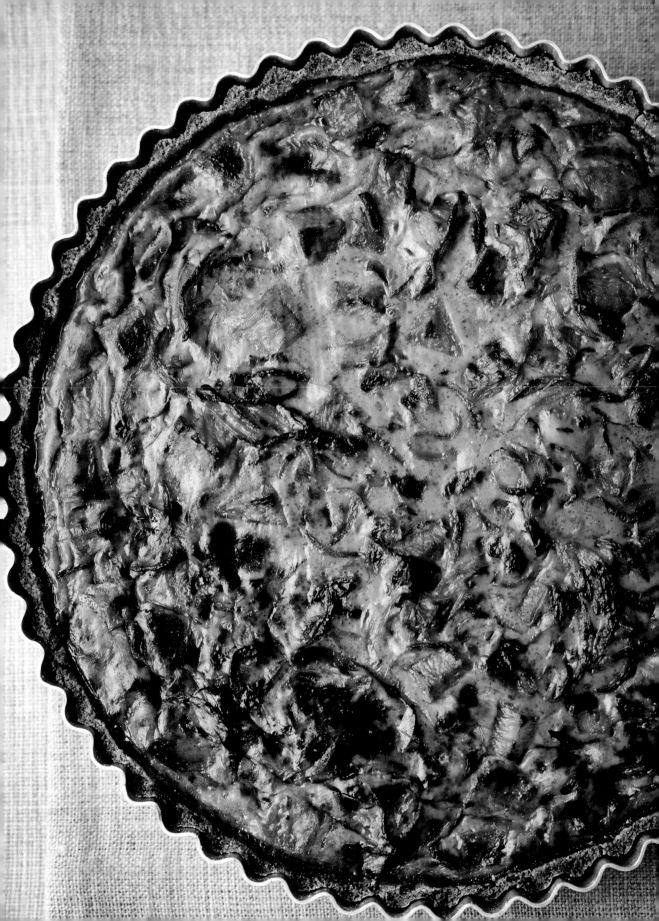

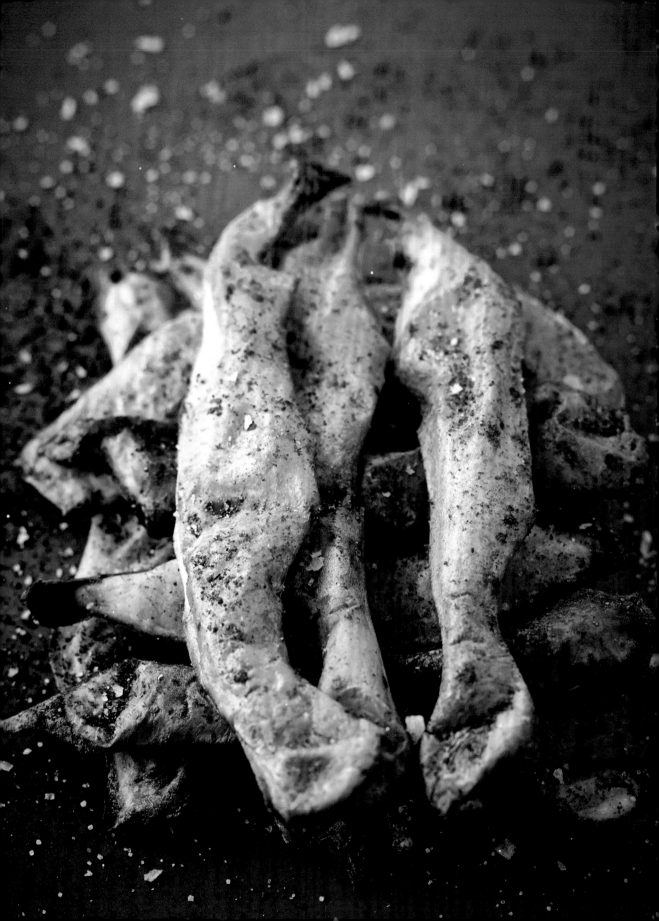

BAKED POTATO CRISPIES

Every Sunday when we have roast potatoes, I have the unenviable task of peeling the tatties and throwing the peel into the bin. One Sunday, I was thinking about these delicious potato skins from one of my favourite restaurants, which they serve with lashings of chive sour cream. So I tossed the peelings onto a tray, spread them out in a single layer, sprayed them with oil and put them into the oven. A short time later, out came these fabulous potato crisps, with more flavour than normal crisps, but with all the goodness of a skin full of fibre. These make great good-priced canapés too, served with a variety of dips.

Makes
Enough for 2 to share as nibbles

100g potato skin peelings (about 1kg potatoes gives roughly this amount of peelings)
1 tbsp olive oil
Sea salt
¼ tsp cayenne or paprika (optional)

Preheat the oven to 200°C, (Fan 180°C), 400°F, Gas Mark 6.

Scatter the potato skins all over a large baking tray in a single layer. Drizzle with the oil (or spray with one of those fabulous spray oil things) and then sprinkle over a little salt and the cayenne or paprika, if using.

Bake in the oven for 10–12 minutes, tossing halfway through, or until the potato skins are crisp and crunchy. I always keep an extra eye on them as they can 'catch' and go too dark quite quickly.

Once baked, remove from the oven and serve warm. They are great with dips and are a totally delicious better-for-you-than-shop-bought-crisps snack. These will keep for a few days in an airtight container.

(PER SERVING)	ENERGY	FAT	SAT FAT	SUGAR	PROTEIN	SALT
LORRAINE'S RECIPE	78 Kcal	5.5g	0.8g	0g	1.3g	0.63g
COMPARISON RECIPE	218 Kcal	18.5g	2.2g	0.1g	4.1g	0.60g

CAULIFLOWER 'COUSCOUS' WITH CHILLI, SESAME & MINT

This is not baked, not in any way, shape or form, but I wanted to include it in the book as an interesting alternative to couscous (the comparison recipe is regular couscous). It is much lower in carbohydrates than regular couscous and you can add whatever bits and pieces you fancy to make it your own tasty, almost guilt-free accompaniment. The sugar content comes from the natural sugars in the onions, cauliflower and red pepper.

Serves

4 (or 6 as an accompaniment)

Food processor

1 large cauliflower
Spray oil
2 large red onions, very finely chopped
2 big garlic cloves, finely chopped
1 red pepper, very finely chopped
2 red chillies, deseeded (if you like it less hot) and very finely chopped
4cm piece of fresh ginger, peeled and very finely chopped
100ml good chicken stock
Juice of 1 lemon
Drizzle (about 1–2 tsp) of sesame oil (optional but really, really good)
Salt and freshly ground black pepper

To serve
Small handful of fresh mint leaves
Small handful of fresh basil leaves

Remove and discard the woody stem and outer leaves from the cauliflower. Chop it up into rough chunks and then blitz it in a food processor using the pulse button, until it resembles couscous then set this aside.

Put a really large frying pan on a medium heat and add a spray of oil. Gently fry the red onion for 3–4 minutes until softened, but not coloured. Then add the garlic and cook for a further minute. Next, add the red pepper, chilli and ginger and cook for a couple of minutes. Tip in the cauliflower and stock and continue to cook for about 10–12 minutes until the cauliflower is just tender and its raw taste has gone. Finish with the lemon juice and season with a little salt and pepper.

Remove the cauliflower mixture from the heat and spoon into a large serving dish. Drizzle over the sesame oil, if using, then rip over the mint and basil leaves and serve.

(PER SERVING – BASED ON 4 SERVINGS)	ENERGY	FAT	SAT FAT	SUGAR	PROTEIN	SALT
LORRAINE'S RECIPE	124 Kcal	3.1g	0.6g	13.1g	7.4g	0.39g
COMPARISON RECIPE	332 Kcal	16.1g	3g	2.9g	5.8g	1.34g

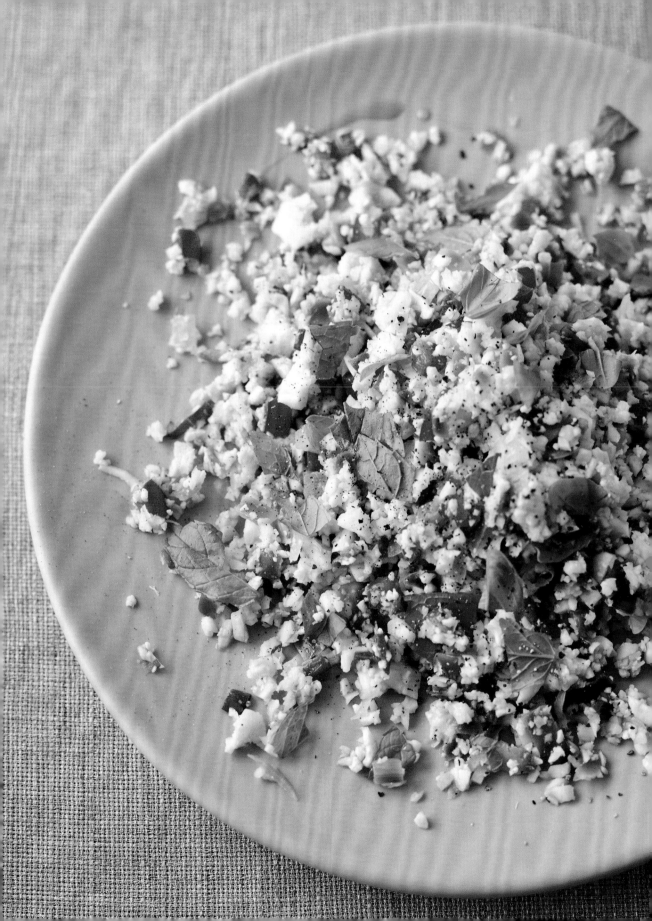

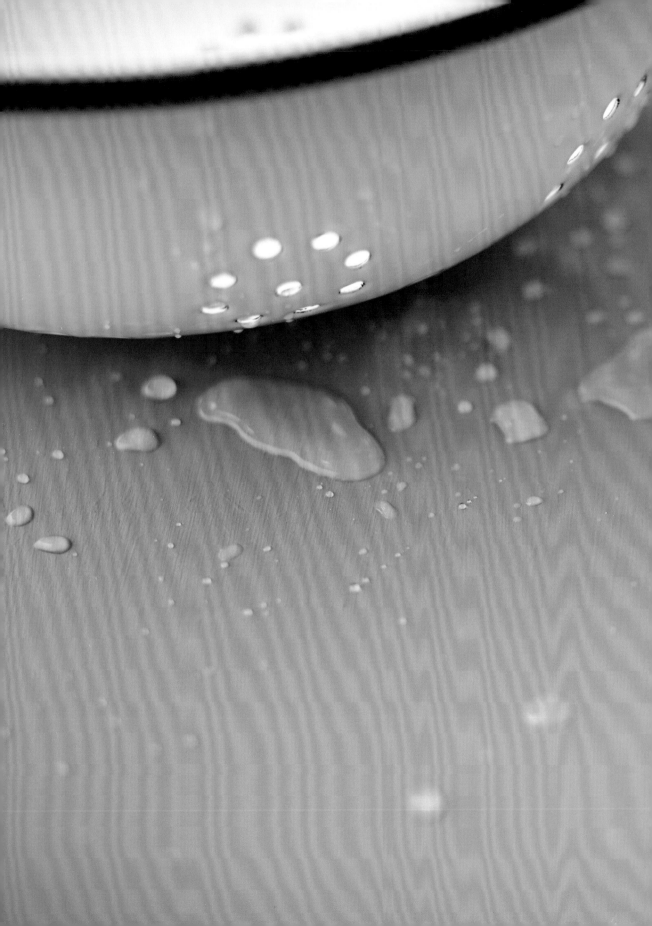

SUCCESS IS GETTING WHAT YOU WANT;
HAPPINESS IS WANTING WHAT YOU GET.
DALE CARNEGIE

PUDDINGS &
DESSERTS

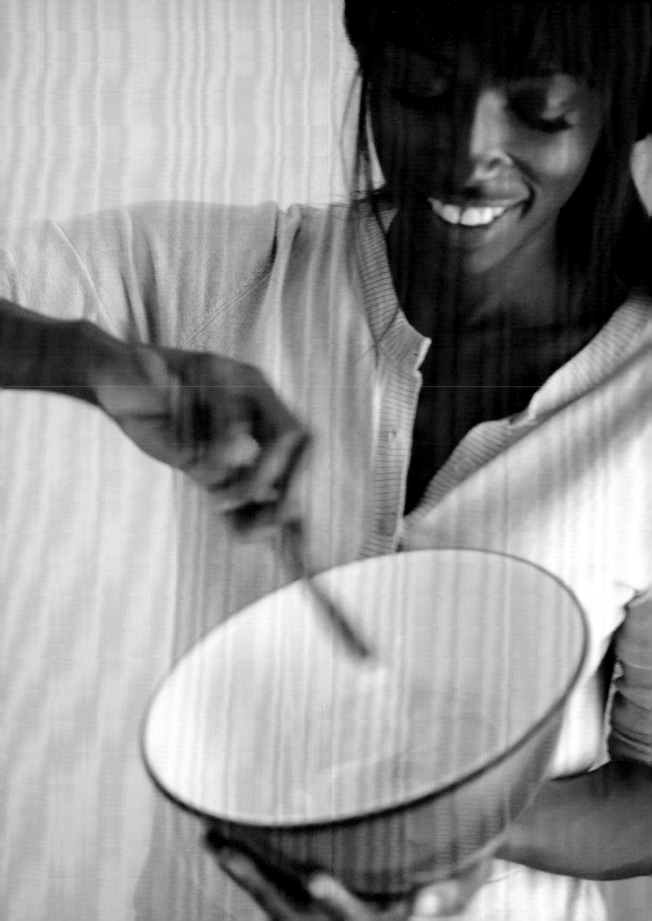

PLUM & ALMOND FRANGIPANE TARTS WITH A STICKY AMARETTO GLAZE

A curiously appetizing concoction of a sponge in a tart, based loosely on the Bakewell which we know, and some of us love. Any leftover bits of filo can be kept and used for something like the Moroccan pie topping (see page 58). These are, I admit, not spectacularly healthy – despite many, many attempts at cutting back the sugar and fat, I couldn't make them taste as good as I wanted them to be. So here's the (nearly) full monty, just fractionally lighter than a full-fat, full-sugar fruity frangipane tart.

Makes
12

Equipment
12-hole muffin tin

Pastry case
Spray oil
6 sheets of filo pastry, defrosted

Frangipane
100g unsalted butter, softened
100g soft light brown sugar
2 eggs
100g ground almonds
25g plain flour
25g wholemeal flour
½ tsp baking powder
Finely grated zest of 1 unwaxed
    lemon
Seeds of 1 vanilla pod or 1 tsp
    vanilla extract
Pinch of salt
1 tbsp Amaretto (optional)

Plums
6 ripe plums, halved and stoned

Vanilla cream
175g crème fraîche
2 tbsp icing sugar, sifted
Seeds of ½ vanilla pod or
    ½ tsp vanilla extract

Glaze
1 tbsp honey
1 tbsp Amaretto

Preheat the oven to 200°C, (Fan 180°C), 400°F, Gas Mark 6. Place a baking sheet into the oven to heat up. This will give extra bottom heat to the tarts so that the bases cook through and are not soggy. Grease a 12-hole muffin tin with a little spray oil and set aside.

Lay four of the filo sheets out on top of each other in a stack. Lay the remaining two on top of each other too, but cut them in half across the width and stack them on top of each other to make another stack four sheets deep. Then, using a 10cm round, straight-sided cutter, stamp out eight circles from the larger sheets and four from the half-sized ones to give 12 round stacks in total. Then line each hole of the muffin tin with a stack of discs, pushing the pastry down well into the 'corners' of each hole. Keep any filo not being worked on under a lightly dampened tea towel so that it doesn't dry out. Spritz each one with a little spray oil and bake in the oven for 10 minutes until crisp and lightly golden.

While the pastry cases are cooking, prepare the frangipane. Beat the butter and sugar together until they are nicely combined and then add the eggs and beat well. Tip in the ground almonds and the flours, baking powder, lemon zest, vanilla seeds or extract, salt and Amaretto (if using), and stir until uniform.

Once the pastry cases are ready, use two spoons to divide the frangipane mixture evenly between them. Place a plum half, cut side down, on top of each mixture. There is no need to push them down, as the plums will sink during cooking. Bake in the oven for about 20 minutes or until the frangipane turns golden and feels springy to the touch.

As the tarts bake, gently stir the crème fraîche, icing sugar and vanilla seeds or extract together with as few stirs as possible until blended. You want to avoid the mixture becoming too loose. Cover with cling film and set aside in the fridge until ready to serve.

Mix the honey and Amaretto in a small bowl and then set aside also.

Once the tarts are ready, remove them from the oven, brush the tops with the honey glaze, and then serve with a spoonful of the vanilla cream.

(PER TART)	ENERGY	FAT	SAT FAT	SUGAR	PROTEIN	SALT
LORRAINE'S RECIPE	312 Kcal	19.2g	9.1g	15.9g	5.5g	0.22g
COMPARISON RECIPE	333 Kcal	22.9g	10g	17.1g	5.9g	0.24g

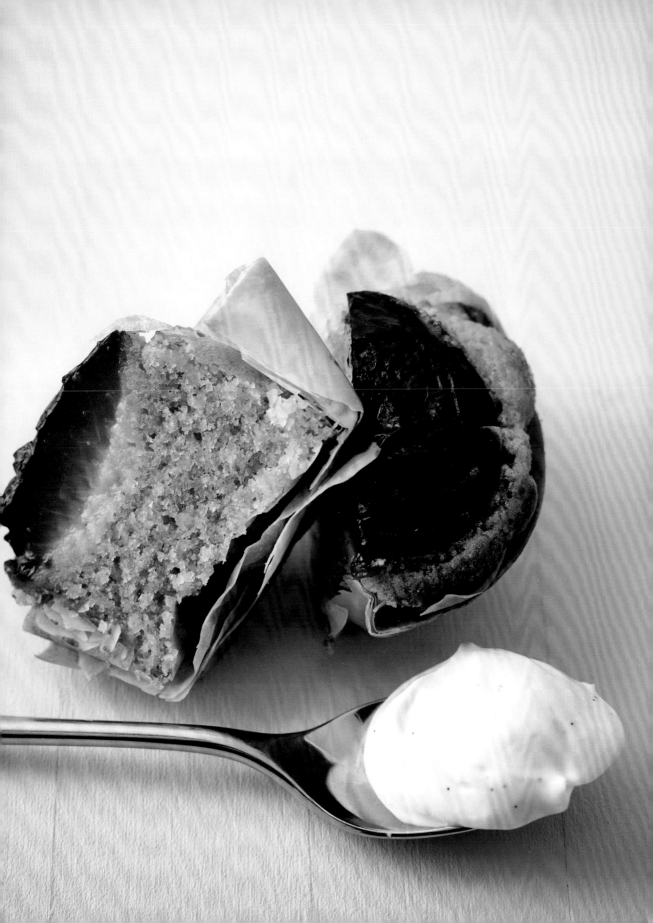

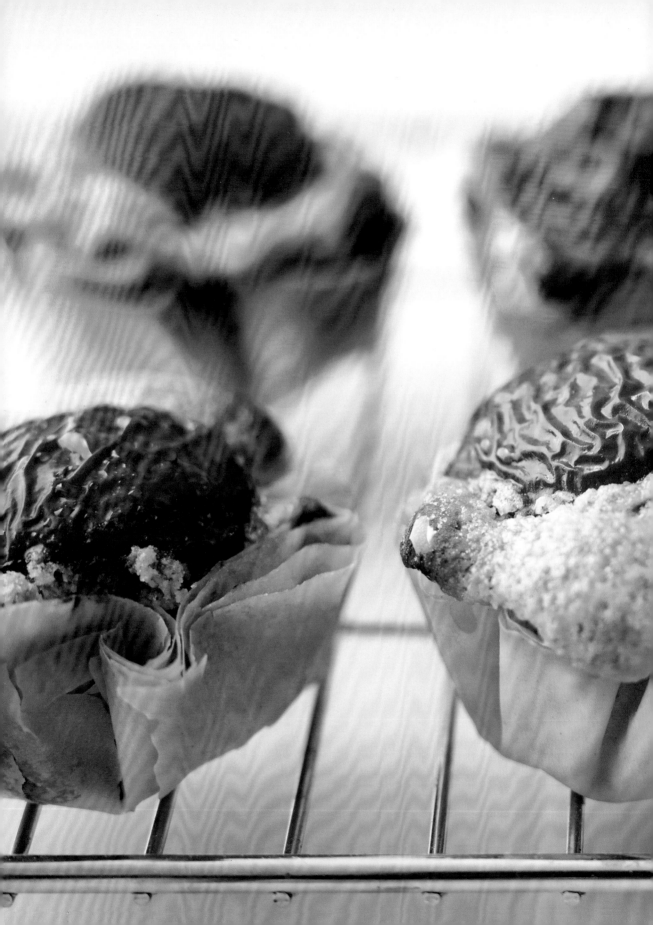

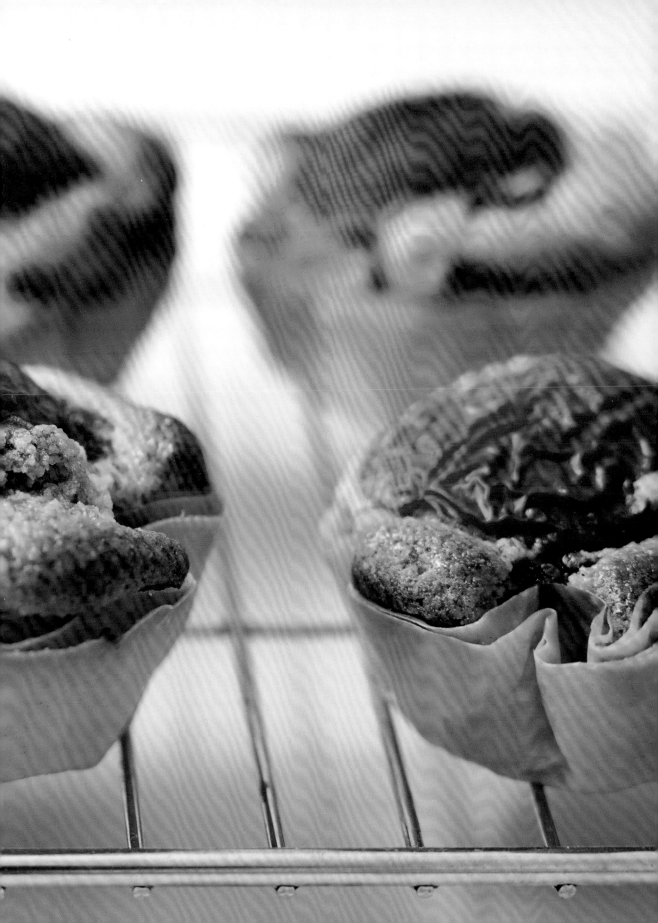

KEY LIME & LEMON CHEESECAKE LOAF

One of the hardest things for me to do as a model was not to eat the gorgeous food they would put on for us during a shoot. The dining area of the studio was always littered with divineness and even when shooting on location the picnics they put on looked like Ottolenghi had waved his magic wand all over them. One sunny day, with a bunch of models down in the Florida Keys, a swimsuit shoot was ensuing. Halfway through, just before lunch, the caterers emerged with the ubiquitous salads, soups and nutty-looking breads and then a key lime pie. I spent the next four hours part smiling at the camera and part staring at the key lime pie (which of course no one else was eating). Once the shoot was finished, I dived straight for that pie and ate the best part of half of it. This lighter recipe is in honour of that most memorable day. It's not easy to find key limes, here – perhaps actually impossible – so regular limes work a treat.

Serves

12

Equipment

1kg loaf tin, food processor

Base

125g light digestive biscuits
50g unsalted butter, melted
1 tsp caster sugar

Topping

6 gelatine leaves
800g low-fat (not the lightest) cream cheese
200g light sour cream
100g soft light brown sugar
Seeds of 1 vanilla pod or 1 tsp vanilla extract
Finely grated zest and juice of 3 unwaxed lemons
Finely grated zest and juice of 3 limes

To serve

Small handful of fresh mint leaves and a few raspberries (optional)

Line a 1kg loaf tin with a piece of cling film much larger than the tin. It's best to have excess cling film hanging over the sides, which you can use to cover the cheesecake once in the tin and also as handles to pull the cheesecake out once set. I find it best to slightly wet the inside of the loaf tin first, and this way the cling film sticks to it more easily. A 1kg loaf tin's size and shape may vary, but as a guide, mine measures 23 x 7.5cm on the bottom (25 x 11.5cm across the top) and 7.5cm high.

Put the digestive biscuits in a food processor and blitz them to fine crumbs. Then, tip them into a medium bowl and mix in the butter and sugar. Tip the mixture into the bottom of the loaf tin and press the crumbs down really firmly but evenly with your hand or the back of a spoon. Refrigerate for at least 15 minutes until firm.

Meanwhile, prepare the filling. Soak the gelatine leaves in a bowl with enough cold water to cover and set aside to soften. Beat the cream cheese, sour cream, sugar, vanilla seeds or extract, lemon and lime zests and lemon juice (reserve the lime juice for now) together in a large bowl until smooth, and set aside.

The gelatine should now be really soft and floppy. Warm the lime juice in a small pan over a gentle heat until it just begins to steam. Then, take it off the heat, squeeze the excess water from the gelatine leaves and stir them into the lime juice until dissolved. Leave this for about 10 minutes until cool.

Once cool, beat this liquid into the cream cheese mixture really well and pour it into the loaf tin. Spread the top evenly with the back of a spoon and then flip the excess cling film up to cover it loosely but completely. You may need an extra piece of cling film if you don't have enough to play with. Place in the fridge to set overnight or for at least 5 hours.

Once the cheesecake is set, carefully peel back the cling film from the top and use this to lift the cheesecake out of the tin. Carefully peel the cling film from the sides and slice the cheesecake into 12 even-sized slices. Scatter the mint and raspberries over, if you are using them, and serve at once.

(PER SERVING)	ENERGY	FAT	SAT FAT	SUGAR	PROTEIN	SALT
LORRAINE'S RECIPE	239 Kcal	14g	8.1g	15g	8.6g	0.89g
COMPARISON RECIPE	444 Kcal	35.1g	21.7g	18.6g	4.8g	0.78g

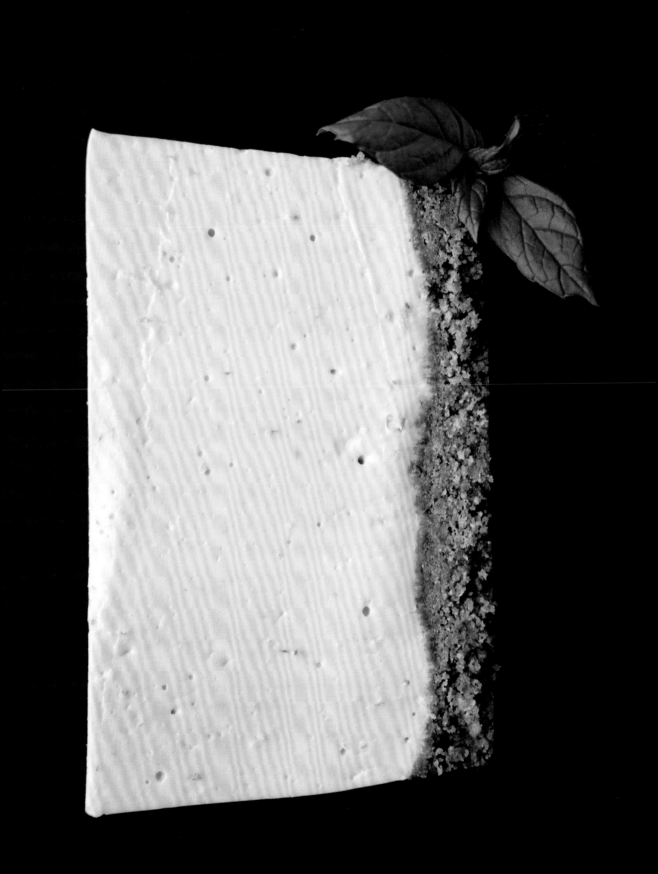

STRAWBERRY OPEN TART WITH LEMON & VANILLA 'CREAM' SERVED WITH BASIL & MINT

This is one of my favourite recipes in the book. I think it became that because it was such a massive challenge to get it right. Initial attempts resulted in a filling which was splitting and not setting, and it was tough to pull away from my patisserie routes and not just add loads of sugar to get it right. After much trial and error I present to you a tasty tart which looks very pretty on the plate.

Serves
6

Equipment
20cm round, loose-bottomed straight-sided tart tin, 3½cm deep

Pastry
Spray oil
A little flour for dusting
425g Oaty Almond and Vanilla Pastry (see page 259)

'Cream' filling
200g low-fat Greek yogurt
200g low-fat cream cheese
25g icing sugar
Finely grated zest of 1 unwaxed lemon
Seeds of 1 vanilla pod or 1 tsp vanilla extract

Strawberries
2 tbsp honey
400g medium-sized strawberries, hulled or just chop the green bit off

To serve
Finely grated zest of ½ unwaxed lemon
Few fresh basil leaves
Few fresh mint leaves

Preheat the oven to 180°C, (Fan 160°C), 350°F, Gas Mark 4. Grease the inside of a 20cm round, loose-bottomed, straight-sided tart tin that is 3½cm deep with a little spray oil and set aside on a baking sheet.

Lightly dust a clean surface with flour and roll the pastry out to the thickness of a £1 coin. Lift the pastry up carefully and drape it over the rolling pin to help lay it into the prepared tin, leaving the excess to hang over. Pinch a little of the excess pastry off, roll it into a ball and then push it down gently into the 'corners' of the tin, so that when the tin is removed after baking, the edges are nice and straight. Trim the excess pastry off with a sharp knife.

The pastry will probably now be a bit soft, so put it in the fridge for about 20 minutes or so or until it is nice and firm. Take a large square of baking parchment, scrunch it up and then open it out to line the pastry with it. This just makes it a little easier to stay sitting in. Then fill the paper-lined pastry with dried beans or ceramic baking beans and bake it for 15 minutes until just firm to the touch and beginning to turn golden. Lift the paper and beans out and return the pastry case to the oven to bake for 5 more minutes. This should dry the bottom out and make it a bit more evenly golden. Then, remove from the oven and leave to cool.

Meanwhile, mix the yogurt and the cream cheese together in a medium bowl until smooth and well blended. Sift the icing sugar over, add the lemon zest and vanilla seeds or extract and really beat it together well so there are no lumps. Cover and refrigerate until ready to use.

Also, prepare the strawberry glaze by simply mixing the honey with 1 tablespoon hot water in a small bowl and setting aside.

Once the pastry case is completely cool, carefully remove it from the tin and place it on a serving plate. Spoon the cream filling into the centre and spread it out with the back of a spoon to fill evenly. Then arrange the strawberries hulled side down all over the top, so the pointy ends are sticking up all over the tart. Of course I do have a problem with this looking messy and need to do it in neat and perfect rows or circles, but throwing them on any way you wish is fine.

Brush the strawberries all over with the honey glaze. Scatter the lemon zest, basil and mint leaves over and serve at once.

(PER SERVING)	ENERGY	FAT	SAT FAT	SUGAR	PROTEIN	SALT
LORRAINE'S RECIPE	410 Kcal	18.8g	8.3g	18.1g	13.5g	0.51g
COMPARISON RECIPE	816 Kcal	57.6g	36.5g	32.5g	9g	0.44g

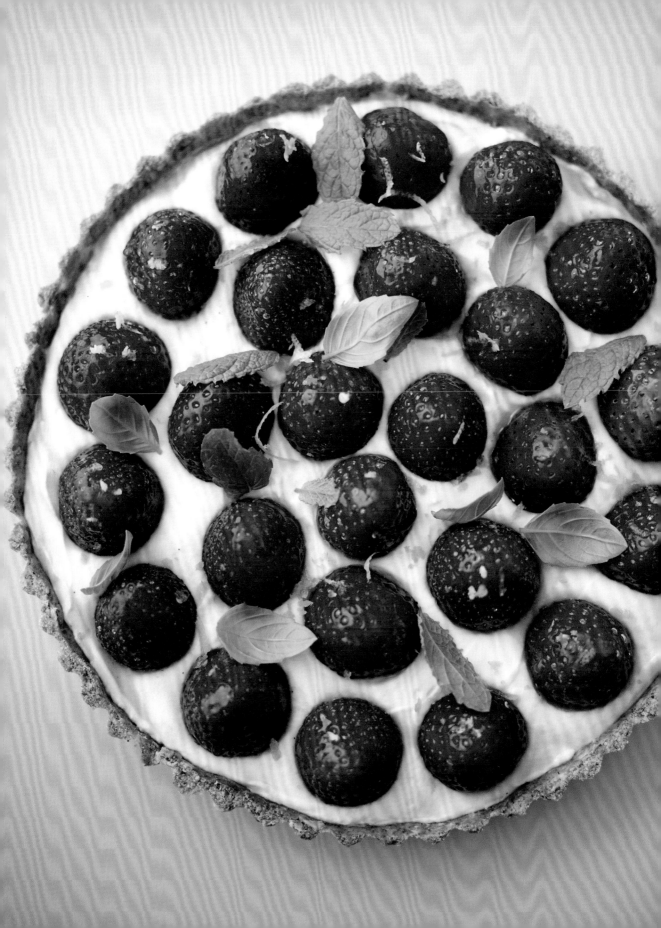

VICTORIA 'MERINGUE' SPONGE WITH MANGO & LIME, & A VANILLA 'CREAM' FILLING

'With that amount of sugar, how did you manage to squeeze this bad boy into a book called *A Lighter Way to Bake*?', you ask? Sadly, a meringue does not work so well scientifically without a certain amount of sugar. And although I have reduced the amount usually required for a meringue of this type, I do acknowledge that there is a lot of sugar in there. (Raises hand and waves white flag.) The less sugar that goes into the meringue compared to the number of egg whites, the more soft and chewy it gets – too little, and it just did not have enough strength to hold itself up as a Vicky sponge. So, justification aside, I really hope you enjoy this messy magical meringue and see it as a little treat now and again when your sweet tooth is crying out for appeasement!

Serves

8

Equipment

2 x 20cm round, loose-bottomed sandwich tins, electric whisk or food processor

Spray oil

Meringue

175g caster sugar
50g soft light brown sugar
5 egg whites

'Cream' filling

100ml 2% fat Greek yogurt
100ml low-fat cream cheese
Seeds of 1 vanilla pod or 1 tsp vanilla extract

Fruit filling

250g prepared mango chunks (or 2 medium mangoes), cut into 2cm square pieces
Finely grated zest and juice of 1 lime
3cm piece of fresh root ginger, peeled and grated (optional)

Preheat the oven to 140°C, (Fan 120°C), 275°F, Gas Mark 1. Grease two 20cm round, loose-bottomed sandwich tins with a little spray oil, line the bases with a disc of baking parchment and set aside on a baking sheet.

You will need to use an electric whisk to make the meringue or, even better, a food processor. Whisk the sugars and two of the egg whites together in the machine until the mixture is really stiff and shiny. Add the remaining egg whites, one at a time, whisking between each addition until the mixture is well whisked up before adding the next. This may take some time, but keep going until the mixture is white and stiff. The beauty of making the meringue this way is that you can leave the eggs to whisk up and you will not over-whisk them, you will just come back to the stiffest, shiniest egg whites ever! (Well, a little bit brown due to the sugar...).

Once the eggs are whisked up, divide the mixture evenly between the sandwich tins and bake for 1 hour or until the meringues are crisp on top and cooked through. Once cooked, remove them from the oven and leave to cool in the tins.

Meanwhile, prepare the 'cream' filling. Mix the Greek yogurt, cream cheese and vanilla seeds or extract in a medium bowl until well blended. If there are lumps, then give the mixture a really quick beat with the spoon and they will go. Cover and refrigerate until ready to use.

Once the meringues have cooled, run a sharp knife around the inside of the tins and the edge of each meringue. They may crack a little and a few bits may fall off, but that is the nature of meringue. Put a plate upside down on top of one of the meringues and then, holding both the sandwich tin and the plate, flip the whole thing over. Remove the tin, peel the baking parchment off and then carefully flip the meringue over, top side up. Repeat with the remaining meringue and then place the less good-looking one on a serving plate.

Spoon two-thirds of the cream filling over in blobs and then spread it out gently with a palette knife. Scatter the mango on top, making sure there are some pieces close to the edge of the meringue so that when the top goes on the golden cubes of mango are visible. Scatter the lime zest and ginger (if using) on top and then drizzle the lime juice over. The citrus will cut through any sweetness and the ginger will add a subtle bit of heat. Dollop the remaining cream filling on top of the fruit and then carefully set the remaining (nicer-looking) meringue on top to finish.

I find this does not need to be served with anything other than a very sweet tooth.

(PER SERVING)	ENERGY	FAT	SAT FAT	SUGAR	PROTEIN	SALT
LORRAINE'S RECIPE	172 Kcal	1.9g	1.2g	33.2g	4.8g	0.15g
COMPARISON RECIPE	345 Kcal	18g	11g	40.6g	3.1g	0.21g

COFFEE & PECAN SWISS ROLL WITH IRISH CREAM FILLING

I have used two egg whites in place of one of the eggs in this recipe. It makes the sponge a little lighter, but I believe just as tasty. The wholemeal flour adds a richer nutty edge – as always, you can just replace it with plain flour if you don't fancy it, but it is worth a try. I actually prefer it in terms of taste and texture. This roll will probably be a little more squidgy and soft than the ones you are used to, because of the reduced sugar (and egg) in it. For a Irish-cream-less version, try a plain cream cheese filling sweetened with icing sugar, and some fresh fruits scattered on top. Or even substitute 15g of the wholemeal flour for 20g of cocoa powder for something a little more wicked.

Serves
6 with 12 skinny slices

Equipment
20.5 x 31cm Swiss roll tin, food processor, electric whisk

Sponge
Spray oil
50g soft dark brown sugar
2 tbsp instant coffee granules
2 eggs
2 egg whites
Seeds of ½ a vanilla pod or ½ tsp vanilla extract
75g wholemeal flour
1 tsp baking powder
Pinch of salt
1 tbsp caster sugar

Filling
150g low-fat cream cheese
1½ tbsp Irish cream liqueur (leave out if you're making this for the kiddies)
1–2 tbsp icing sugar, or to taste
Pinch of finely grated unwaxed lemon zest (this lifts the whole cake and makes a big difference)
25g pecans, chopped up quite small, just to add some crunch

Coffee sugar syrup
2 tbsp caster sugar
1 tbsp instant coffee granules

Preheat the oven to 190°C, (Fan 170°C), 375°F, Gas Mark 5. Lightly grease a 20.5 x 31cm Swiss roll tin with spray oil and line with baking parchment. I just cut a long strip of paper to cover the bottom and come up on opposite sides of the tin and leave the excess hanging over a little – this makes it easier to lift the baked cake out of the tin.

First make the sponge. Blitz the sugar and coffee in a food processor for a few seconds to give a finely chopped mixture. This is really worth doing to help bring out the coffee flavour in the cake.

The only way to conquer this meringue mixture is with an electric whisk. Put the eggs, egg whites and vanilla seeds or extract in a large bowl and whisk for a good 3–4 minutes, until the eggs are mousse-like and have increased in size somewhat. Add the coffee and sugar mixture gradually in stages and keep whisking for another 3–4 minutes or so. To test to see if the eggs are whisked up enough, take a spoonful of the mixture and drop it back into the bowl. The egg mix should sit on the surface for a second before it disappears back into the mixture. This does take some time and it will never be as frothy as 3 eggs (the egg whites just don't give it bulk) but it should still be really light and really fluffy.

Once the eggs are ready, lightly scatter the flour, baking powder and salt over the top and use a spatula to fold everything in very gently so as to retain all of that air which has been whisked into it. Gently pour the mixture into the Swiss roll tin from a low height so you don't knock any air out, and level it out with a palette knife or the back of a spoon. Bake in the oven for 15–20 minutes or until springy to the touch. Then remove from the oven and leave to cool completely.

Meanwhile, mix the cream cheese and cream liqueur together in a small bowl until well blended and lump free. Sift the icing sugar in bit by bit, tasting as you go until it tastes just right for you. You may feel it does not need the extra sugar. However, if you are making this a non-alcoholic version then just leave the cream liqueur out and definitely add the icing sugar. Finally, stir in the lemon zest, and cover and refrigerate until needed.

When the Swiss roll is almost cool, make the coffee sugar syrup. Put the sugar, coffee granules and 2 tablespoons of water in a small pan over a low heat, stirring until the sugar and coffee dissolves. Then turn up the heat and let it bubble away for 30–60 seconds until syrupy, before removing from the heat.

Once the Swiss roll is cool, put a piece of baking parchment a little larger than the Swiss roll tin on the work surface and sprinkle the tablespoon of caster sugar evenly over it. Lift the Swiss roll out of the tin with the help of the overhanging baking parchment, and place it upside down on the sugar-sprinkled baking parchment. If the sponge is a bit stuck around the edges of the tin, just carefully run a small sharp knife around the inside edge to release it. Peel the paper off the base of the sponge, which is now facing upwards, and brush the surface all over with the coffee syrup.

Then, using a palette knife or a large flat knife, spread the cream cheese mixture evenly all over the Swiss roll. When I did it, it felt as if I was spreading mayonnaise on a giant piece of bread! Scatter over the pecans and then, with one of the shorter sides facing you, roll the first bit of the Swiss roll up nice and tightly. Then continue to roll the whole thing up, again quite tightly and not worrying about anything squidging out of the sides.

Place the Swiss roll seam side down on a serving plate and then serve! I have allowed two 2cm pieces per serving here, as it is quite rich.

(PER SERVING - 2 SLICES)	ENERGY	FAT	SAT FAT	SUGAR	PROTEIN	SALT
LORRAINE'S RECIPE	223Kcal	8.9g	3.2g	20.3g	7.8g	0.39g
COMPARISON RECIPE	363Kcal	25.8g	11.7g	18.1g	7.2g	0.27g

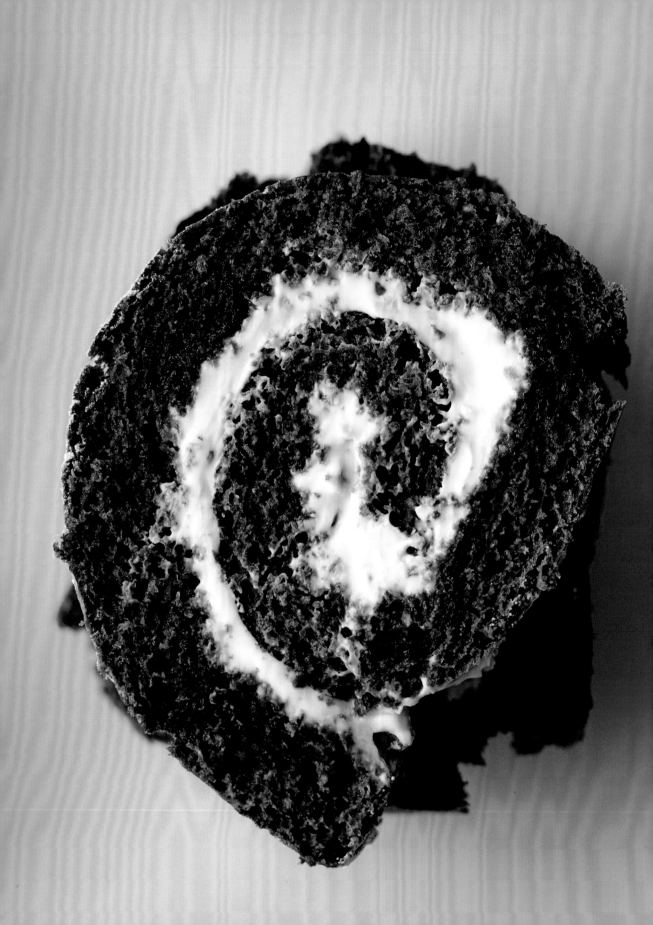

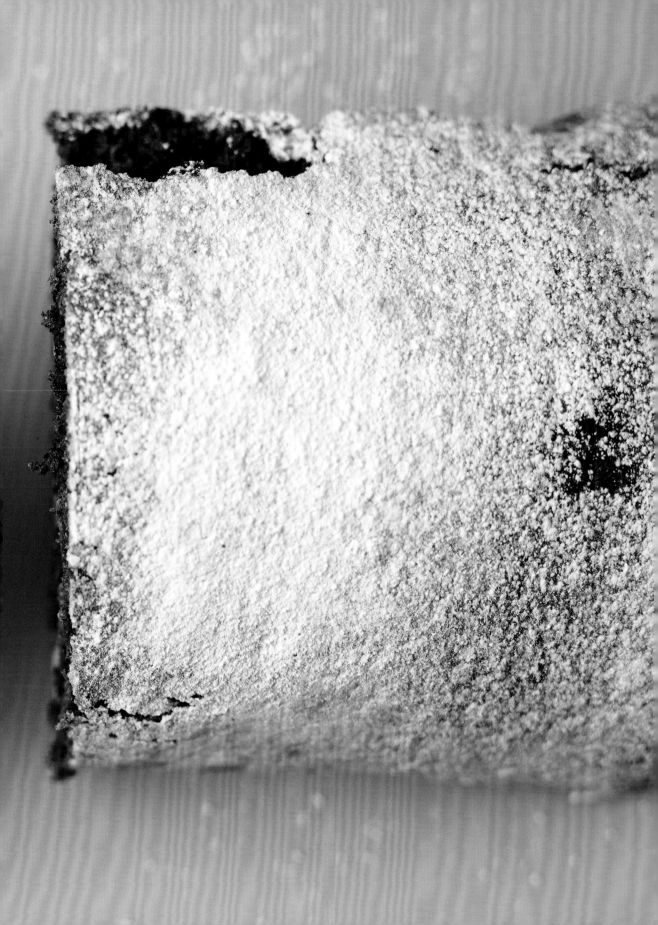

RASPBERRY, RHUBARB & CARDAMOM GALETTE WITH A HAZELNUT & VANILLA CREAM

If you can't find ground cardamom, take two cardamom pods, bash them to open them, discard the shells and grind up the seeds inside until fine.

Serves
8

Filling
4 sticks of rhubarb, trimmed and cut into 2cm pieces
2 tbsp soft light brown sugar
Good pinch of ground cardamom (see recipe intro)
Seeds of 1 vanilla pod or 1 tsp vanilla extract
Finely grated zest of ½ an orange
150g raspberries

Pastry
400g Sweet Honey Shortcrust Pastry (see page 258) or Sweet Shortcrust Spelt Pastry (see page 262)
1 egg, lightly beaten

Hazelnut and vanilla cream
200g low-fat crème fraîche
50g hazelnuts, toasted and roughly chopped
4 tsp icing sugar, sifted
Seeds of ½ a vanilla pod or ½ tsp vanilla extract

To serve
Few mint leaves (optional)

Preheat the oven to 180°C, (Fan 160°C), 350°F, Gas Mark 4.

Toss the rhubarb, sugar, cardamom, vanilla seeds or extract and orange zest together in a medium bowl and then set aside for a moment.

Roll the pastry out on a large sheet of baking parchment to a 25cm circle about 4mm thick. Spoon the rhubarb into the centre of the pastry, leaving a border of about 4cm all the way around. Fold the edges of the pastry up onto the rhubarb all the way around as in the picture. It is like folding up the corners of a book to mark your place (taboo, I know – folding corners of a book is frowned upon by the literati but is something I do). Then, glaze the pastry edge with the egg, slide the baking parchment and galette onto a baking sheet and bake in the oven for 30–35 minutes.

Meanwhile, make the hazelnut crème fraîche. Simply mix the crème fraîche, hazelnuts, icing sugar and vanilla seeds or extract together until well blended. Cover and set aside in the fridge until ready to use. So easy!

Once cooked, the galette pastry should be crisp and golden and the rhubarb tender when pierced with a knife. Remove it from the oven and carefully stir the raspberries through the rhubarb. This is a bit fiddly but it is nice to see both fruits mixed together. The raspberries only need a moment or two in the oven, so pop the galette back into the oven for, er, a moment or two. Then, remove from the oven, cut into eight wedges and serve with a dollop of the hazelnut cream.

Finish with some fresh mint for a splash of green, if you like.

(PER SERVING)	ENERGY	FAT	SAT FAT	SUGAR	PROTEIN	SALT
LORRAINE'S RECIPE	297 Kcal	17.1g	8.1g	9.2g	7.4g	0.11g
COMPARISON RECIPE	334 Kcal	21g	13.6g	23.2g	2.7g	0.07g

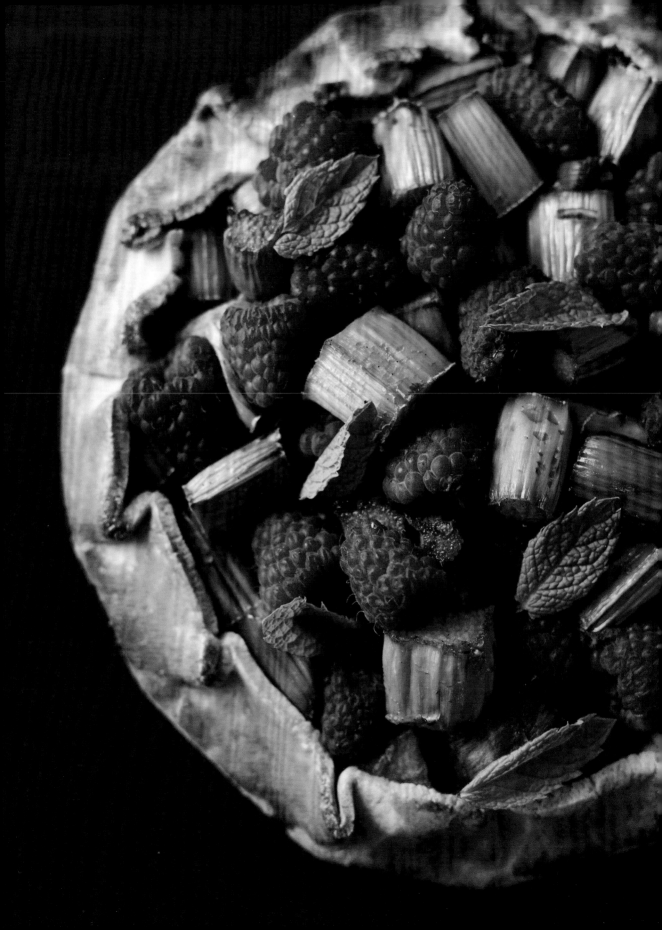

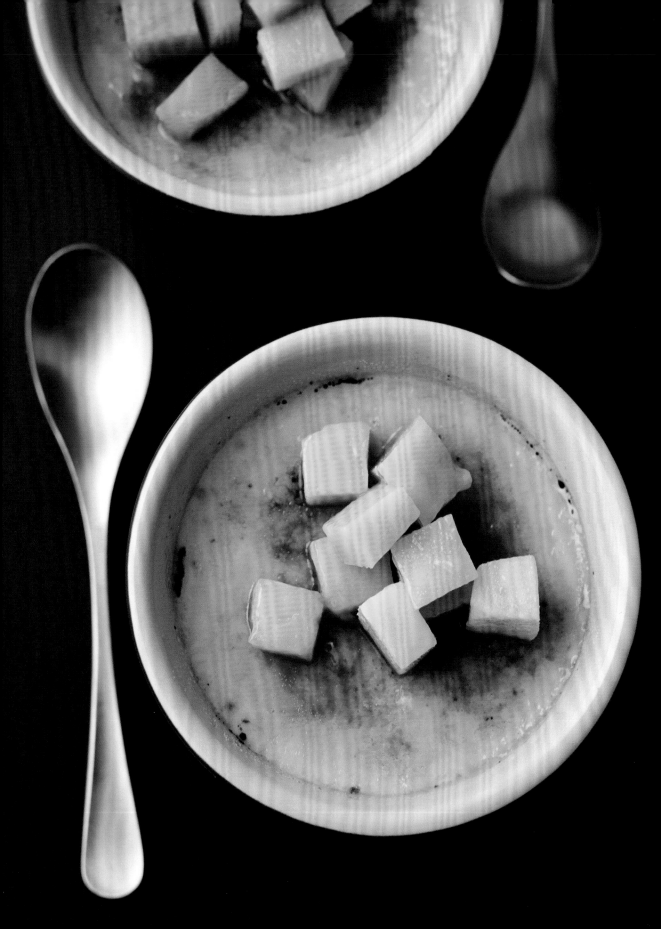

LEMON & VANILLA CRÈME BRÛLÉE WITH FRESH MANGO TOPPING

So my default position when making crème brûlées would be to use double cream and even a touch of mascarpone to give a deliciously deep and creamy texture with lots of body and flavour. Here, to enable the flavour to stay the same and yet cut the fat by a substantial margin, I have used a combination of single cream and semi-skimmed milk. Experiments with Greek yogurt and half-fat Greek yogurt did not turn out at all well, resulting in something which I could not possibly call a crème brûlée. Therefore yes, there is cream still in the dish, but it is greatly reduced. The texture will not be quite as silky smooth as the full-fat version, but I find the flavours very pleasing on the palette!

Makes

6

Equipment

6 x 125ml ramekins, cook's blowtorch

Filling

250ml single cream
350ml semi-skimmed milk
Seeds of 2 vanilla pods or 2 tsp vanilla extract
3 eggs
50g caster sugar
1 tbsp cornflour
Finely grated zest of 1 unwaxed lemon

Brûlée topping

1 tbsp caster sugar
100g prepared mango chunks, or 1 small mango, cut into 1cm pieces (or smaller if you can!)

Preheat the oven to 150°C, (Fan 130°C), 300°F, Gas Mark 2. Arrange six 125ml ramekins in a deep-sided roasting tin and set aside. My ramekins were deep (4cm, to be precise) rather than shallow. Crème brûlées cooked in shallow but wide ramekins will require a shorter cooking time. Pop the kettle on to boil.

Put the cream, milk and vanilla seeds (and pod) or extract into a small pan and set over a medium heat until it is just starting to steam.

Meanwhile, put the eggs, sugar, cornflour and lemon zest into a large jug and mix them together well.

Once the milk mixture is steaming, stir a little bit of it into the egg mixture. Then gradually add the remaining milk mixture while stirring all the time. Divide the brûlée mixture evenly between the ramekins and pour enough boiling water into the roasting tin to come a third of the way up their sides. This will act as a temperature control and will stop the crème brûlées from getting too hot. If the eggs get too hot, they will curdle rather than cook into a smooth and creamy custard. Carefully transfer them to the oven to bake for about 30 minutes or until the mixture has almost set, but still has a little wobble in the centre. The wobble is so important, as if they are cooked beyond this the mixture inside may go grainy (but will still taste nice!).

Once the custards reach this stage, remove them from the oven and carefully lift the ramekins out of the roasting tin to cool down completely. Once cool, arrange them on a tray, cover with cling film and refrigerate for at least 1 hour or until needed. You can prepare them to this stage and leave them in the fridge for several hours if you like. These are great for when guests are coming and you want to be super prepared in advance!

Once the crème brûlée is nice and cold, sprinkle the tablespoon of caster sugar evenly between the tops in an even layer. Use a blowtorch to caramelize the sugar, passing it back and forth across the tops until the crème brûlées go a good golden brown. Top with about 1 tablespoon of mango chunks just in the centre of the brûlées, and serve.

(PER SERVING)	ENERGY	FAT	SAT FAT	SUGAR	PROTEIN	SALT
LORRAINE'S RECIPE	220 Kcal	12.3g	6.6g	16.4g	7.2g	0.22g
COMPARISON RECIPE	678 Kcal	53.8g	31.3g	47.2g	5.4g	0.12g

TARTE AU CITRON

The trick with this tart is to not over-cook it, otherwise the top can crack and the texture will not be as smooth as it could be. But if it is slightly over-cooked (which I have done many times, I admit) it still tastes totally divine and those pesky cracks can be covered up with a light sprinkling of icing sugar. I did try this with the lower-fat crème fraîche, but the only way I could be satisfied with the mouthfeel and texture was with the full-fat version. In spite of this, the tart is still much friendlier on the tum than a lot of other versions.

Serves
8

Equipment
22cm round, loose-bottomed, fluted tart tin (3cm deep), dried beans or ceramic baking beans

Pastry
Spray oil
400g Rich Sweet Wholemeal Shortcrust Pastry (see page 260)
A little plain flour for dusting

Lemon filling
4 eggs
2 egg whites
125ml full-fat crème fraîche
100g caster sugar
Finely grated zest and juice of 5 unwaxed lemons, or 4 if they are big (to give about 200ml juice)
Seeds of ½ a vanilla pod or ½ tsp vanilla extract
1 tsp cornflour

2 tsp icing sugar, for dusting

Preheat the oven to 180°C, (Fan 160°C), 350°F, Gas Mark 4. Lightly grease a 22cm round, loose-bottomed, fluted tart tin (3cm deep) with the spray oil and set aside on a baking sheet.

Roll the pastry out on a lightly floured surface to about the thickness of a £1 coin. Drape it over the rolling pin and transfer it carefully to the tin. Line the tin with the pastry, being careful not to stretch or pull the pastry otherwise it will shrink during baking. The pastry might be a bit crumbly but don't worry, just patch any tears or holes back together and they will be fine once cooked. Use a little ball of pastry to push it down right into the 'corners' of the tin – I like to press the handle of a wooden spoon all the way around into the fluted edge to give a good shape once finished. Trim the excess pastry with a sharp knife. The pastry will probably now be a bit soft, so put it into the fridge for about 20 minutes or so or until it is nice and firm.

Meanwhile, start on the filling. Whisk the eggs and egg whites in a large bowl to combine them a little. Then mix in the crème fraîche, caster sugar, lemon zest and juice, vanilla seeds or extract and cornflour until well blended and smooth. Set aside to infuse.

Take a large square of baking parchment, scrunch it up and then open it out to line the pastry case. This makes it a little easier for it to stay put. Fill the paper-lined pastry with dried beans or ceramic baking beans and bake it for 15 minutes until just firm to the touch and beginning to turn golden. Then lift the paper and beans out and return the pastry case to the oven to bake for 5 more minutes. This should dry the bottom out and make it a bit more evenly golden. Remove from the oven (but keep it close by) and leave for 10–15 minutes until just cool to the touch.

Preheat the oven to 150°C, (Fan 130°C), 300°F, Gas Mark 2, which is a nice gentle temperature to cook the eggs. Once the tart case is cool, pour the infused lemon mixture in to come right to the top. Then carefully transfer the tart back to the oven (now you see why it was handy to keep it close by!) and bake for 25–30 minutes or until the centre of the tart still has a very slight wobble. Check the tart at 20 minutes and just keep an eye on it, as although it will look molten at the beginning of its oven journey, it can set quite quickly. Once cooked, remove from the oven and leave to cool in the tin.

Once cold, carefully remove from the tin. Dust the icing sugar over, cut into eight wedges and serve.

(PER SERVING)	ENERGY	FAT	SAT FAT	SUGAR	PROTEIN	SALT
LORRAINE'S RECIPE	358 Kcal	20.6g	11.6g	17.6g	9g	0.17g
COMPARISON RECIPE	404 Kcal	22.4g	12.2g	32.7g	7.2g	0.19g

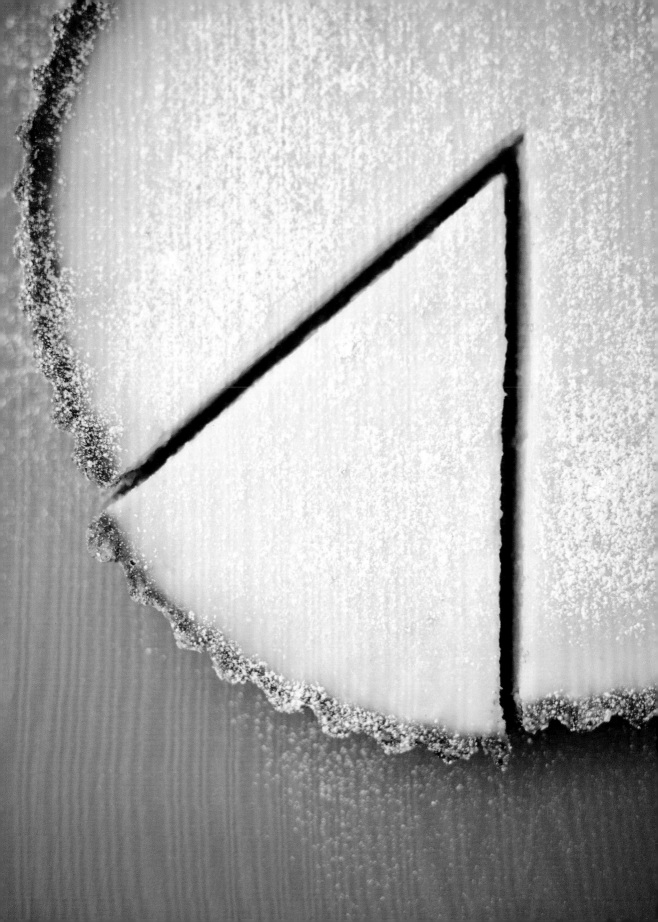

NO-BAKE MANGO, PASSION FRUIT & LIME CHEESECAKE BARS

So, why is there a non-baked cheesecake in a book called *A Lighter Way to Bake*? Well, I had a bit of battle with this one. I tried again and again to bake it, but just could not get the right texture and mouthfeel. I felt it was due to the low-fat filling ingredients, which sometimes do not take too kindly to being heated. I was happy with other 'baked custards' such as the crème brûlée and the lemon tart, but the cheesecake bars only felt right when they were fridge set. So, I have slipped this one in the book (and the other cheesecake recipe, on page 98). However, if you want to bake it, just add three eggs and a tablespoon of cornflour to the filling and pop the tin into a deep-sided roasting tin. Put some water into the roasting tin so that it comes halfway up the sides of the cheesecake tin, then bake in the oven for 30 minutes at 150°C, (Fan 130°C), 300°F, Gas Mark 2, or until there is just a little wobble in the centre of the cheesecake. It still tastes totally scrumptious, but I prefer my cheesecakes unbaked.

Makes
10 bars or 20 bite-sized pieces

Equipment
20cm square cake tin at least
  7.5cm deep, food processor

Base
Spray oil
50g unsalted butter
150g ginger nut biscuits

Filling
6 gelatine leaves
800g low-fat cream cheese
  (low, not lightest)
200g sour cream
100g caster sugar
Seeds and juice of 6 passion fruit
Finely grated zest and juice of
  2 limes
Seeds of 1 vanilla pod or 1 tsp
  vanilla extract
250g prepared mango chunks
  (or 2 medium mangoes, diced)

To serve
Small handful of fresh mint leaves

Lightly grease a 20cm square cake tin at least 7.5cm deep with spray oil, and line the base with baking parchment. I cut a long strip that will run across the bottom and up opposite sides with a little overhang at each end. This makes it easier to lift the cheesecake out of the tin once set.

To prepare the base, melt the butter in a medium pan over a low heat. Meanwhile, put the biscuits into a food bag, secure it closed and bash them with a rolling pin until they resemble fine breadcrumbs. Alternatively, you can whizz them to fine crumbs in a food processor. Once the butter has melted, tip the crushed biscuits in and mix together well. Then tip the mixture into the base of the lined tin, spreading it out evenly with the back of a spoon. It will be a fairly thin layer so spread it out well, making sure that the base is covered and really packing it down tightly. Then pop it into the fridge for about 30 minutes until set firm.

Meanwhile, prepare the filling. Place the gelatine leaves in a small bowl, pour over enough cold water to cover and leave to soak for 5–10 minutes, until soft. Stir the cream cheese, sour cream, sugar, passion fruit seeds and juice, lime zest and juice and vanilla seeds or extract together until well blended. Blend the mango in a food processor until really smooth. Pour it into a small pan and set it over a low heat to bring just to the boil. Remove from the heat, squeeze the excess water from the now-softened gelatine leaves and stir them through until dissolved. Set aside to cool completely before stirring through the cream cheese mixture until well blended.

Pour this mixture on top of the now-set biscuit base and gently bang the tin on the work surface to settle it down evenly and level. Cover with cling film and pop it in the fridge overnight or for at least 5 hours, until set.

Once it is set, carefully lift the cheesecake out of the tin using the overhanging bits of paper. Carefully peel the paper from the sides and then cut into 10 generous bars or 20 bite-sized pieces. Scatter with the mint if using, and serve.

(PER SERVING – BASED ON 10 BARS)	ENERGY	FAT	SAT FAT	SUGAR	PROTEIN	SALT
LORRAINE'S RECIPE	332 Kcal	19.3g	12.1g	24g	10.2g	0.98g
COMPARISON RECIPE	756 Kcal	69g	44.1g	16.3g	7.7g	0.67g

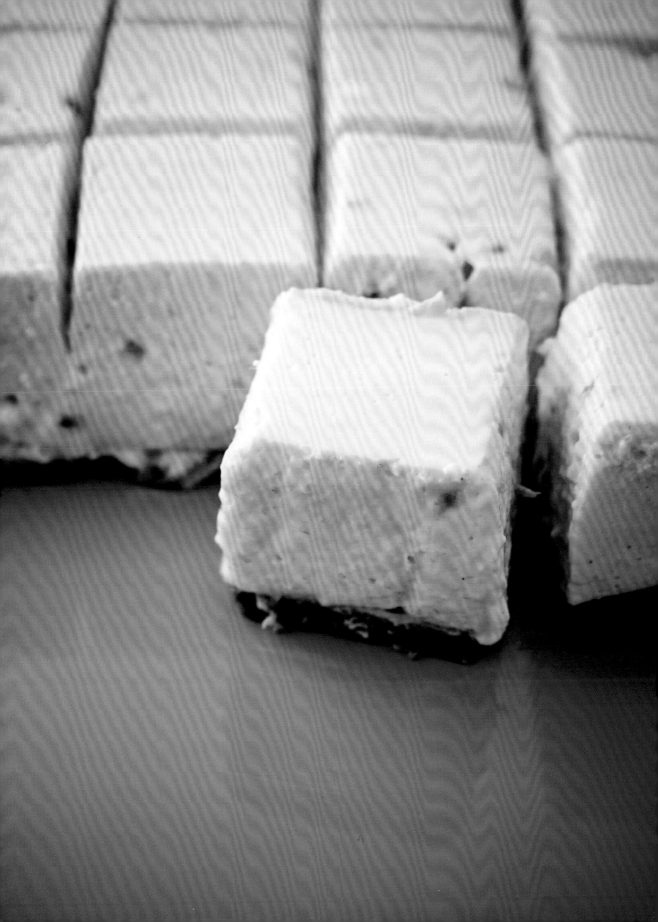

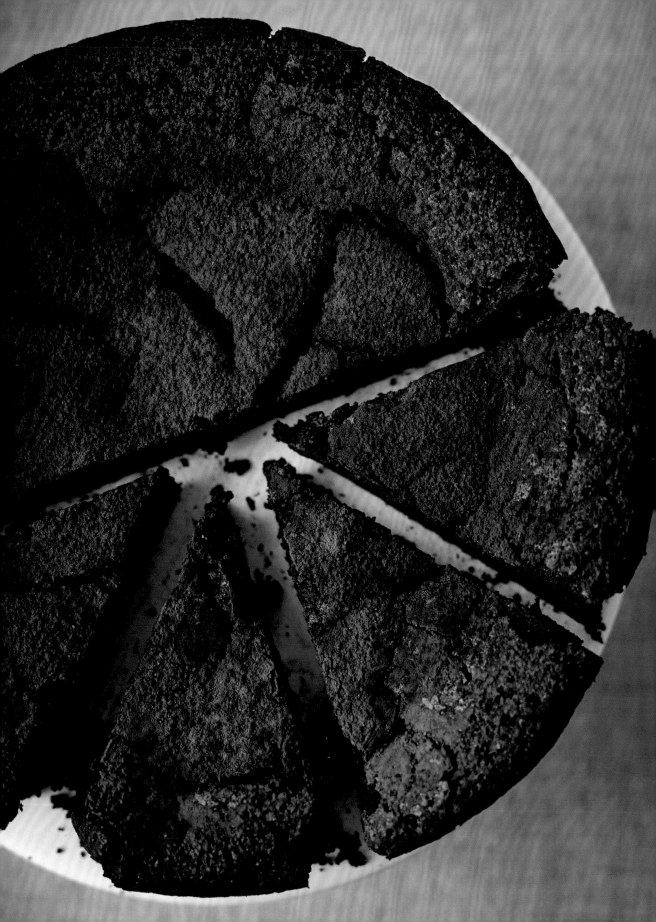

CHOCOLATE, CHOCOLATE TORTE

A torte in the true sense of the word is a multi-layered gâteau covered in icing and/or a glaze – like the ones you see when peering through a French patisserie window, glistening in their exquisite perfection. The Chocolate, Chocolate Torte here is one which may not dazzle you visually with its precise edges and shiny top, but with one mouthful I am hoping you – like me – will be transported to the chocolate, chocolate land which just makes you smile as the rich taste settles on your tongue. There's no getting away from the sugar in a torte recipe, with less it just won't be as palatable, but a little torte goes a long way.

Serves

8

Equipment

18cm round, loose-bottomed or springform cake tin, electric whisk

Spray oil

4 tsp cocoa powder

100g unsalted butter, diced

1 tsp instant coffee granules

200g dark chocolate, snapped into small pieces

200g milk chocolate, snapped into small pieces

4 eggs, separated, plus one extra egg white

75g caster sugar

Preheat the oven to 180°C, (Fan 160°C), 350°F, Gas Mark 4. Cut out a disc and a strip of baking parchment the correct sizes to line the base and sides of an 18cm round, loose-bottomed or springform cake tin, and lay them out flat. Grease them and the insides of the tin with a little spray oil. Dust half of the cocoa over the paper in an even layer and then carefully line the tin with it, cocoa side up, and set aside on a baking sheet.

Melt the butter in a medium pan, add the coffee granules and stir until dissolved. Then remove from the heat, add the two kinds of chocolate and set aside to allow them to slowly melt.

Meanwhile, put the egg yolks in a large bowl and whisk up until they begin to go a bit lighter in colour. This will probably take 2–3 minutes with an electric whisk and longer by hand. They won't get really fluffy but will just be nice and creamy.

Once the chocolate has melted, give the mixture a good stir to combine, pour it into the egg yolks and stir together gently.

Next, whisk the egg whites up in a large clean bowl until they start to go white but not yet foamy. Then, while still whisking, add the sugar and allow the mixture to form a foamy meringue (rather than the usual stiff glossy mixture).

Add a big dollop of this meringue into the chocolate mixture and mix everything together well. Then gently fold in half of the remaining meringue, trying to keep as much air in the mixture as possible. Finally, add the final bit of meringue, again folding it in gently until all is combined.

Gently pour the torte mixture into the prepared tin from a low height so you don't knock out any of that lovely air which has just been whisked in. Smooth the top with the back of a spoon and bake in the oven for 45–50 minutes, or until the cake is soft to the touch but a knife comes out clean when inserted into the centre.

Once baked, remove from the oven and leave to cool in the tin. It will collapse in the centre but don't worry too much – that's the nature of it and it will still taste amazing. Once cool, carefully remove from the tin and place on a serving plate. Dust the remaining cocoa over and serve. It should be gratifyingly gooey inside.

(PER SERVING)	ENERGY	FAT	SAT FAT	SUGAR	PROTEIN	SALT
LORRAINE'S RECIPE	443 Kcal	28.9g	16.6g	39.8g	7.9g	0.26g
COMPARISON RECIPE	470 Kcal	30.5g	15.3g	41g	6.4g	0.17g

LOW-FAT LEMON YOGURT ICE-CREAM

I must confess, I am not an ice-cream lover. When the ice-cream van came wobbling down the street with its music blaring out from the speakers just that little bit out of tune, I would dash in to get my coins and it would be an Orange Maid which would get me all excited, much to the horror of my Mr Whippy-loving friends. But when it comes to the perfect accompaniment for a bake, a scoop of ice-cream is hard to beat. I've broken the rules to let this recipe into a book about baking, because it's extremely low fat, ticks all the taste boxes, and also is infinitely better for you than a dollop of cream. There are so many good ice-creams in the shops nowadays, but making your own is still a very special thing.

Serves

6

Equipment

Ice-cream machine

350g 0% fat Greek yogurt
50ml semi-skimmed milk
25g icing sugar
3 tbsp honey
Zest and juice of 1 unwaxed lemon

Place all the ingredients in a bowl and mix together thoroughly.

Tip into your ice-cream machine to churn. Alternatively, if you don't have an ice-cream machine, pour the mixture into a container, put it in the freezer and every 30 minutes fork the mixture through, or use an electric whisk to churn it over. This will break up the big ice crystals so that when you eat it the mixture is nice and smooth. Do this every 30 minutes for 2–3 hours until the mixture is frozen. Once it is, you are there!

(PER 2-SCOOP /112G SERVING)	ENERGY	FAT	SAT FAT	SUGAR	PROTEIN	SALT
LORRAINE'S RECIPE	122 Kcal	0.2g	0.1g	22.5g	8.8g	0.1g
COMPARISON RECIPE	471 Kcal	38.2g	23.7g	32.4g	1.2g	0.05g

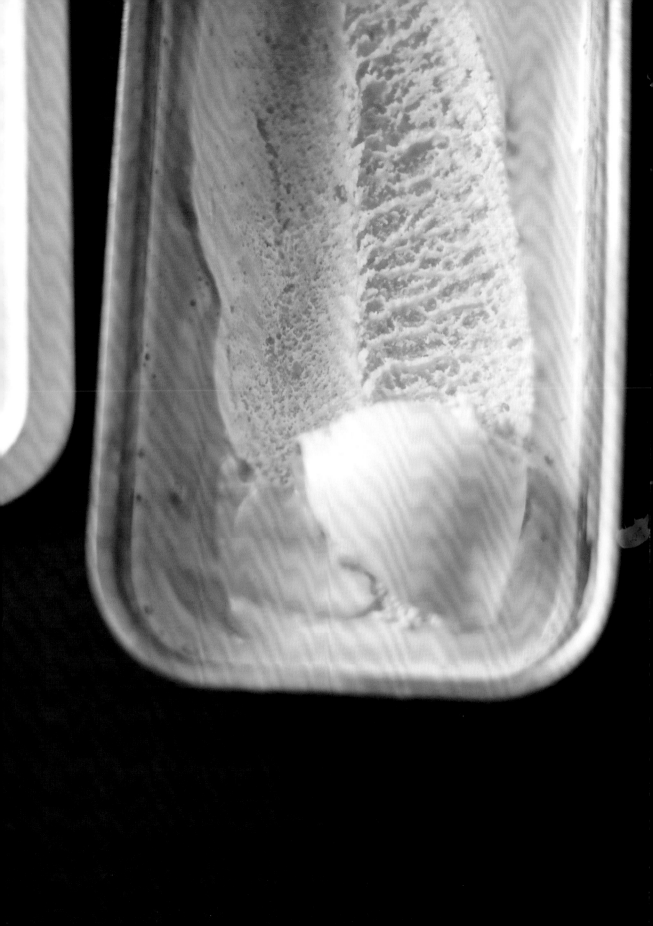

GET A GOOD IDEA AND STAY WITH IT.
DO IT, AND WORK AT IT UNTIL IT'S
DONE RIGHT.
WALT DISNEY

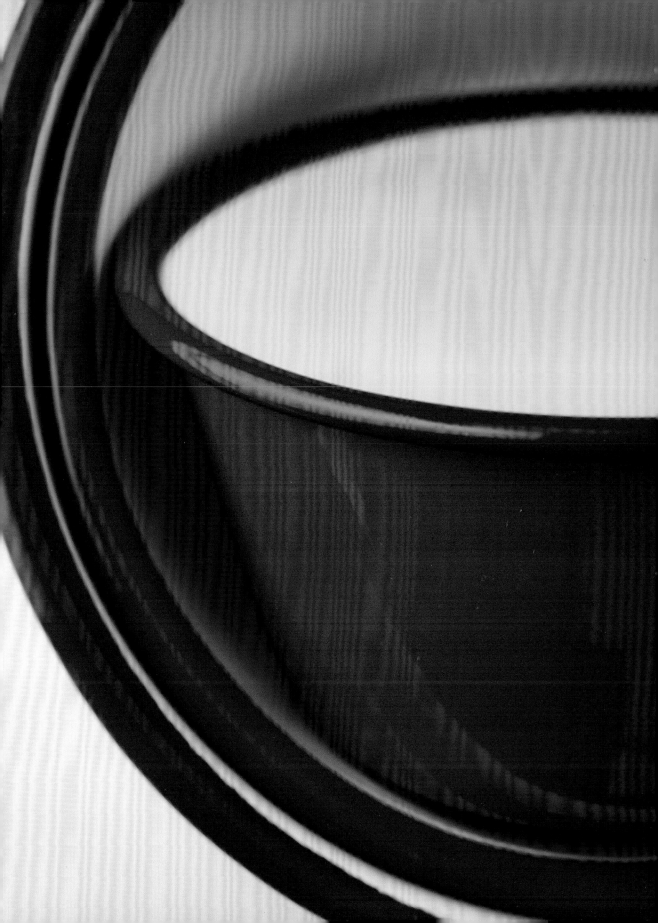

CAKES

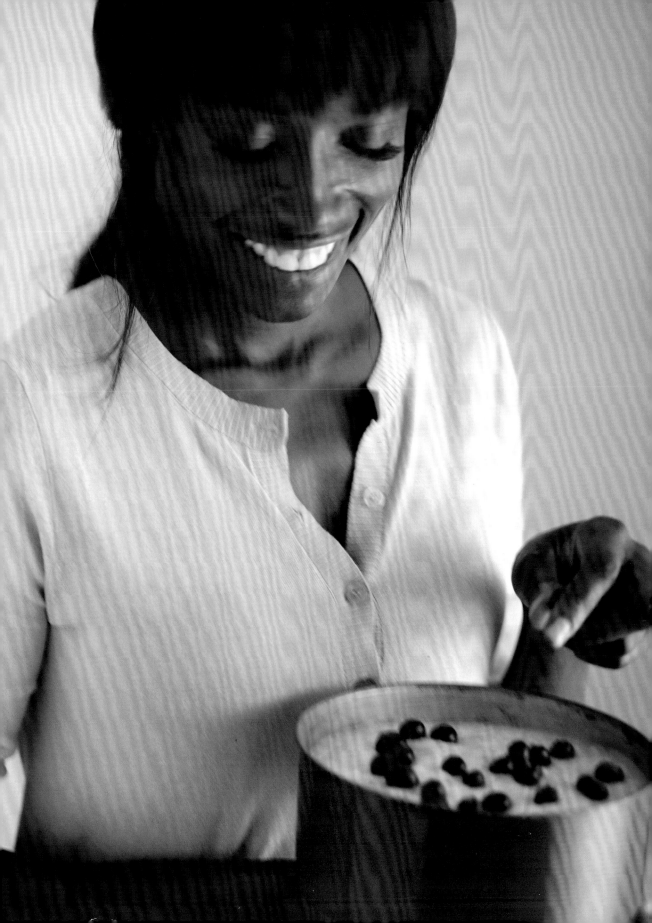

BLUEBERRY & LIMONCELLO DRIZZLE CAKE

I was talking to the lady from the management company I'm with, the very gorgeous Nicola, about my forthcoming (this one) book and she said to me, and I remember this quite clearly, 'A baking book is not a baking book without a good lemon drizzle cake in, don't you think? You have a good one in there don't you?' Having handed in the book already without a drizzle cake recipe, I quickly cobbled this one together with what I feel are very pleasing results. Nicola, my love, this one is for you.

Serves
12

Equipment
20cm round, loose-bottomed deep
    cake tin, food mixer or electric
    whisk

Sponge
Spray oil
125g caster sugar
100g unsalted butter, softened
100g full-fat Greek yogurt
2 eggs, lightly beaten
250g self-raising flour
4 egg whites
2 tsp baking powder
½ tsp vanilla extract
Finely grated zest of 2 unwaxed
    lemons (if waxed, wash them in
    hot, soapy water and dry them to
    get rid of the wax before using)
200g blueberries

Topping
50g icing sugar, sifted
2 tbsp limoncello (or lemon juice
    for an alcohol-free version)

Preheat the oven to 170°C, (Fan 150°C), 325°F, Gas Mark 3 and set the shelf in the middle. Spray a 20cm round, loose-bottomed deep cake tin with oil, line the bottom with baking parchment and then set it aside on a baking sheet.

Put the sugar, butter and yogurt into a large bowl and beat like mad with a whisk until well combined. A food mixer would be great for this job, otherwise get your whisk, roll up your sleeves and just go for it. Now, this mix is not going to go all light and fluffy and pretty like its full-fat cousin, but you are just looking for some semblance of uniformity (it will have quite a few little lumps in, but that is okay).

Next, add the whole eggs and half of the flour and beat for a good few minutes, until the mixture is well blended and starts to look a little smoother. Whisk the egg whites until light and frothy then fold them into the mixture with the rest of the flour, the baking powder, vanilla extract and lemon zest and beat until you have a smooth batter. Finally, stir half of the blueberries through.

Pour the mixture into the tin and smooth it down evenly with the back of a spoon. Arrange the remaining blueberries, flat side down, on the top in a few lines across the centre. Pop into the oven for about 25–30 minutes until a knife inserted into the centre comes out clean. The top should be quite a light golden brown and the sponge will feel firm to the touch.

Meanwhile, to make the topping, put the icing sugar into a small bowl. Stir in the limoncello (or lemon juice) to give a smooth, runny mixture and set aside until ready to use.

Once the cake is cool, place it on a serving platter or cake stand. Slowly spoon the topping all over the sponge and allow it to pour over the edges beautifully. Cut into 12 wedges and serve! If making in advance, keep it in the fridge.

(PER SERVING)	ENERGY	FAT	SAT FAT	SUGAR	PROTEIN	SALT
LORRAINE'S RECIPE	233 Kcal	9g	5.2g	18.3g	4.8g	0.5g
COMPARISON RECIPE	270 Kcal	10.2g	6.2g	28.7g	3.6g	0.39g

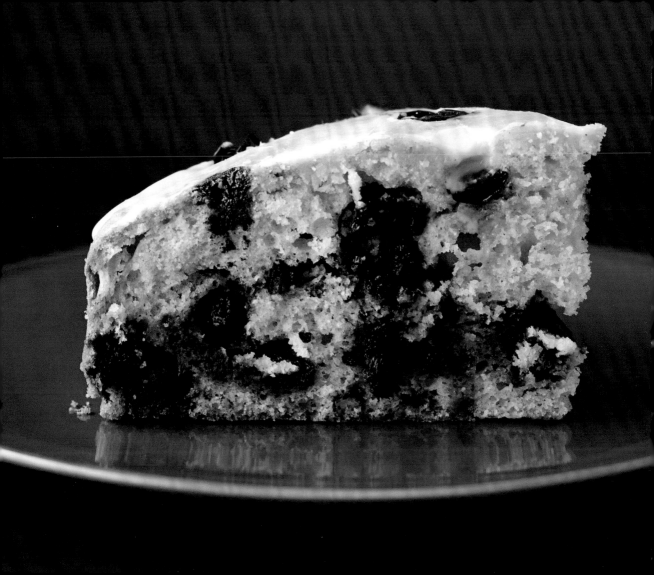

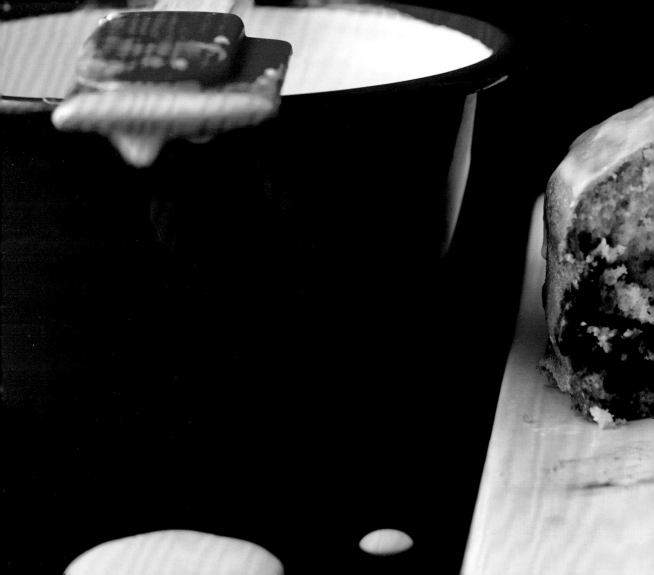

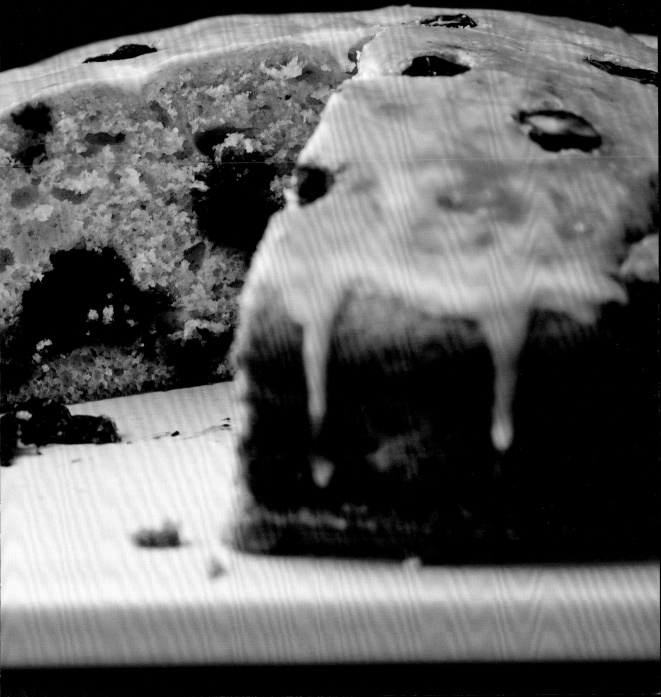

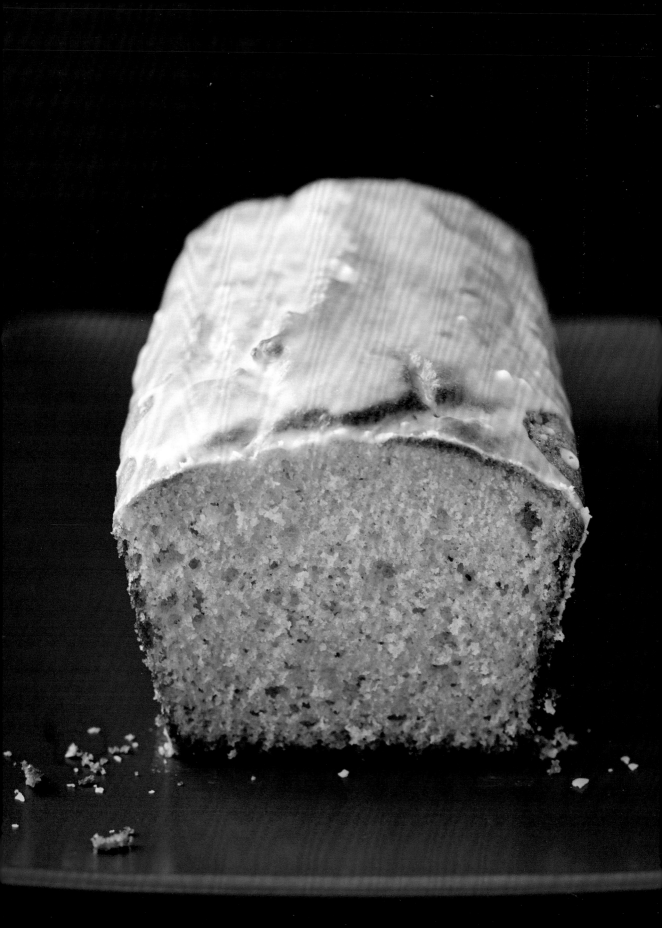

LEMON 'YOGURT' POUND CAKE WITH A TANGY CITRUS GLAZE

So, I did battle with this cake. I tried it with pretty much everything as a substitute for butter. Low-fat cream cheese produced a very weird mouthfeel. Lots of yogurt and oil produced the kind of cake one finds in the back of a village health food shop (grainy and bread-like). So I took my old lemon drizzle cake recipe from *Fast, Fresh and Easy Food* and made it with the least amount of butter and sugar possible. I got there. In the end. A lovely, lemony yogurt cake, full of fabulous flavour and topped off with a tasty, zesty glaze.

Makes
1 loaf with 12 slices

Equipment
22 x 10cm loaf tin, large bowl or freestanding electric mixer set with the beater

Sponge
75g unsalted butter, softened
100g caster sugar
2 eggs
1 egg white
2 tbsp low-fat Greek yogurt
150g self-raising flour
1 tsp baking powder
1 tsp vanilla extract or the seeds of 1 vanilla pod
Finely grated zest of 2 unwaxed lemons (if waxed, wash in hot, soapy water and dry to get rid of the wax before using)

Glaze
50g icing sugar
2 tbsp lemon juice

Preheat the oven to 180°C, (Fan 160°C), 350°F, Gas Mark 4. Lightly grease and line a 22 x 10cm loaf tin with baking parchment. I make sure that the paper overlaps a little bit, which makes it much easier to remove the loaf from the tin once it is cooked.

Beat the butter and sugar in a large bowl (or in a food mixer set with the beater) until well combined. Beat in the eggs, egg white and Greek yogurt. The mixture will start to look, well a bit curdled, but keep on beating it for a moment or two and then add the flour, baking powder, vanilla extract or seeds and lemon zest. Stir everything together until it is all combined and spoon it into the loaf tin.

Pop into the oven to bake for 20–25 minutes or until a skewer inserted into the centre comes out clean. Once baked, remove from the oven and leave the cake to cool in the tin for a few minutes. Use the baking parchment to pull the cake out of the tin, peel the paper off and leave on a wire rack until completely cool.

Meanwhile, to make the glaze, put the icing sugar in a small bowl. Stir in the lemon juice to give a smooth, runny mixture and set aside until ready to use.

Once the cake is cool, place it on a serving plate. Slowly spoon the glaze all over the top and allow to just pour over the edges beautifully. Cut into 12 slices and serve!

(PER SLICE)	ENERGY	FAT	SAT FAT	SUGAR	PROTEIN	SALT
LORRAINE'S RECIPE	159 Kcal	6.4g	3.6g	13.7g	3.4g	0.27g
COMPARISON RECIPE	198 Kcal	9.9g	5.7g	17g	2.9g	0.43g

WHITE CHOCOLATE & CHERRY TORTE WITH A CRÈME FRAÎCHE CHANTILLY

The white chocolate in this cake adds a touch of extra flavour and a whole lot of moistness and texture.

Serves
10

Equipment
23cm round springform cake tin

Sponge
Spray oil
150g white chocolate, snapped into small pieces
100g caster sugar
100g low-fat Greek yogurt
75g unsalted butter, very soft
3 eggs, lightly beaten
175g self-raising flour
2 tsp baking powder
Seeds of 1 vanilla pod or 1 tsp vanilla extract
1 tbsp kirsch for soaking the cake (can leave out for kiddies)

Crème fraîche Chantilly
200g low-fat crème fraîche
25g icing sugar, sifted
Seeds of 1 vanilla pod or 1 tsp vanilla extract

To serve
250g fresh cherries

Preheat the oven to 180°C, (Fan 160°C), 350°F, Gas Mark 4.

Lightly grease a 23cm round springform cake tin with a little spray oil. Line the base with baking parchment and set aside on a baking sheet.

Tip the chocolate into a small heatproof bowl. I like to melt chocolate in a microwave in 30-second blasts, stirring between each blast. Alternatively, melt the chocolate in a bowl that just sits on top of a medium pan with a little bit of boiling water. Just make sure the bowl doesn't touch the water as this could make the chocolate grainy. Leave the chocolate to sit until it melts, then stir, remove from the heat and set aside.

Next, beat the sugar, Greek yogurt and butter together in a large bowl until well combined. The mixture may have a few lumps and bumps in it, but that is okay. Add two-thirds of the beaten egg along with half of the flour and beat the mixture together until it looks uniform. Add the remaining egg and flour, the baking powder and vanilla seeds or extract and mix it all together, then fold the melted chocolate through thoroughly. Pour the mixture into the tin and level the top with the back of a spoon. Bake in the oven for about 30–35 minutes or until the cake is golden brown, spongy to the touch and a knife inserted into the centre comes out clean.

Meanwhile, prepare the crème fraîche Chantilly. Mix the crème fraîche, icing sugar and vanilla seeds or extract in a medium bowl with as few stirs as possible until blended. Cover and refrigerate until ready to use.

Once the cake is baked, remove it from the oven, brush the kirsch over evenly and leave to cool in the tin. Once cooled, carefully remove it from the tin and place on a serving plate. Spread the crème fraîche Chantilly on top of the cake and pile the cherries into the centre. I like to remove the stalks from about two-thirds of the cherries, pile them on first and then top with the remaining cherries with the stalks sticking upwards. Serve at once, remembering to warn your guests about the stones in the cherries.

(PER SERVING)	ENERGY	FAT	SAT FAT	SUGAR	PROTEIN	SALT
LORRAINE'S RECIPE	321 Kcal	16.2g	9.4g	26.2g	6.4g	0.54g
COMPARISON RECIPE	384 Kcal	23.1g	13.8g	30.9g	5.8g	0.5g

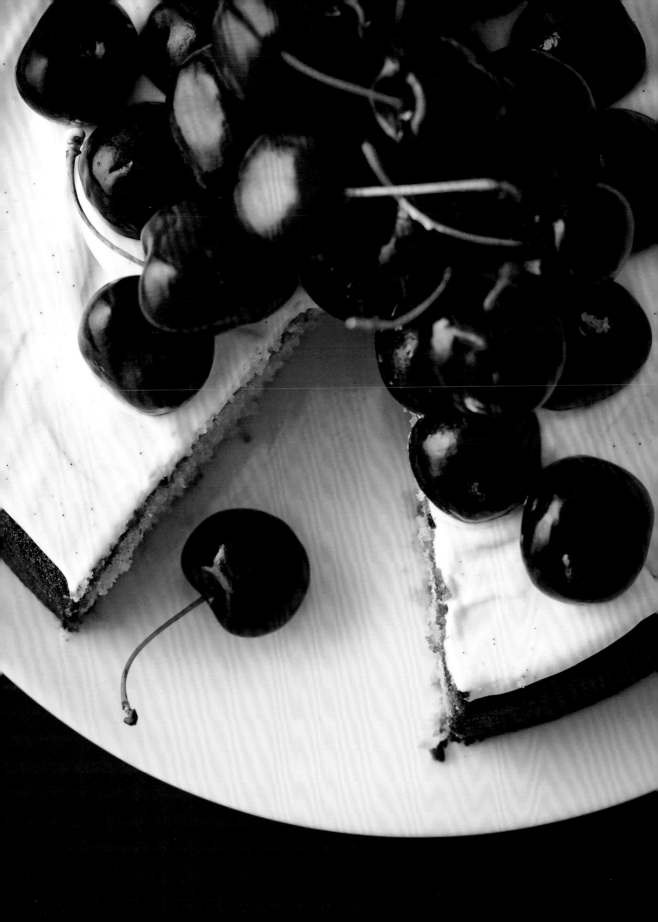

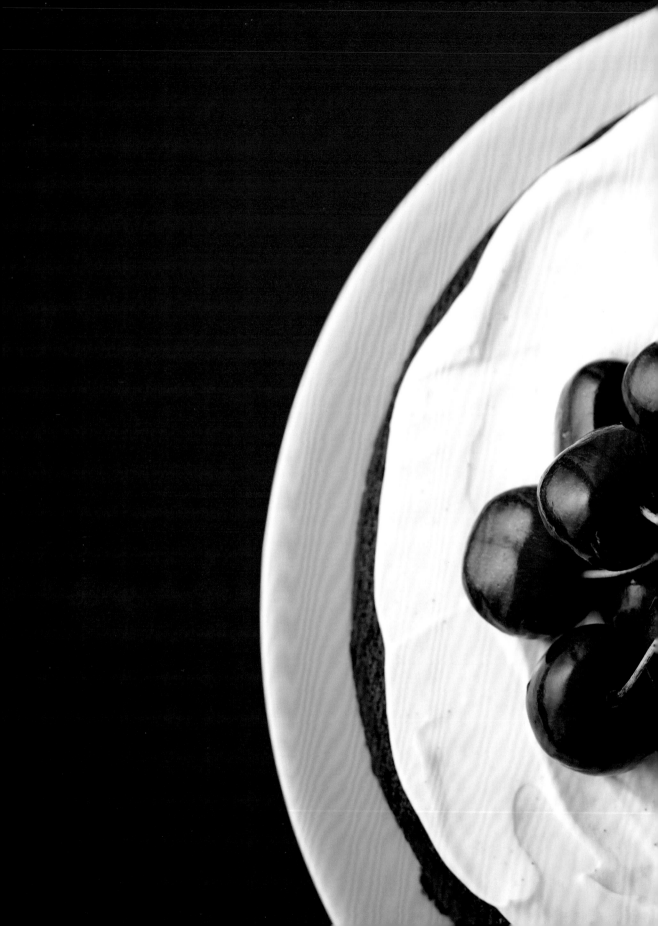

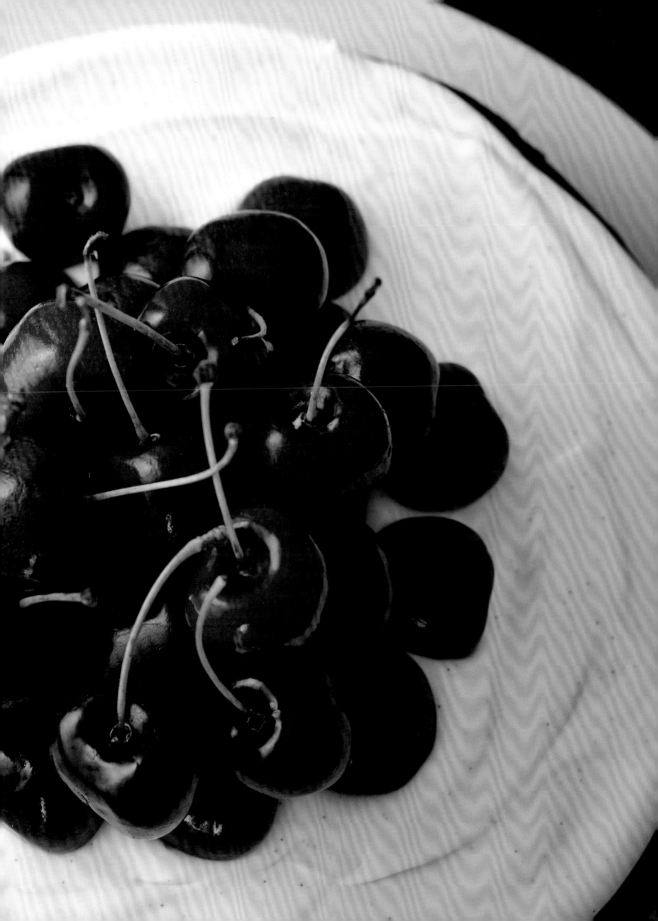

APRICOT & GINGER CHIFFON CAKE

You will for sure read a few recipe blurbs containing the words 'cry' and 'did not want to carry on' in this book because that was very much my experience with some of the recipes. I have a recipe for a chiffon cake from catering school, which contained more sugar than you would care to shake a stick at. However, as we know, sugar is the purveyor of all things sweet and it became increasingly hard to make this cake taste as sweet as I wanted it to without large amounts of the white stuff. Progress was made with a small addition of maple syrup (also very calorific, but less is needed to give the same sweet effect), and then the addition of apricots, packed full of sugar, but again, less of the fruit was needed to make the cake nicely sweet. I do hope you enjoy this.

Makes

16 slices

Equipment

20cm tube pan

Spray oil
200g plain flour
1½ tbsp ground ginger
2 tsp baking powder
100g dried apricots, very finely chopped
100ml vegetable oil
50ml maple syrup
3 egg yolks
Seeds of 1 vanilla pod
8 egg whites
75g soft light brown sugar

Preheat the oven to 170°C, (Fan 150°C), 325°F, Gas Mark 3. Lightly grease a 20cm tube pan with a few spritzes of spray oil.

Toss the flour, ginger and baking powder together in a large bowl and make a well in the centre. Add the apricots, vegetable oil, maple syrup, egg yolks and vanilla seeds, and then mix together to give a fairly stiff consistency.

Place the egg whites in another large bowl and whisk them until they begin to firm up. Then, while continuing to whisk, gradually add the sugar, bit by bit, until it forms a nice fluffy meringue mixture, a bit like shaving foam.

Bit by bit, add about half of the meringue mixture to the cake mixture, beating it in well before adding another. The aim here is to loosen the mixture to a dropping consistency. Once you have achieved this, carefully fold in the remaining meringue, trying to retain as much air as possible in the mixture. Once all of the meringue has been added, pour the cake mixture into the tube pan and level it out a little by shaking the tin very gently. Wipe away any splashes of mixture on the inside of the tin and then bake the cake for 40–45 minutes or until a skewer inserted into a centre part of the cake comes out clean.

Once cooked, remove the cake from the oven and leave in the tin for a few minutes until cool enough to handle. Put a plate upside down on top of the tin and, holding the plate and the tin with oven gloves, flip the whole lot over and give it a shake to allow it to pop down onto the plate. If it is a bit stubborn coming out, then carefully run a knife around the edge of the cake and around the tube in the middle and try again.

Allow it to cool a little, but this cake is so, so good served slightly warm.

(PER SLICE)	ENERGY	FAT	SAT FAT	SUGAR	PROTEIN	SALT
LORRAINE'S RECIPE	156 Kcal	7.2g	0.8g	10.2g	3.9g	0.26g
COMPARISON RECIPE	162 Kcal	6.6g	1.2g	14.9g	3.4g	0.33g

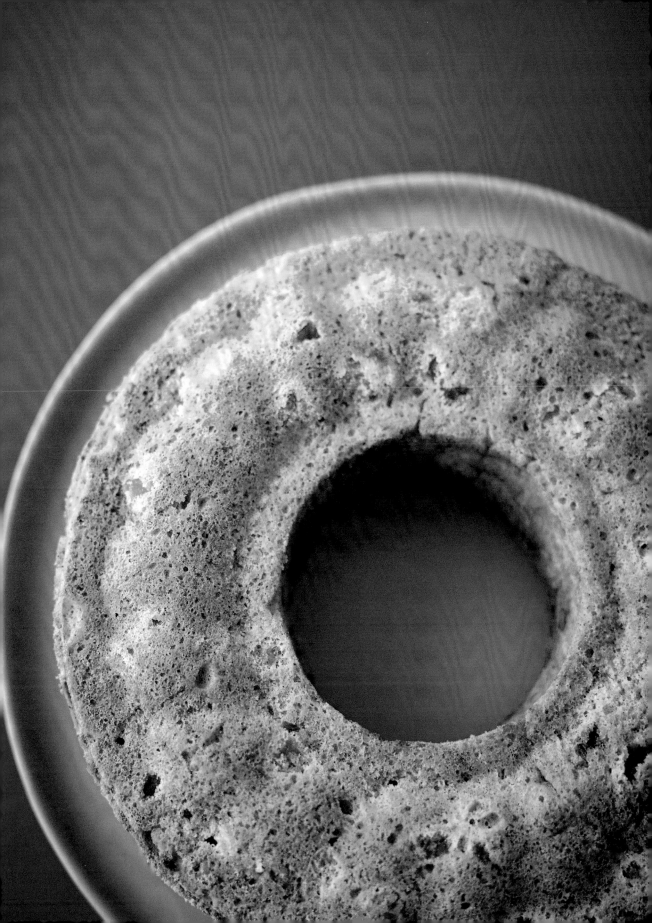

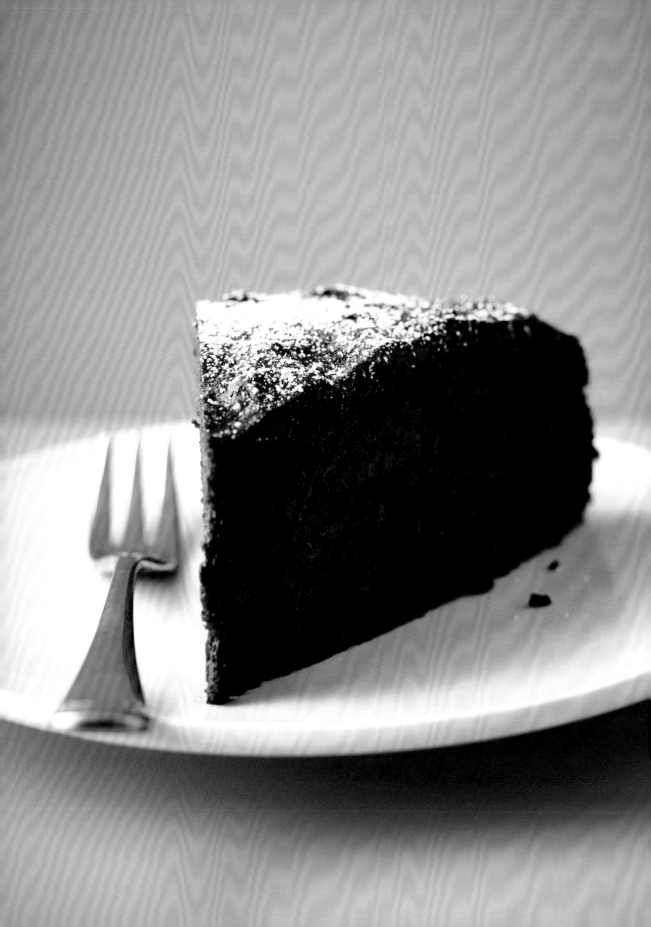

REALLY TASTY CHOCOLATE FUDGY ORANGE & BEETROOT CAKE

Ignore that beetroot does not usually go into a cake and give this a little go. The beetroot adds a wicked sweet and moist twist, which is really quite surprising in the best possible way. The pickled stuff you can buy in packets is not right at all for this recipe, so to cook the raw beetroot, either boil them for about 30 minutes to 1 hour (depending on their size) or wrap in tin foil and roast at 180°C, (Fan 160°C), 350°F/Gas Mark 4 for 1½ to 2 hours until tender. Either way, peel and grate them once cold. I have been told some places sell cooked beetroot that have not been soaked in vinegar; if you can find those, then everyone is a winner!

Serves

10

Equipment

18cm round, loose-bottomed, deep cake tin, food mixer or electric whisk

100g unsalted butter, softened
150g dark chocolate (minimum 70% cocoa solids), snapped or chopped into small pieces
3 eggs
4 egg whites
Seeds of 1 vanilla pod or 1 tsp vanilla extract
150g soft light brown sugar
150g wholemeal flour
1½ tsp baking powder
2 tsp ground ginger
Finely grated zest of 1 orange
200g fresh cooked beetroots (see recipe intro), peeled and roughly grated
1 tbsp icing sugar, to finish

Preheat the oven to 170°C, (Fan 150°C), 325°F, Gas Mark 3. Use the spray oil to grease an 18cm round, loose-bottomed, deep cake tin. Line the base with baking parchment and set on a baking sheet.

Melt the butter in a pan and once it has melted, remove from the heat, add the chocolate and set it aside to melt.

Meanwhile, put the eggs, egg whites and vanilla seeds or extract into a large bowl and whisk them up until mousse-like and white. This can be done by using a whisk or a food mixer. Then, working in two batches, add the sugar, whipping it up well between each addition until stiff.

Once melted, stir the chocolate and butter together and pour it around the edge of the whisked eggs. Then, gently fold it in until well blended and the mixture turns dark brown. Really scoop up the chocolate, which will fall to the bottom of the bowl, to get it nicely folded in. Gently sprinkle the flour, baking powder, ground ginger and orange zest over and then gently fold this in well also. Finally, gently fold the beetroot in and carefully pour the mixture into the prepared tin.

Bake in the oven for 40–45 minutes until firm on top and a knife comes out still a little sticky from the centre of the cake. I like to undercook this cake ever so slightly so that it stays nice and moist. It will still cook a little further in its own heat when out of the oven, so just trust me on this.

Once it has reached this stage, remove the cake from the oven. Leave to cool in the tin.

Once the cake is cooled, sprinkle over the icing sugar and serve.

(PER SERVING)	ENERGY	FAT	SAT FAT	SUGAR	PROTEIN	SALT
LORRAINE'S RECIPE	298 Kcal	14.7g	8.3g	27.4g	6.7g	0.33g
COMPARISON RECIPE	380 Kcal	21.3g	12.5g	31g	5.3g	0.34g

WALNUT, HONEY & WHITE CHOCOLATE CAKES

Gorgeous, sticky, small and naughty luscious little cakes. Though they are a teeny bit higher in fat than the comparison recipe, they are a smidgen lower in saturated fat and impressively each cake is just over 2 teaspoons lower in sugar.

Makes
12 petite cakes

Equipment
12-hole cupcake tin, mechanical ice-cream scoop

Sponge
75g unsalted butter, softened
75g caster sugar
1 tbsp honey
2 eggs
1 egg white
2 tbsp low-fat crème fraîche
Seeds of 1 vanilla pod or 1 tsp vanilla extract
150g self-raising flour
75g walnuts, roughly chopped

White chocolate glaze
200g white chocolate chips, roughly chopped
50ml semi-skimmed milk, at room temperature

Preheat the oven to 180°C, (Fan 160°C), 350°F, Gas Mark 4. Line a 12-hole cupcake tin with cupcake cases and set aside.

Beat the butter, sugar and honey together well in a large bowl until well blended and lighter in colour. Add the eggs, egg white, crème fraîche and vanilla seeds or extract and mix together well. It will not look that appetizing yet, but it soon will! Add the flour and two-thirds of the walnuts and mix to combine.

Then, using a mechanical ice-cream scoop, divide the mixture evenly between the 12 paper cases. Pop them into the oven to bake for 20–25 minutes or until they feel springy to the touch and a skewer inserted into the centre of one of the cakes comes out clean. Once the cakes are cooked, remove them from the oven and the tin and leave to cool completely for 10 minutes or so.

Meanwhile, tip the chocolate chips into a small heatproof bowl. I like to melt chocolate in a microwave in 30-second blasts, stirring between each blast. Alternatively, melt the chocolate in a bowl that just sits on top of a medium pan with a little bit of boiling water. Just make sure the bowl doesn't touch the water as this could make the chocolate grainy. Leave the chocolate to sit until it melts, then remove from the heat and leave it to cool to room temperature.

Sit a wire cooling rack on top of a flat baking sheet. Then, once the cupcakes are cool, carefully peel and discard the paper case from each one and sit them on the wire rack.

Stir the milk through the now-cooled chocolate until well blended and loosened a little. Spoon this chocolate mixture generously over each cake, scatter the remaining walnuts on top to stick and then leave to one side for the chocolate to set before serving.

(PER CAKE)	ENERGY	FAT	SAT FAT	SUGAR	PROTEIN	SALT
LORRAINE'S RECIPE	272 Kcal	16.3g	7.4g	18.5g	5.1g	0.22g
COMPARISON RECIPE	290 Kcal	14.7g	8.8g	27.7g	3.5g	0.30g

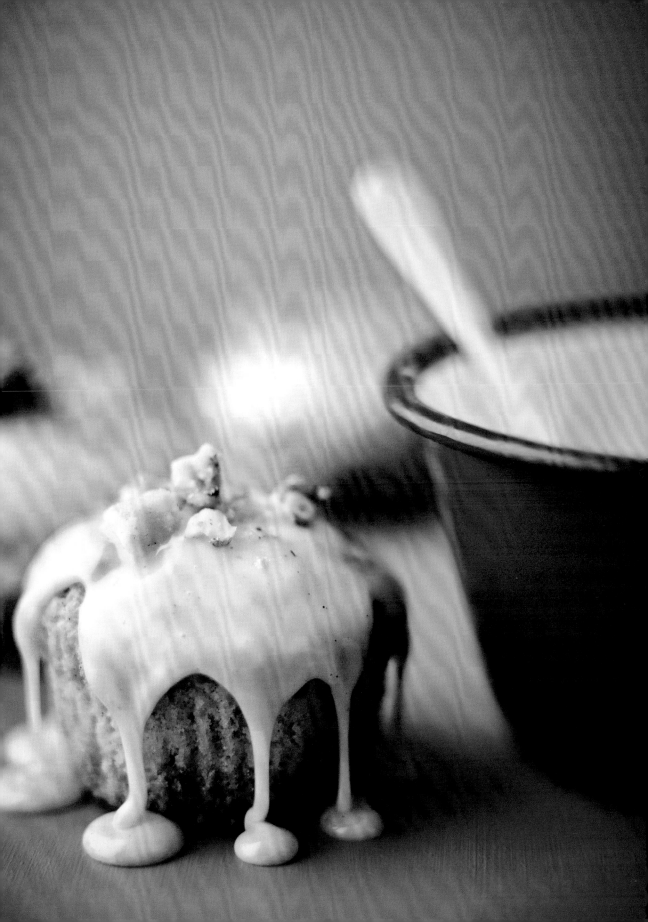

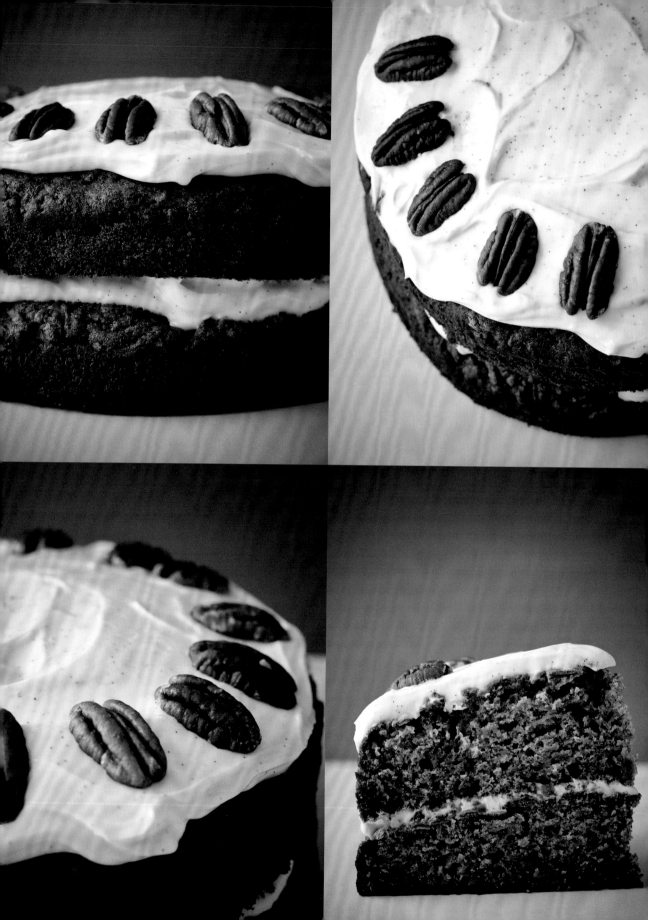

CARROT & APPLE CAKE

Carrot cakes are often more healthy than regular cakes due to things like the addition of, errr, carrots! They also often include other fruit and use oil rather than butter, which cuts the saturated fats and adds fibre. So the task with this recipe was just to gently reduce the sugar and try to reduce the oil, while still ensuring that the cake is as tasty and as yummy as ever.

Serves
10 (small slices)

Equipment
2 x 20cm sandwich tins

Sponge
Spray oil
150g wholemeal flour
150g self-raising flour
150g carrots, peeled and roughly grated
125g soft light brown sugar
175ml sunflower oil
2 apples, peeled, cored and roughly grated
3 eggs
1 egg white
1 tsp baking powder
1 tsp bicarbonate of soda
1 tsp ground ginger
18 pecan nuts

Cream cheese frosting
300g low-fat cream cheese
3 tbsp icing sugar, sifted
1 tbsp crème fraîche
Seeds of 1 vanilla pod or 1 tsp vanilla extract

Preheat the oven to 180°C, (Fan 160°C), 350°F, Gas Mark 4 and get the middle shelf at the ready. Grease two 20cm sandwich tins with a light spray of oil, line the bottoms with discs of baking parchment and set them on a baking sheet.

Put all of the cake ingredients (except the pecan nuts) into a large bowl and mix everything together until well combined. Divide the mixture evenly between the two tins. Bake in the oven for 30 minutes or until the sponges feel springy to the touch and they are shrinking a little from the edges of the tins. Once the cakes are baked, remove from the oven and leave to cool in the tins.

Next, to make the frosting put the cream cheese, icing sugar, crème fraîche and vanilla seeds into a medium bowl and mix together until smooth and well combined. Then, cover and pop into the fridge to firm up a little while waiting for the cakes to cool.

Once the cakes have cooled, carefully remove them from their tins. Sandwich the cakes together with half of the frosting, then put the rest of the frosting on top. Arrange the pecans around the outer edge of the top frosting and serve. If making in advance, keep it in the fridge.

(PER SLICE)	ENERGY	FAT	SAT FAT	SUGAR	PROTEIN	SALT
LORRAINE'S RECIPE	479 Kcal	31.3g	6.7g	19.8g	10g	0.63g
COMPARISON RECIPE	574 Kcal	32.8g	10.4g	46.5g	7g	0.83g

COCONUT & LIME LOAF

I nearly fell down and fainted when I read about the nutritional content of coconut. Wowzers, no wonder it tastes so very, very good! A little bit is all that is needed in this loaf for a totally tropical taste. The slices are small, so I often treat myself to two!

Makes
1 loaf with 8 skinny slices

Equipment
22 x 10cm loaf tin

Sponge
175g plain flour
50g desiccated coconut
1 tsp baking powder
Tiny pinch of salt
1 egg
200g 0% fat Greek yogurt
75g soft light brown sugar
Zest and juice of 1 lime (wash in hot, soapy water and dry to get rid of the wax before using)
Seeds from 1 vanilla pod or 1 tsp vanilla extract

Lime sugar syrup
2 tbsp caster sugar
Zest and juice of 1 lime (washed and dried)

Preheat the oven to 180°C, (Fan 160°C), 350°F, Gas Mark 4 and line a 22 x 10cm loaf tin with baking parchment. I make sure that the paper overlaps a little bit, which makes it much easier to remove the loaf from the tin once it is cooked.

Toss the flour, coconut, baking powder and salt together in a large bowl and make a well in the centre. Beat the egg lightly in a medium bowl, and then whisk in the yogurt, sugar, lime juice and zest and the vanilla seeds or extract. Mix the wet mixture into the dry ingredients to give a wet dropping consistency. It is important to do this with as few stirs as possible so the flour doesn't get overworked, which would result in quite a tough loaf. Pour the mixture into the tin and spread and smooth the top with the back of a spoon. Bake in the oven for 35–40 minutes or until a skewer inserted into the centre comes out clean.

Make the lime sugar syrup about 5 minutes before the loaf is baked. Put the sugar and lime juice in a small pan over a low heat, stirring until the sugar dissolves. Then turn up the heat and let it bubble away for 30–60 seconds until syrupy. Remove from the heat, stir the lime zest in and set aside to infuse and thicken up a little more.

Once the loaf is cooked, remove from the oven and brush the top with the lime sugar syrup. Leave the loaf to stand in the tin for a few minutes before lifting out and allowing to cool completely on a wire rack. Enjoy warm or cold.

(PER SLICE)	ENERGY	FAT	SAT FAT	SUGAR	PROTEIN	SALT
LORRAINE'S RECIPE	192 Kcal	5g	3.6g	16.5g	5.9g	0.25g
COMPARISON RECIPE	300 Kcal	18.1g	11.2g	20.2g	5.4g	0.58g

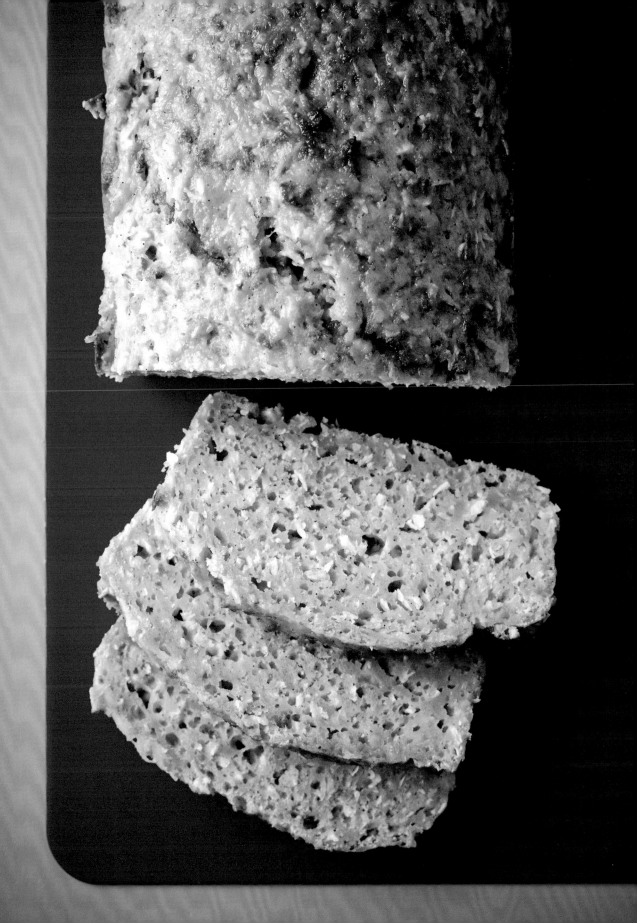

HASSELBACK APPLE & CINNAMON CAKE

The word 'hasselback' is usually saved for the potato. Rumour has it that the name comes from the restaurant for which they were invented in Sweden sometime in the 1940s. A hasselback potato is quite simply one that has been cut into a fan-like shape with a knife making thin slices. When presented with a glut of apples, and being all apple-crumbled out, I wanted to use the flavours of an autumnal day in a cake but with a bit of visual difference. I hope the restaurant in Djurgården can forgive me for using some artistic licence on their invention!

Serves
10

Equipment
23cm springform or loose-bottomed cake tin

Sponge
Spray oil
250g self-raising flour
150g low-fat crème fraîche
75g wholemeal flour
75g soft light brown sugar
75ml rapeseed or sunflower oil
50g unsalted butter, softened
3 eggs
2 tbsp semi-skimmed milk
2 tsp ground cinnamon
1 tsp baking powder
Seeds of ½ a vanilla pod or ½ tsp vanilla extract

Decoration
2 eating apples, peeled, cut in half and cored
1 tbsp maple syrup

Preheat the oven to 180°C, (Fan 160°C), 350°F, Gas Mark 4. Grease a 23cm springform or loose-bottomed cake tin with a little spray oil and line the base with baking parchment. Set aside on a baking sheet.

Put all of the ingredients for the cake into a large bowl and mix everything together until well combined. Then simply pour the mixture into the prepared tin.

Take half an apple and place it cut side down on the work surface, and slice it into 1cm slices. Place the slices lightly on top of the cake, retaining the half apple shape. Repeat with the rest of the apple.

There is no need to press the apple down into the mix. Bake the cake in the oven for 40–45 minutes until golden on top and a skewer inserted into a centre part of the cake comes out clean.

Once the cake is ready, remove it from the oven and brush it all over with the maple syrup. Set it aside for a few minutes to cool a little before carefully removing the cake from the tin and putting it on a serving plate to cool completely.

(PER SERVING)	ENERGY	FAT	SAT FAT	SUGAR	PROTEIN	SALT
LORRAINE'S RECIPE	282 Kcal	15.5g	5.2g	12.1g	5.3g	0.43g
COMPARISON RECIPE	286 Kcal	14.2g	8.2g	23.7g	4.1g	0.49g

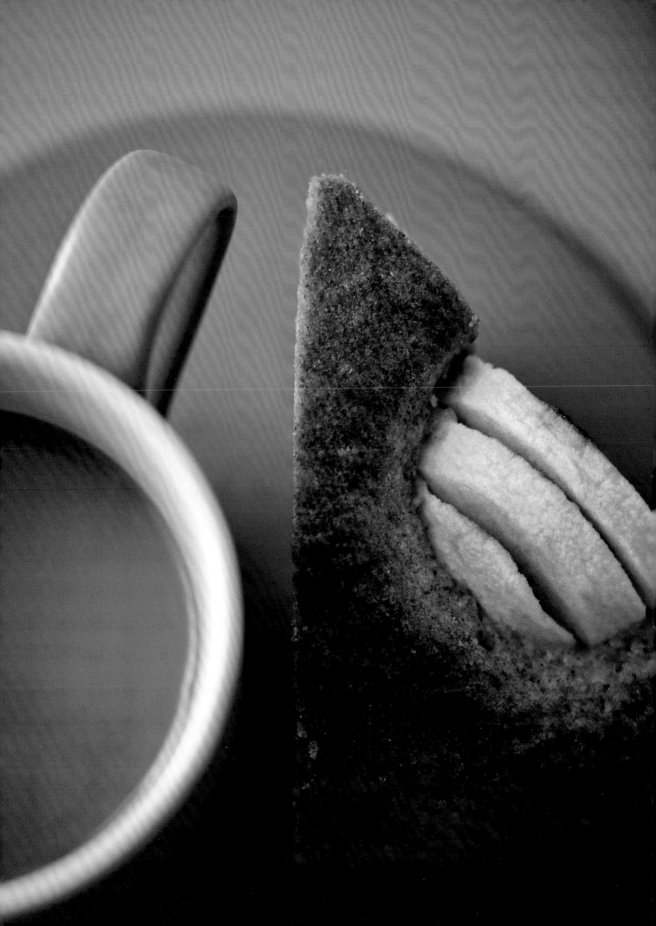

VICTORIA SPONGE

This cake was my nemesis. I kept trying and trying and not getting anywhere. One balmy April night, I was in the kitchen testing this little sponge with *The Real Housewives of New York City* on my laptop to keep me company when, boom, I opened the oven and there she was. A Victoria sponge — fluffy, light and tasty. When you mix the butter, yogurt and sugar together it does not look pretty and no matter how soft the butter is, it stills insists on going into lumps, but persevere with this national treasure because I can attest that it is worth it.

Makes
10 (slimmish slices)

Equipment
2 x 20cm loose-bottomed sandwich tins, food mixer or electric whisk

Sponge
Spray oil
125g caster sugar
100g unsalted butter, softened
100g full-fat Greek yogurt
2 eggs, lightly beaten
250g self-raising flour
4 egg whites
2 tsp baking powder
½ tsp vanilla extract
Icing sugar, to decorate

Sugar syrup
4 tbsp caster sugar
2 tbsp lemon juice

Filling
100g low-fat cream cheese
100g no-fat natural yogurt
4 tbsp icing sugar, sifted
Seeds from 1 vanilla pod
125g raspberries

Preheat the oven to 170°C, (Fan 150°C), 325°F, Gas Mark 3 and set the shelf in the middle. Spray two 20cm loose-bottomed sandwich tins with oil, line them with baking parchment and then set them on a baking sheet.

Put the sugar, butter and yogurt into a large bowl and beat like mad with a whisk until well combined. A food mixer would be great for this job, otherwise get your whisk, roll up your sleeves and just go for it. Now, this mix is not going to go all light and fluffy and pretty like its full-fat cousin, but you are just looking for some semblance of uniformity (and it will have quite a few little lumps in, but that is okay).

Next, add the whole eggs and half of the flour and beat for a good few minutes until the mixture is well blended and starts to look a little more smooth. Whisk the egg whites until light and frothy and fold them into the mixture with the rest of the flour, the baking powder and vanilla extract and beat until you have a smooth batter. Divide the mixture evenly between the tins and then pop them into the oven for about 20 minutes. The top should be quite a light golden brown and the sponge will feel firm to the touch.

About 5 minutes before the end of the cooking time, prepare the sugar syrup. Put the sugar and lemon juice in a small pan with 2 tablespoons of water and allow to simmer over a low heat, stirring until the sugar dissolves. Turn the heat up and allow it to bubble away for 30–60 seconds until it reaches a syrupy consistency. Remove from the heat and allow it to cool and thicken up a little more.

Once the sponges are cooked, remove them from the oven. Pierce the cakes all over with a skewer inserted halfway through and then pour the sugar syrup over slowly, allowing it to seep through. Leave the cakes to cool completely in the tins before carefully removing.

Meanwhile, prepare the filling. Whisk the cream cheese, yogurt, icing sugar and vanilla seeds together in a medium bowl until smooth and refrigerate until ready to use. Tip the raspberries into a small bowl and crush them lightly with a fork.

To assemble the cake, set the best-looking top aside and sit the other (top side up) on a serving plate or cake stand as the base. Spread the crushed raspberries evenly over, followed by the cream cheese filling to just come to the edge. Sit the reserved cake half, nice side up, on top and serve, dusting with a little icing sugar.

(PER SLICE)	ENERGY	FAT	SAT FAT	SUGAR	PROTEIN	SALT
LORRAINE'S RECIPE	315 Kcal	12.1g	7.1g	27.9g	7.2g	0.61g
COMPARISON RECIPE	501 Kcal	25.3g	14.9g	53.8g	5.1g	0.8g

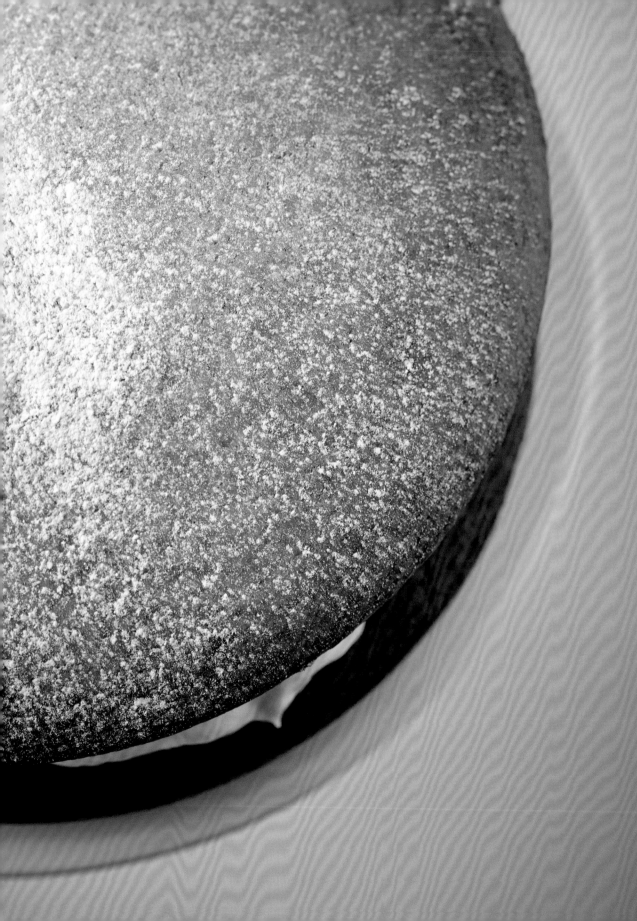

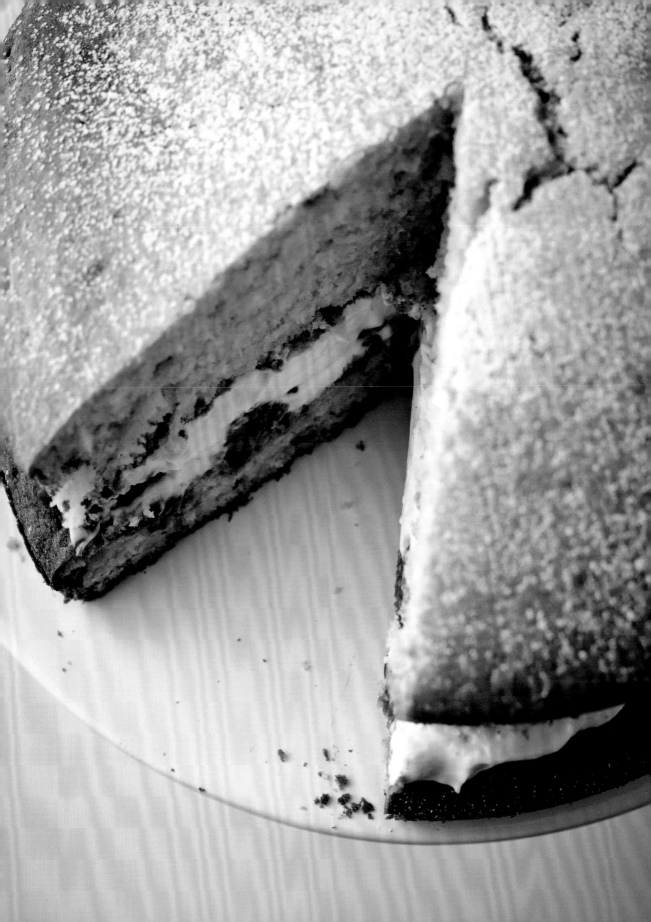

RIGHT ACTIONS IN THE FUTURE ARE THE BEST
APOLOGIES FOR BAD ACTIONS IN THE PAST.
TYRON EDWARDS

COOKIES & TRAYBAKES

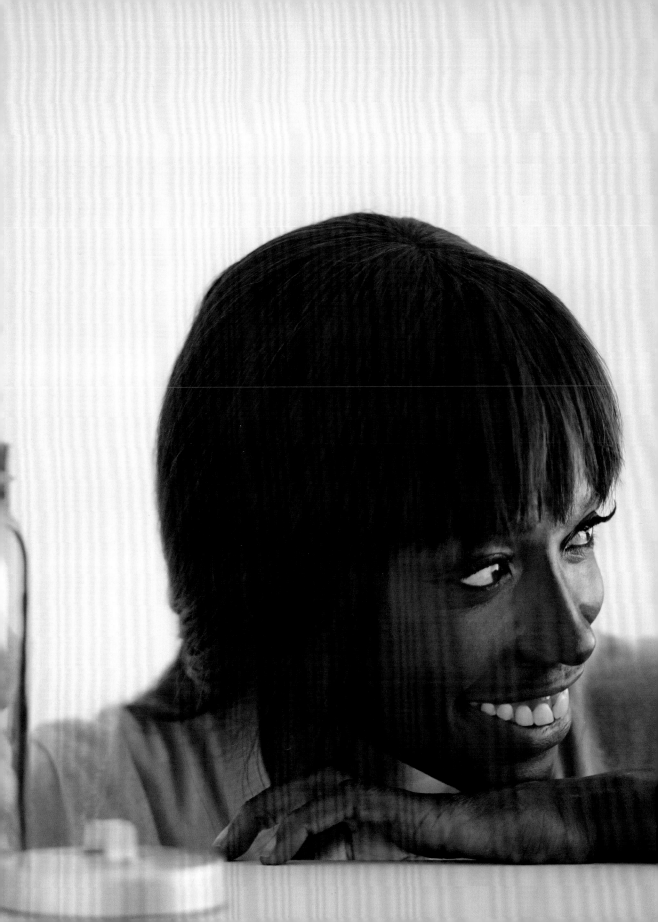

LEMON, RASPBERRY & BLUEBERRY THUMBPRINT COOKIES

So as I write this, I am lying in bed propped up by various pillows, my daughter next to me on Facebook, Twitter and Tumblr, while I am stuck with what to say about our American import, the thumbprint cookie. The thumbprint is traditionally filled with jam (or even Nutella), but for a fresher, less sugary alternative (even the no added sugar jams have lots of sugar in, even if it is fruit sugar), I settled on lashings of colourful fresh fruit.

Makes

12 cookies

50g butter
50g caster sugar
2 eggs, lightly beaten
200g plain flour
Zest of 2 unwaxed lemons (if waxed, wash in hot soapy, water and dry to get rid of the wax before using)
Pinch of salt
1 tbsp lemon juice
12 raspberries
24 blueberries

Preheat the oven to 200°C, (Fan 180°C), 400°F, Gas Mark 6 and line a large baking sheet with baking parchment.

Cream the butter and sugar in a large bowl until well combined. Add the eggs, beating them in well. Then add the flour, lemon zest and salt and mix again until combined. The mixture will be slightly wet and sticky.

Using damp hands, divide the mixture into 12 even-sized balls, placing them spaced apart on the baking sheet as you go. Squish each one down with the palm of your hand to about 1cm in thickness, then make a thumbprint in the centre of each cookie. Wiggle your finger about a bit to make the dip wide enough to fit three berries in. Put one raspberry and two blueberries into each thumbprint and press them down lightly to really nestle them in. Bake in the oven for 8–10 minutes until very lightly golden and cooked through.

Once cooked, remove from the oven and leave to cool a little before transferring to a wire rack to cool completely.

(PER COOKIE)	ENERGY	FAT	SAT FAT	SUGAR	PROTEIN	SALT
LORRAINE'S RECIPE	121 Kcal	4.7g	2.5g	5.1g	2.9g	0.13g
COMPARISON RECIPE	181 Kcal	9.3g	5.6g	12.1g	1.9g	0.23g

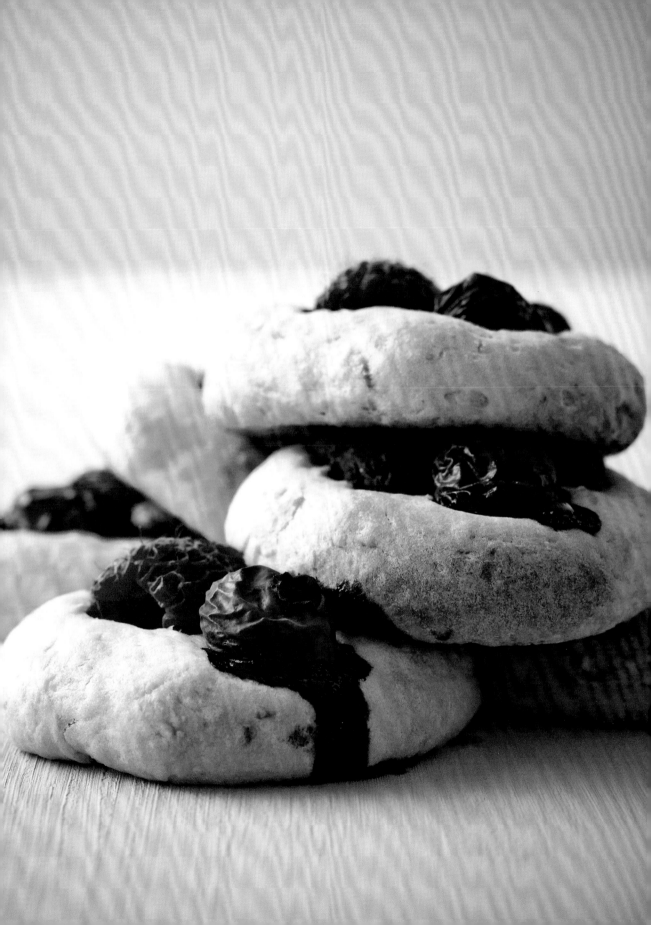

CHOCOLATE & ALMOND COOKIES

It's so, so easy to make cookies with lashings of sugar and butter, which, of course, we love, but how nice to also have some cookies in the jar to snack on and feel just a little bit better about.

Makes

12 cookies

50g unsalted butter, softened
50g soft light brown sugar
1 egg
100g wholemeal flour
50g ground almonds
50g cocoa powder
1 tsp baking powder
1 tsp bicarbonate of soda
1 tsp vanilla extract
Handful of flaked almonds

Preheat the oven to 180°C, (Fan 160°C), 350°F, Gas Mark 4 and line a large baking sheet with baking parchment.

Blend the butter and sugar together in a large bowl until smooth and well combined. Then add the egg and mix together well. Finally, add the flour, ground almonds, cocoa powder, baking powder, bicarbonate of soda and the vanilla extract and mix together to give quite a crumbly mixture. Now get your hands stuck in to bring the mixture together to give a slightly sticky dough ball.

Divide the dough into 12 equal-sized pieces and, using damp hands, roll each one into a ball, placing them spaced apart on the baking sheet as you go. Use the palm of your hand to squash each ball down to about 6cm wide and about a 5mm thick. Decorate the tops however you wish with the flaked almonds, laying them down and pressing them in slightly. Bake the cookies in the oven for 10–12 minutes until cooked, but still just soft to the touch.

Remove from the oven and leave to cool slightly before transferring the cookies to a wire rack to cool completely. These are also delicious eaten warm.

(PER COOKIE)	ENERGY	FAT	SAT FAT	SUGAR	PROTEIN	SALT
LORRAINE'S RECIPE	140 Kcal	9.3g	3.2g	4.8g	4.1g	0.45g
COMPARISON RECIPE	154 Kcal	11.1g	4.1g	9g	3.2g	0.04g

PEANUT BUTTER COOKIES

It is tough in all honesty to make peanut butter cookies that are truly light. There are quite a few recipes out there with a lot less peanut butter in, but even if you harnessed the best will in the world, you would not be able to taste the peanuts at all. So whilst I am not saying these peanut butter cookies are better for you then eating a stick of celery, I am saying that I have worked hard to reduce the peanut butter, sugar and butter content in them as best I can so that they still have that scrumbunctious flavour. I also found some no-added-sugar peanut butter, which will cut down the sugar content even further.

Makes

12 cookies

175g crunchy peanut butter
  (no-added sugar if you can find it)
50g caster sugar
1 egg
1 tsp vanilla extract
50g wholemeal flour
50g oats

Preheat the oven to 190°C, (Fan 170°C), 375°F, Gas Mark 5 and line a large baking sheet with baking parchment.

Beat the peanut butter and sugar together in a large bowl. The mixture just needs to be well mixed together rather than light and fluffy. Beat in the egg, vanilla extract and 1 tablespoon of water until well combined. Then add the flour and oats and mix together to give a soft dough ball.

Get your hands stuck in and shape the mixture into 12 even-sized balls, arranging them spaced apart on the tray as you go. Squish them down with the palm of your hand to about 5mm thick. Bake for 10–12 minutes until lightly golden and cooked through, but still slightly soft to the touch.

Remove from the oven and set aside to cool a little before transferring to a wire rack to cool completely and firm up.

(PER COOKIE)	ENERGY	FAT	SAT FAT	SUGAR	PROTEIN	SALT
LORRAINE'S RECIPE	142 Kcal	8.5g	2.1g	5.5g	5.2g	0.15g
COMPARISON RECIPE	154 Kcal	9.7g	3.9g	8.1g	3.5g	0.25g

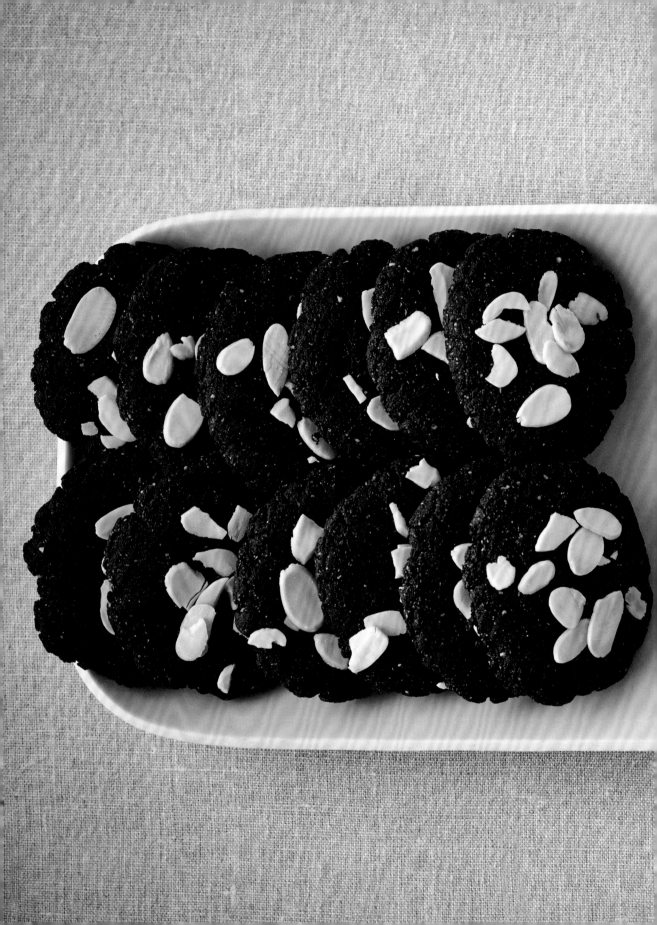

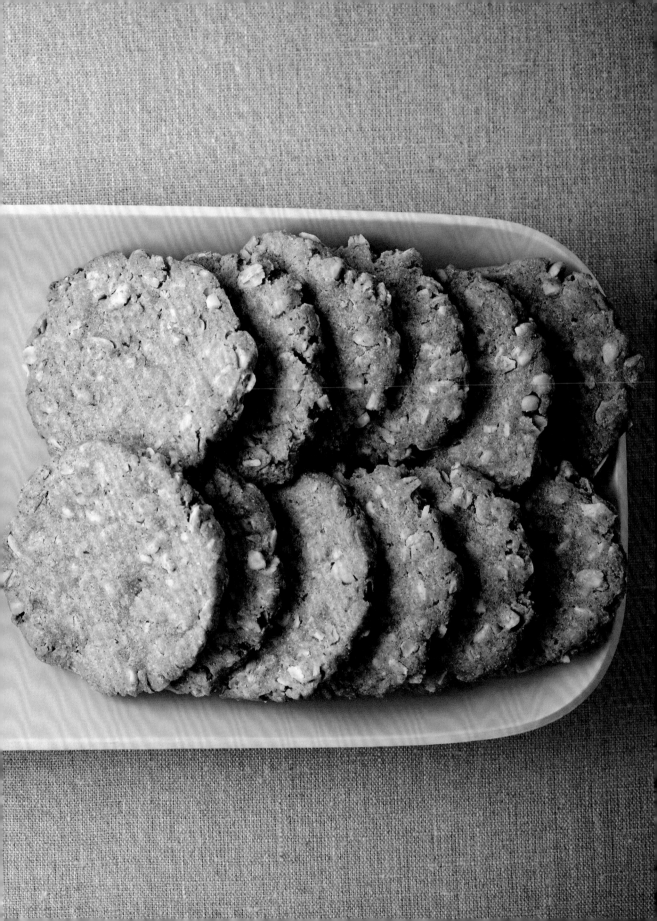

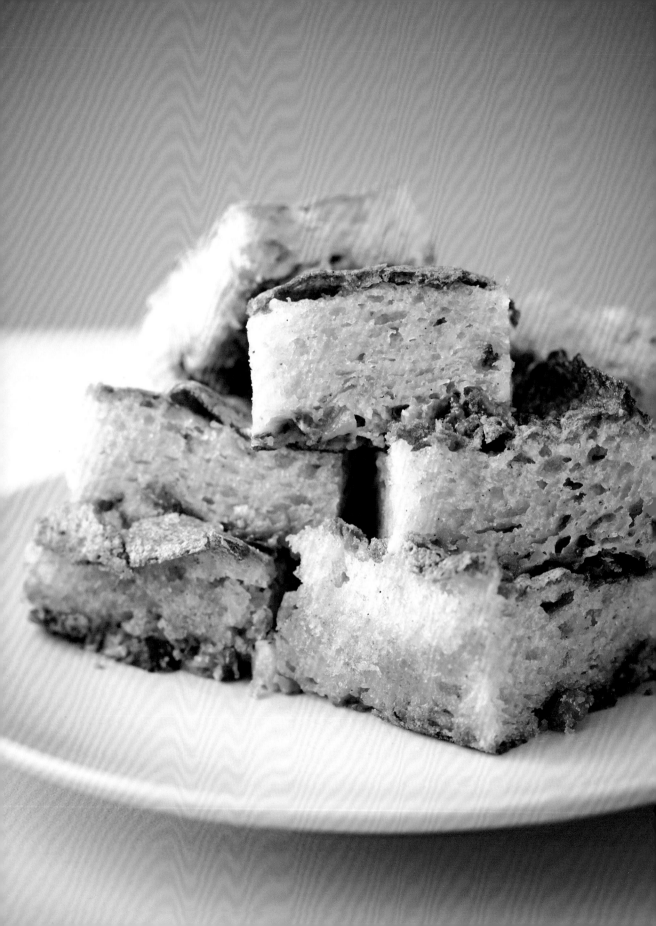

WHITE CHOCOLATE & PISTACHIO SPONGE BLONDIES

It must have been the Americans that came up with the name 'blondies'. Otherwise the brownies would have all the fun?! Do use the green pistachios, which you can usually find in the cooks' or special ingredients section of the supermarket. If you struggle to find these, my suggestion would be to leave them out altogether, as the dried old ones in their shells are simply no substitute whatsoever. Try a different nut, like a walnut or pecan, for that added textural crunch.

Makes

16 bite-sized squares or
8 rectangular bars

Equipment

20cm square cake tin, electric mixer fitted with a whisk attachment

Spray oil
75g unsalted butter
150g white chocolate, roughly chopped
3 eggs
Seeds of ½ a vanilla pod or ½ tsp vanilla extract
75g caster sugar
3 tbsp plain flour
1 tsp baking powder
Pinch of salt
100g strawberries, hulled and chopped into 1cm cubes
50g green pistachio nuts, roughly chopped

Preheat the oven to 170°C, (Fan 150°C), 325°F, Gas Mark 3. Grease a 20cm square cake tin with a little spray oil and then line it with baking parchment. I just cut a long strip of paper to cover the bottom and come up on opposite sides of the tin with the excess hanging over a little. This makes it easier to lift the baked cake out of the tin.

To prepare the blondies, melt the butter in a small pan over a low heat. Then remove from the heat, add the white chocolate and set aside to allow it to melt.

Put the eggs and vanilla seeds or extract in a large bowl and, using a hand whisk or a mixer fitted with a whisk attachment, give them a good whisk up. They will become really light, fluffy and mousse-like. Add the sugar and keep whisking. The sugar will make the eggs increase in bulk even more. To test if the eggs are whisked up enough, use a spoon to pick up some of the egg mixture and then drop it back down. If they are whisked up enough, the spoonful will sit on the surface for about 5 seconds (if it sits for longer, that's brilliant too!) before disappearing back into the mixture. Once the egg mixture reaches this stage, it is ready.

Give the now-melted chocolate a little stir into the butter to blend and pour it around the edges of the egg mixture. Do this from a low height so you don't knock out all of that wonderful air which you have just beaten in. Then, using a spatula, fold them together, scooping right down to the bottom of the bowl, as the chocolate tends to sink down there. Sprinkle the flour, baking powder and salt over and fold the mixture in using as few 'folds' as possible so you keep all that air in, but enough folds to make sure there are no lumps of flour in there. Finally, gently fold in the strawberries and pistachios.

Gently pour the mixture into the prepared tin from a low height and level it out with the back of a spoon. Bake for 30–35 minutes until a knife inserted into the centre comes out clean. Once cooked, remove from the oven and leave to cool in the tin. It will collapse in the centre a little, but don't worry – it will taste great. Once cooled, carefully remove from the tin, peel off the paper and cut into eight rectangular bars or 16 bite-sized squares and serve. The pistachios will sink to the bottom along with the strawberries – all meant to happen and all very tasty.

(PER SERVING, BASED ON 16 SQUARES)	ENERGY	FAT	SAT FAT	SUGAR	PROTEIN	SALT
LORRAINE'S RECIPE	152 Kcal	9.7g	4.7g	11g	3.1g	0.2g
COMPARISON RECIPE	168 Kcal	10.7g	5.7g	10.9g	2.5g	0.1g

OATMEAL & GINGER COOKIES

I have a large bowl of oats most mornings when it is cold in Blighty. Which means that most mornings, I have a bowl of oats. They are the only thing I find that fills me up from breakfast to lunch with no need for a mid-morning snack. This is due, I am told, to their ability to release energy slowly. But these cookies contain fast-energy-releasing sugar too, I hear you say, pointing at the book? Apparently, if the two are combined together, the oats have a way of slowing down the fast bouncing-off-the-walls quality of the sugar (things like nuts and whole grains can do this too).

Makes

12 cookies

50g unsalted butter
100g soft light brown sugar
1 egg, lightly beaten
2 tsp olive oil
125g wholemeal flour
100g rolled oats
1 tbsp ground ginger
1 tsp baking powder
¼ tsp bicarbonate of soda
Pinch of salt

Preheat the oven to 170°C, (Fan 150°C), 325°F, Gas Mark 3. Line a large baking sheet with baking parchment.

Cream together the butter and sugar. I kind of smoosh it against the side of the bowl until it starts to come together. It doesn't need to be all light and fluffy, just combined is good. Stir in the egg and olive oil until well mixed.

Add the flour, oats, ginger, baking powder, bicarbonate of soda and salt. Mix everything together to give a wettish mixture. Using damp hands, roll the mixture up into 12 even-sized balls and place them on the baking sheet as you go. They need to be spaced apart as they will spread a little while baking. Squish them down to about 1cm in thickness with a fork and then bake in the oven for 10–12 minutes until cooked through, but still soft to the touch.

Once cooked, remove them from the oven and leave to cool a little before carefully moving to a wire rack. These are delicious served warm, but do become more crispy once completely cool. Also, the gingeriness comes through even more once cold.

(PER COOKIE)	ENERGY	FAT	SAT FAT	SUGAR	PROTEIN	SALT
LORRAINE'S RECIPE	143 Kcal	5.6g	2.6g	8.8g	3.4g	0.2g
COMPARISON RECIPE	172 Kcal	8.1g	4.8g	10.1g	2.4g	0.26g

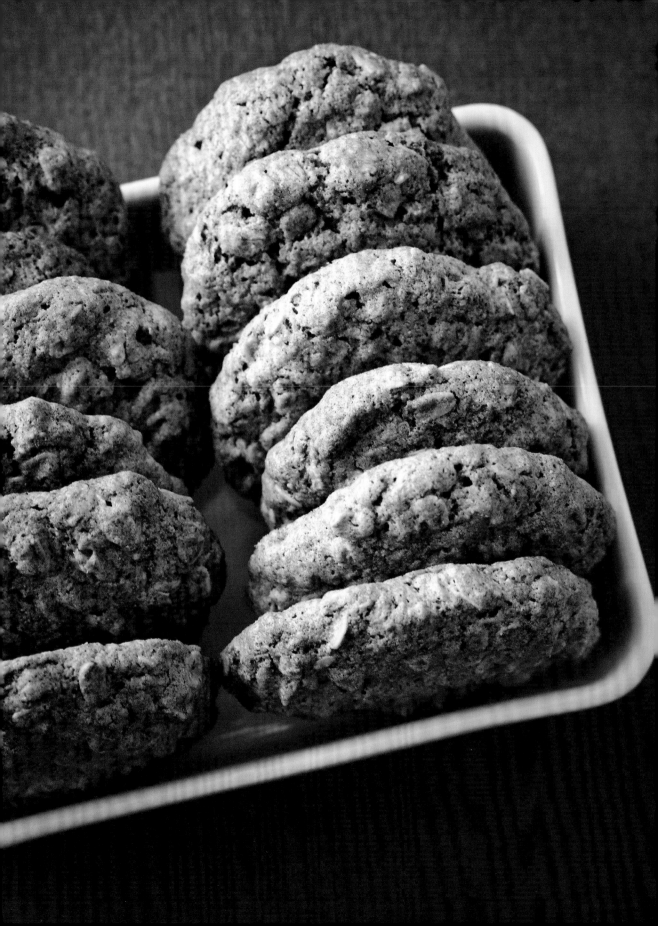

BLOOMING BROWNIES

I have used my own recipe from *Baking Made Easy* to compare with this lighter version (omitting the Oreos in the comparison table to make the analysis fair and just). The cookies and cream fudge brownies from my very first book will always have a place in my heart, but friends have said to me that if they want to eat brownies a little more often, then in their words, 'something's gotta give'. The outcome is a much lighter brownie, with a slightly more cakey taste, but still just the right amount of naughtiness to feel that you are getting a tasty treat.

Makes

16 brownie squares

Equipment

20cm square tin, electric mixer with a whisk attachment

100g unsalted butter
100g dark chocolate (at least 70% cocoa solids), roughly chopped
75g milk chocolate, roughly chopped
3 eggs
2 egg whites
100g soft light brown sugar
3 tbsp wholemeal flour
Pinch of salt
50g cocoa powder
1 tsp bicarbonate of soda

Preheat the oven to 180°C, (Fan 160°C), 350°F, Gas Mark 4 and line a 20cm square tin with baking parchment.

Melt the butter in a small pan over a low heat. Then add the chocolate, remove the pan from the heat and set aside so that the chocolate can melt.

Meanwhile, put the eggs and the egg whites into a large bowl and whisk them up until they go pale and fluffy. An electric mixer is best for this, but you can do it by hand if you like. Add the sugar bit by bit, whisking between each addition until all is combined and the mixture is really light and mousse-like.

Once the chocolate is melted, give it a little stir and then carefully pour it around the whisked-up eggs so that you don't knock out any of the air. Lightly scatter the flour, bicarbonate of soda and salt over, and then sift the cocoa powder on top, gently folding everything together really well. The melted chocolate has a habit of sinking to the bottom of the pan, so really get underneath the egg mixture to ensure everything is well combined.

Carefully pour the mixture into the lined tin from a low height so you don't knock any air out. There is no raising agent in this, so the only way it will puff up in the oven is down to the air that you have whisked into it. Smooth the mixture out evenly with the back of a spoon.

Bake the brownies in the oven for 20–25 minutes until springy to the touch, but crusty on top and until a skewer pierced into the centre comes out clean. Remove from the oven and leave in the tin until cool enough to handle. Remove the brownie from the tin and leave to cool completely on a wire rack before cutting into 16 even-sized squares to serve.

(PER BROWNIE)	ENERGY	FAT	SAT FAT	SUGAR	PROTEIN	SALT
LORRAINE'S RECIPE	165 Kcal	10.3g	5.9g	13g	3.5g	0.34g
COMPARISON RECIPE	203 Kcal	13.5g	7.8g	17.4g	2.6g	0.23g

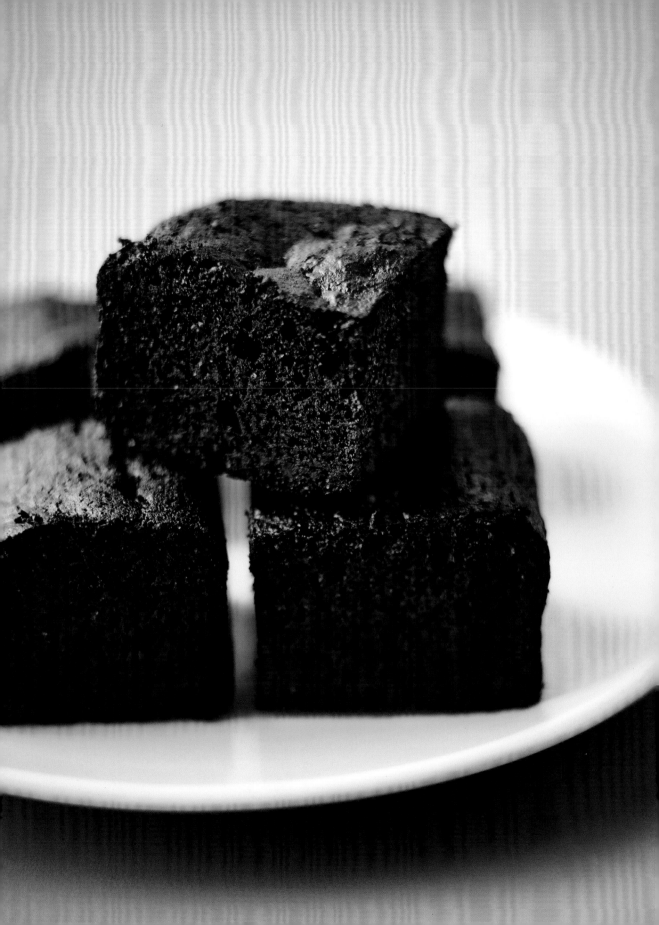

WHITE CHOCOLATE CHUNK COOKIES

During my degree course at the University of West London, one of the modules was all about chocolate. I was surprised to learn that white chocolate is not really chocolate at all, but basically just a mass of sugar, milk stuff and cocoa butter. NO cocoa solids whatsoever. In short, the lighter the chocolate, the less actual cocoa solids are in it and, sadly, the more sugar. I managed to get in 100g of white chocolate for proper chocolate satisfaction, so it's sweet, but with reduced fat and calories, and the addition of wholemeal flour, it's a big improvement on standard white chocolate cookies.

Makes

12 cookies

80g unsalted butter, softened
80g caster sugar
1 egg
150g wholemeal flour
100g white chocolate chips
50g plain flour
1 tsp baking powder
1 tsp bicarbonate of soda
1 tsp vanilla extract

Preheat the oven to 180°C, (Fan 160°C), 350°F, Gas Mark 4 and line a large baking sheet with baking parchment.

Blend the butter and sugar in a large bowl until smooth and well combined. Next, add the egg and mix together well. Finally, add the wholemeal flour, chocolate chips, plain flour, baking powder, bicarbonate of soda and the vanilla extract and stir everything together to give quite a crumbly mixture. Get your hands stuck in to bring this mixture together until you have a soft dough ball.

Next, divide the dough into 12 equal-sized pieces and using damp hands, roll each one into a ball, placing them spaced apart on the baking sheet as you go. Use the palm of your hand to squash each ball down to about 6cm wide and about 5mm thick. Bake in the oven for 10–12 minutes until cooked, but still just soft to the touch.

Once cooked, remove from the oven and leave to cool a little before moving to a wire rack to cool completely (although these are most delicious served warm).

(PER COOKIE)	ENERGY	FAT	SAT FAT	SUGAR	PROTEIN	SALT
LORRAINE'S RECIPE	163 Kcal	6.9g	3.9g	12.3g	3.3g	0.37g
COMPARISON RECIPE	178 Kcal	8.5g	5g	12g	2.8g	0.22g

SOFT CHOC, CHOC CHIP COOKIES

I started cooking this at 6.30am on a Saturday morning, pyjamas on, whilst the rest of the house slumbered. At 6pm I was still in my jim jams, with a glass of Aussie Chardonnay, and about to have a freak-out moment as I could not get the recipe right. By 7pm and after a bit of a cry and a walk around the block (I did change out of my pjs), I came back and developed this recipe for Soft Choc, Choc Chip Cookies. They don't have the solid crunch that you may be accustomed to, due to the reduction of butter and sugar (they are almost cake like), but they are still very much a tasty, chocolaty, satisfying munch.

Makes

12 cookies

75g unsalted butter, softened
100g soft light brown sugar
25ml olive oil
2 eggs, lightly beaten
100g wholemeal flour
100g plain flour
50g milk chocolate chips
25g rolled oats
1 tsp baking powder
¼ tsp bicarbonate of soda
25g cocoa powder

Preheat the oven to 190°C, (Fan 170°C), 375°F, Gas Mark 5 and line a baking sheet with baking parchment.

Put the butter and sugar into a bowl and cream everything together well for a minute or two. Add the olive oil and eggs and mix together well. Add the wholemeal flour, plain flour, chocolate chips, oats, baking powder, bicarbonate of soda and cocoa powder and mix it all together. I tend to squish it up on the sides of the bowl to get it all mixed in well. The mixture should be stiff, but slightly sticky.

Using damp hands, roll the mixture into 12 equal-sized balls, placing them on the baking sheet slightly spaced apart as you go. Squish them down to about 1cm in thickness with the palm of your hand.

Bake the cookies in the oven for 8–10 minutes until just soft to the touch, but cooked through. Once ready, remove from the oven and leave to cool a little. They will be very soft when they come out of the oven, but will firm up on cooling. Carefully transfer them to a wire rack to cool completely (although these are actually most delicious when eaten warm).

(PER COOKIE)	ENERGY	FAT	SAT FAT	SUGAR	PROTEIN	SALT
LORRAINE'S RECIPE	200 Kcal	10.3g	4.9g	11.2g	4.2g	0.26g
COMPARISON RECIPE	227 Kcal	10.9g	6.5g	21.5g	2.5g	0.57g

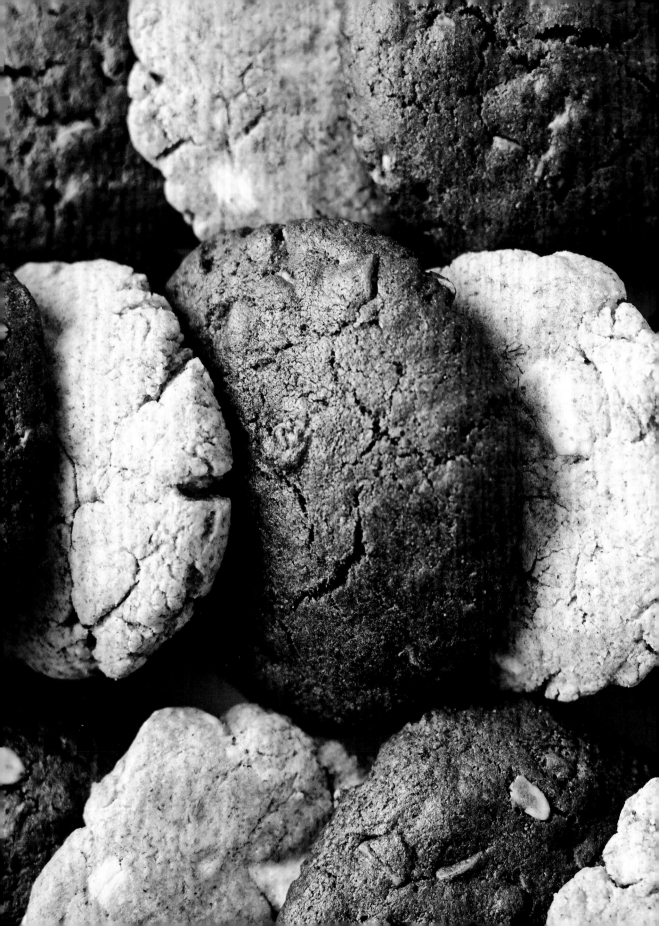

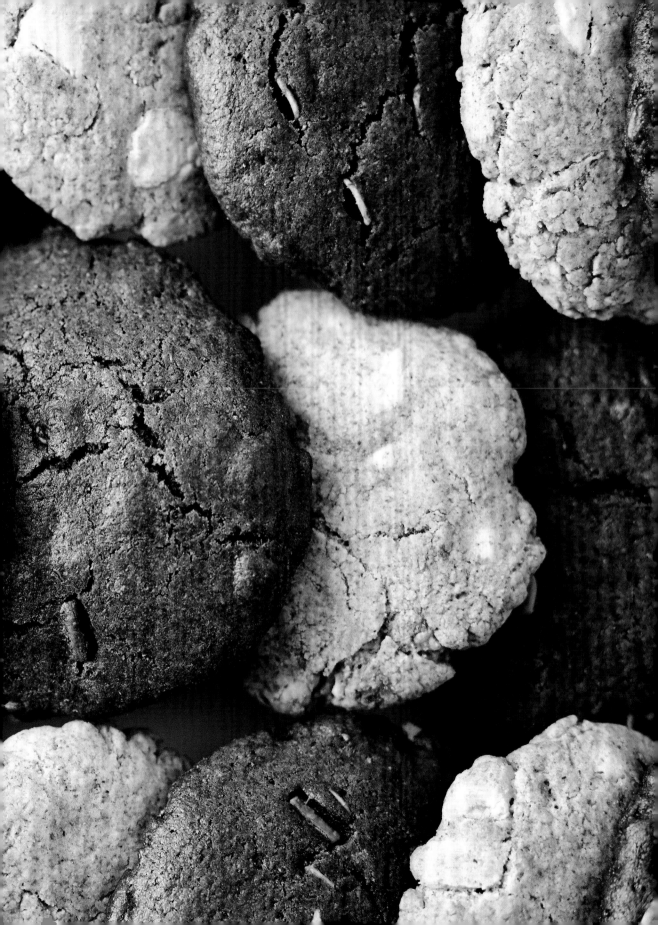

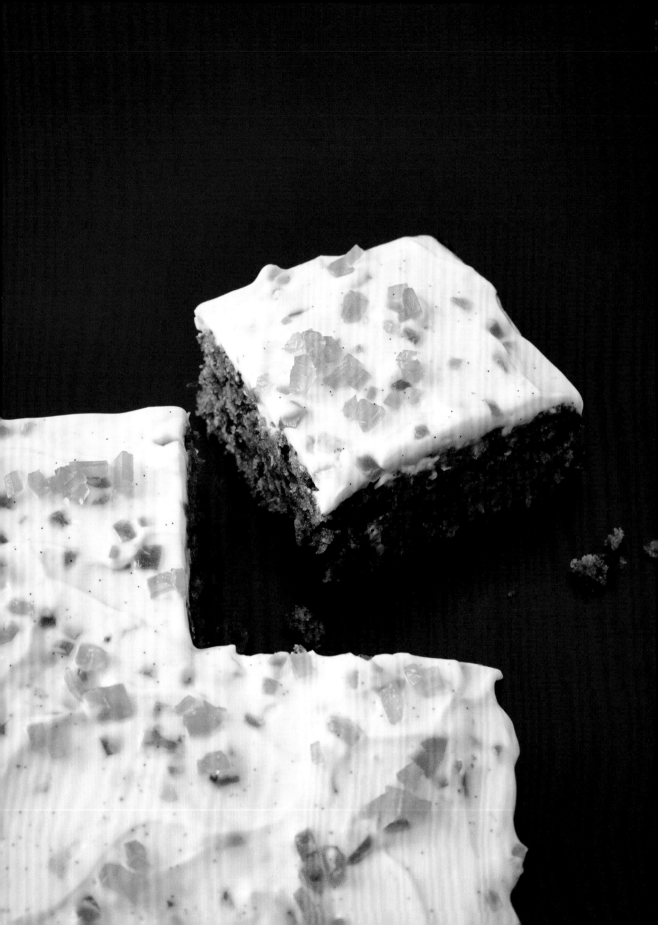

PARSNIP & PECAN TRAYBAKE CAKE WITH STEM GINGER TOPPING

A drum roll played inside my rather large head over Sunday lunch and I thought parsnips, in a cake.... Would I? Should I? Well, I did and you know what? Your baked-in-a-cake goodness has just gone and knocked the tangoed carrot right off its perch. Compared to a full-fat, high-sugar parsnip traybake recipe, this has much less saturated fat, more than half the quantity of sugar and more fibre by way of wholemeal flour.

Makes

8 rectangular portions or 16 smaller bite-sized squares

Equipment

20cm square baking tin

Sponge

Spray oil
225g parsnips (about 3 medium parsnips), peeled and roughly grated
200g wholemeal or wholemeal spelt flour
100g soft dark or light brown sugar
75g unsalted butter, very soft
50ml sunflower oil
50g pecan nuts, roughly chopped
5 tbsp semi-skimmed milk
2 tbsp honey
2 eggs
1 egg white
2 tsp baking powder
1 tbsp ground ginger
Big pinch ground cinnamon
½ tsp freshly grated nutmeg
Seeds of 1 vanilla pod or 1 tsp vanilla extract
Good pinch of salt

Stem ginger frosting

200g low-fat cream cheese
4 tbsp icing sugar, sifted
2 knobs of stem ginger, finely chopped
Seeds of 1 vanilla pod or 1 tsp vanilla extract

Preheat the oven to 180°C, (Fan 160°C), 350°F, Gas Mark 4. Spray a little oil all over the inside of a 20cm square baking tin and line with baking parchment. I don't line all the sides, but do one strip, which covers the base and two opposite sides of the tin. I like to leave this a bit longer so it overhangs the edges, making it easier to remove the cake from the tin once it is baked.

Put all of the ingredients for the sponge into a large bowl and mix together until well combined. Then spoon the mixture into the tin and smooth the top with the back of a spoon. Bake in the oven for 30–35 minutes or until the cake is springy to the touch and a skewer inserted into the centre comes out clean. Once cooked, remove from the oven and leave to cool completely in the tin.

Meanwhile, make the frosting by simply mixing all of the ingredients together in a medium bowl until smooth. Cover and set it aside in the fridge until ready to use.

Remove the cooled cake from the tin, peel the paper off and sit it on a serving plate. Spread the frosting evenly over the cake using a palette knife to give a nice wavy effect and serve.

(PER SERVING – BASED ON 8 PORTIONS)	ENERGY	FAT	SAT FAT	SUGAR	PROTEIN	SALT
LORRAINE'S RECIPE	410 Kcal	23.4g	8.5g	25g	9.2g	0.74g
COMPARISON RECIPE	539 Kcal	24.2g	14.3g	60.2g	5.1g	1.57g

CARDAMOM AND GINGER SHORTBREAD

I just had to tackle this recipe head on. I knew by the very nature of its title — 'short' — that it would be a challenge to replicate a full-fat and sugar version. Initial attempts were really dry and crumbly. Low-fat cream cheese gave a product that was just very chewy and it was only when I added a bit of water and the egg white that things started to come together. This is not a massive change from a normal everyday shortbread because, as I have discovered, shortbread is not shortbread without a certain amount of sugar and fat, but it is a tinsey-winsey bit better than my shortbread recipes of the past!

Makes
10 shortbreads

Equipment
20cm loose-bottomed round sandwich tin, food mixer fitted with the beater attachment

Spray oil
100g unsalted butter, softened
80g soft light brown sugar
200g plain flour
1 tsp ground cardamom
1 piece of stem ginger, finely chopped
Seeds of 1 vanilla pod or 1 tsp vanilla extract
1 tbsp egg white (fiddly I know, but a whole egg white is too much!)
Pinch of salt
2 tbsp semi-skimmed milk

Preheat the oven to 170°C, (Fan 150°C), 325°F, Gas Mark 3. Lightly grease a 20cm loose-bottomed round sandwich tin with a bit of spray oil and then line the base with baking parchment.

Using a food mixer fitted with the beater attachment or by hand with a wooden spoon and in a large bowl, cream the butter and the sugar together until combined. Add the flour, ground cardamom, stem ginger, vanilla seeds or extract, egg white, salt, milk and 1 tablespoon cold water and mix everything together. The mixture is quite dry so I find it best to get my hands in and squash it against the side of the bowl to bring it together.

Tip the mixture into the sandwich tin and squish it tight and flat with the back of a spoon. Once the shortbread is level, press the tip of your index finger all the way around the edge of the shortbread to make a fluted pattern and then use a sharp knife to mark the shortbread into 10 even-sized triangular pieces. Bake in the oven for 35–40 minutes or until the shortbread is a light golden brown and firm, but with a slight softness to the touch.

Once cooked, remove it from the oven and use the sharp knife to cut through the 10 wedges. Leave to cool completely before carefully removing from the tin. Arrange the wedges on a plate and serve.

(PER SHORTBREAD)	ENERGY	FAT	SAT FAT	SUGAR	PROTEIN	SALT
LORRAINE'S RECIPE	177 Kcal	8.6g	5.3g	9g	2.2g	0.05g
COMPARISON RECIPE	220Kcal	12.6g	7.8g	8.6g	1.9g	0.27g

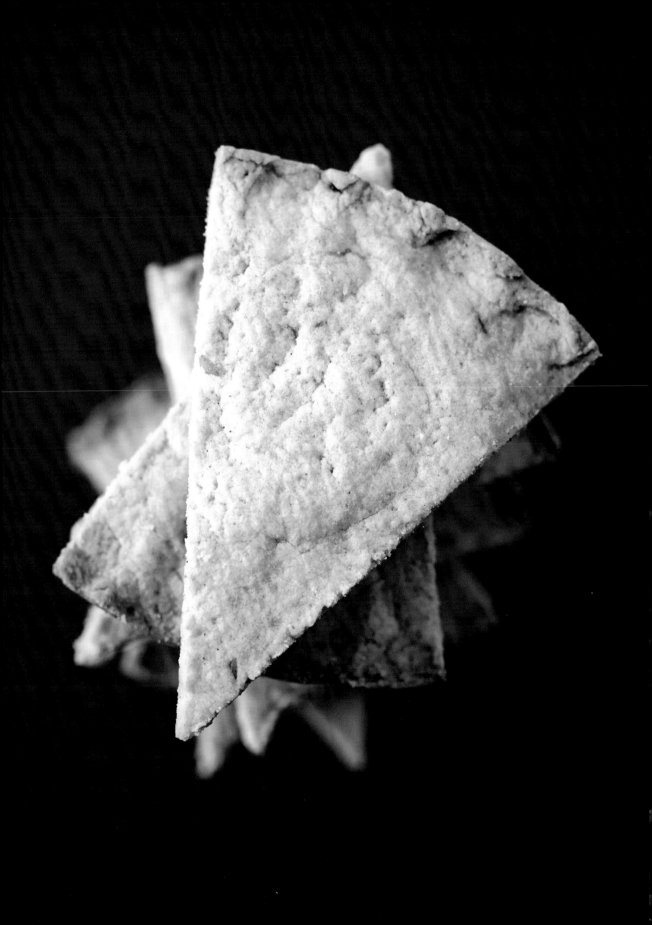

STICKY DATE, MAPLE & CINNAMON TRAYBAKE BITES

I first tried this using regular dates, but it just didn't taste of very much. Medjool dates make all the difference.

Makes
16 bite-sized squares

Equipment
20cm square cake tin, mini blender

1 tea bag (English breakfast is fine)
250g pitted Medjool dates
Spray oil
300g plain flour
100g rolled oats
100g unsalted butter, melted
100g soft light brown sugar
2 tsp ground cinnamon
Seeds of 1 vanilla pod or 1 tsp
   vanilla extract
1 tbsp maple syrup

First make the tea by popping the tea bag into a large jug with 400ml boiling water. Leave it to infuse for about 5 minutes before discarding the tea bag. Add the dates to the tea and set aside for 10 minutes to soak.

Preheat the oven to 180°C, (Fan 160°C), 350°F, Gas Mark 4. Lightly grease a 20cm square cake tin with spray oil and then line it with baking parchment. I just cut a long strip of paper to cover the bottom and come up on opposite sides of the tin with the excess hanging over a little. This makes it easier to lift the baked loaf out of the tin.

After they have soaked, drain the liquid from the dates and blitz them in a mini blender until as smooth as possible. Tip the date purée into a large bowl, then add the flour, oats, butter, sugar, cinnamon and vanilla seeds or extract and mix everything together well to give a soft dough mixture. Press the mixture into the base of the prepared tin so it is nice and compact, flat and even. Bake in the oven for 25–30 minutes, brushing the maple syrup evenly over for the last 5 minutes of cooking. The traybake should be just soft to the touch and turning golden at the edges.

Once cooked, remove from the oven and leave to cool before cutting into 16 bite-sized squares or eight equal-sized rectangles, and serve.

(PER SQUARE)	ENERGY	FAT	SAT FAT	SUGAR	PROTEIN	SALT
LORRAINE'S RECIPE	201 Kcal	5.9g	3.2g	17.9g	3.1g	0.02g
COMPARISON RECIPE	280 Kcal	16.2g	1.7g	23.1g	4.7g	0.16g

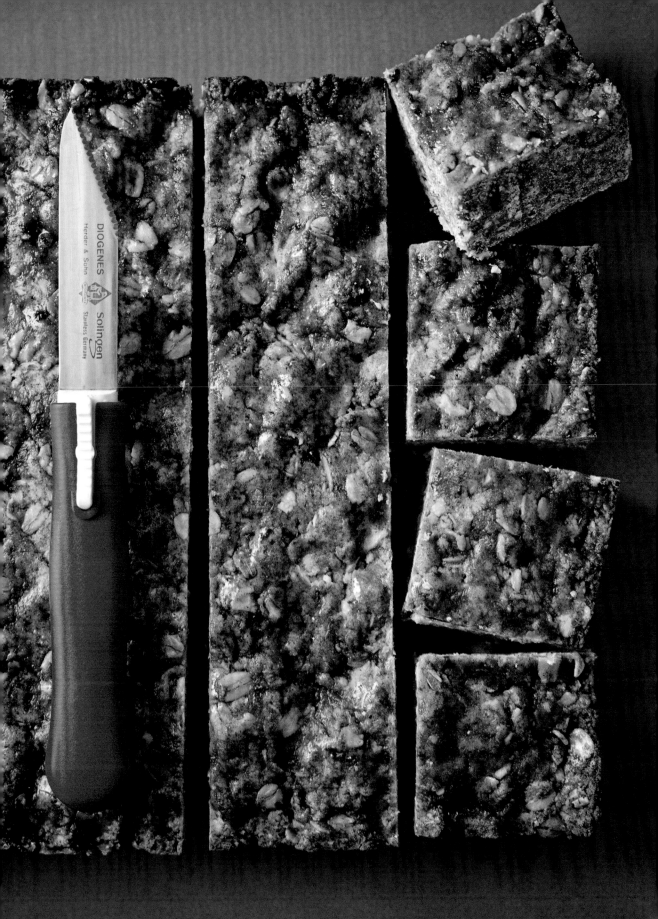

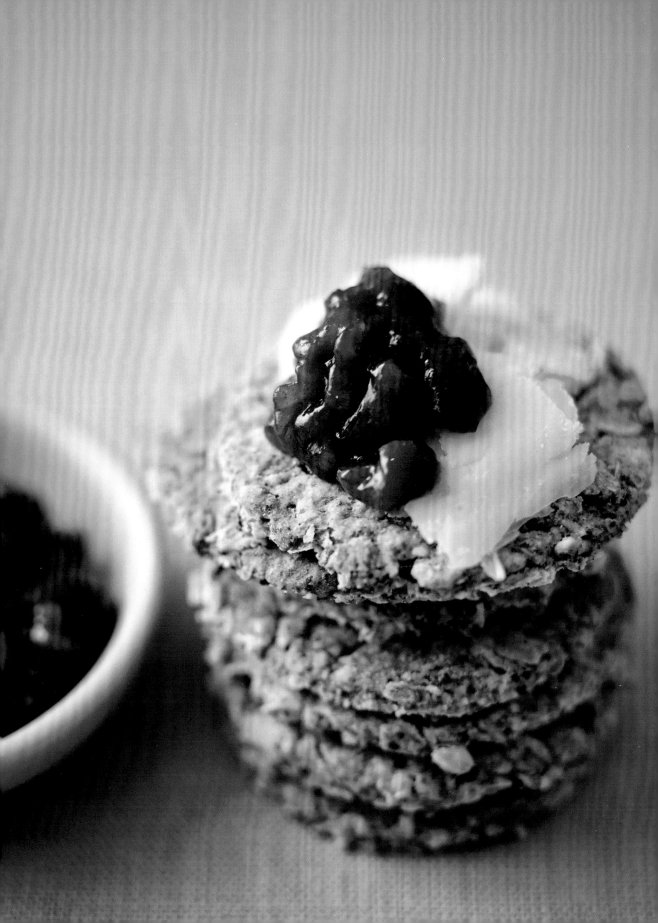

BLACK PEPPER & ROSEMARY OATCAKES

One of my favourite places for a snack is the bar at Fortnum and Mason. Great to visit for lunch or after work, with fabulous wines, hams, cheeses and other fine fancies. The best thing of all is the cheese trolley, expertly laden with an array of smelly cheeses to suit all tastes. The little crackers, biscuits and oatcakes they give you are divine and I have made these to enable me to enjoy a little Fortnum-style snack at home. Bake these very easy oatcakes (oatcakes are a healthy option whichever recipe you use, so the savings here are minimal), go to your local supermarket, buy cold meats, cheese and other yummy goodies, pour yourself and your mate a glass of rosé if the summer weather holds or a rich glass of red if not. Kick back, relax and enjoy.

Makes

20

200g rolled oats
75g wholemeal flour, plus a little
    extra for dusting
Leaves from 4 sprigs of fresh
    rosemary, finely chopped
Large pinch of bicarbonate of soda
A few twists of black pepper
Pinch of salt
25g unsalted butter, cold and cut
    into cubes
125ml cold water (from the tap)

Preheat the oven to 180°C, (Fan 160°C), 350°F, Gas Mark 4. Line two baking sheets with baking parchment and set aside.

Toss the oats, flour, rosemary, bicarb, black pepper and salt together in a large bowl. Add the butter, then pick up bits of the ingredients with the tips of your fingers and rub them between your fingers and thumbs, until all of the butter has been 'rubbed in' to give a uniform crumb mixture.

Gradually add the cold water, stirring the flour mix with a small knife all the time, until you get a thick, quite solid and not-too-soft dough. Tip the dough out onto a surface lightly dusted with flour and knead it into a ball. Roll the dough out to the thickness of just less than a £1 coin. The mixture is quite crumbly, but just squish it back together if it breaks up. Stamp out 20 oatcakes with a 6cm round, straight-sided cookie cutter, placing them onto the baking sheets as you go.

Bake the oatcakes in the oven for 25–30 minutes or until they are going golden brown and are firm to the touch. Once baked, remove from the oven and leave to cool. They are totally delicious served with cheese and chutney. These will keep in an airtight container for a couple of weeks.

(PER OATCAKE)	ENERGY	FAT	SAT FAT	SUGAR	PROTEIN	SALT
LORRAINE'S RECIPE	49 Kcal	1.5g	0.6g	0.1g	1.8g	0.03g
COMPARISON RECIPE	43 Kcal	1.8g	0.6g	0g	1.3g	0.07g

YOUR TIME IS LIMITED, SO DON'T WASTE
IT LIVING SOMEONE ELSE'S LIFE.
STEVE JOBS

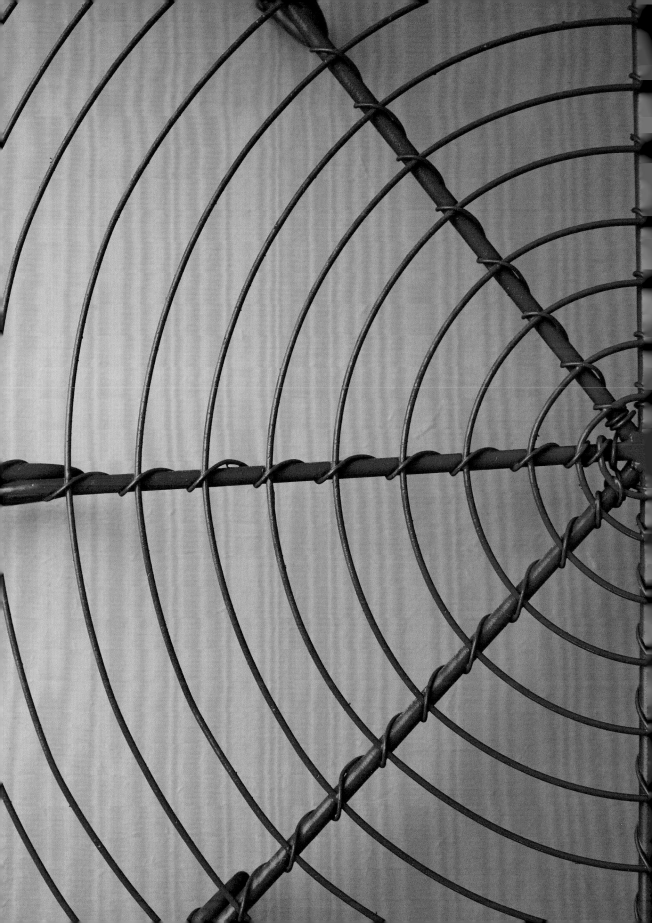

TEATIME
TREATS

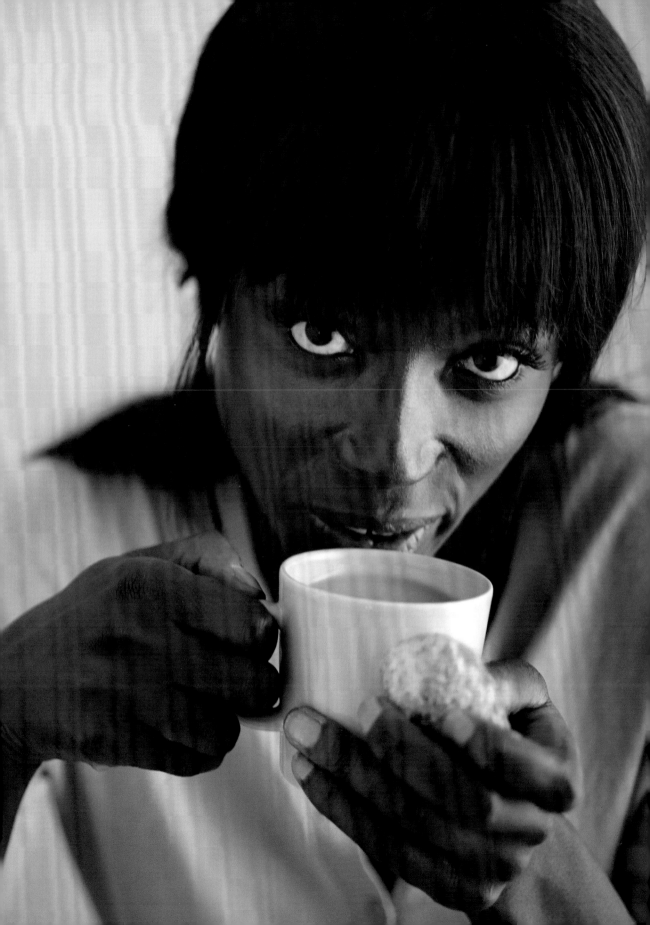

PUMPKIN & SPICE CUPCAKES WITH CREAM CHEESE FROSTING

I went to LA this year and was totally jet-lagged, lashing about in my bed at 3am. So I got in the car, drove to Malibu and came across a posh little beachside boutique hotel. The receptionist kindly let me sit on the balcony for a good hour or so to watch the sun come up over the City of Angels. By the time the wait staff came over, people were already walking their dogs and running up and down the shoreline and I was completely starving. The waitress put down a complimentary plate of pumpkin bread, which was the inspiration for these cute little cupcakes.

Makes
12 cupcakes

Equipment
12-hole muffin tin, muffin cases, electric mixer fitted with a beater attachment or a large bowl, piping bag fitted with a star nozzle

Sponge
175g canned pumpkin
100g wholemeal flour
100g self-raising flour
100g soft light brown sugar
75g unsalted butter, melted
2 eggs
2 tbsp maple syrup or honey
2 tsp baking powder
1 tsp ground ginger
½ tsp mixed spice
½ tsp ground cinnamon
Seeds of 1 vanilla pod or 1 tsp vanilla extract
Pinch of salt
2 satsumas, segmented, to decorate (optional)

Frosting
300g low-fat cream cheese
1 tbsp crème fraîche
3 tbsp icing sugar, sifted
Finely grated zest of 1 orange
Seeds of 1 vanilla pod or 1 tsp vanilla extract

Preheat the oven to 180°C, (Fan 160°C), 350°F, Gas Mark 4 and line a 12-hole muffin tin with paper muffin cases.

Put all of the sponge ingredients (except the satsumas, if using) into a large bowl and beat everything together really well (by hand or machine). Pouring the mixture into a jug or using two spoons (or I like to use a mechanical ice-cream scoop), divide it among the 12 cases.

Bake in the oven for 25–30 minutes or until a skewer inserted into the centre of the cupcakes comes out clean and the cakes feel springy to the touch. Once the cupcakes are cooked, remove them from the oven and leave to cool in the tray.

Meanwhile, make the frosting. Beat the cream cheese and crème fraîche together in a medium bowl until smooth. Add the icing sugar, orange zest and vanilla seeds or extract and mix together well. Cover the frosting and pop it into the fridge to firm up a little until ready to use.

Once the cupcakes are cool, remove them from the tray and arrange on a serving plate. Spoon the frosting into a piping bag fitted with a star nozzle and pipe a small rosette on each one. Alternatively, you can just spoon and spread the frosting on top of each cake. Either way, top each one with a satsuma segment if you fancy it and then serve.

(PER CUPCAKE)	ENERGY	FAT	SAT FAT	SUGAR	PROTEIN	SALT
LORRAINE'S RECIPE	211 Kcal	9.7g	5.7g	14.5g	5.4g	0.34g
COMPARISON RECIPE	269 Kcal	11g	6.7g	34.1g	2.8g	0.44g

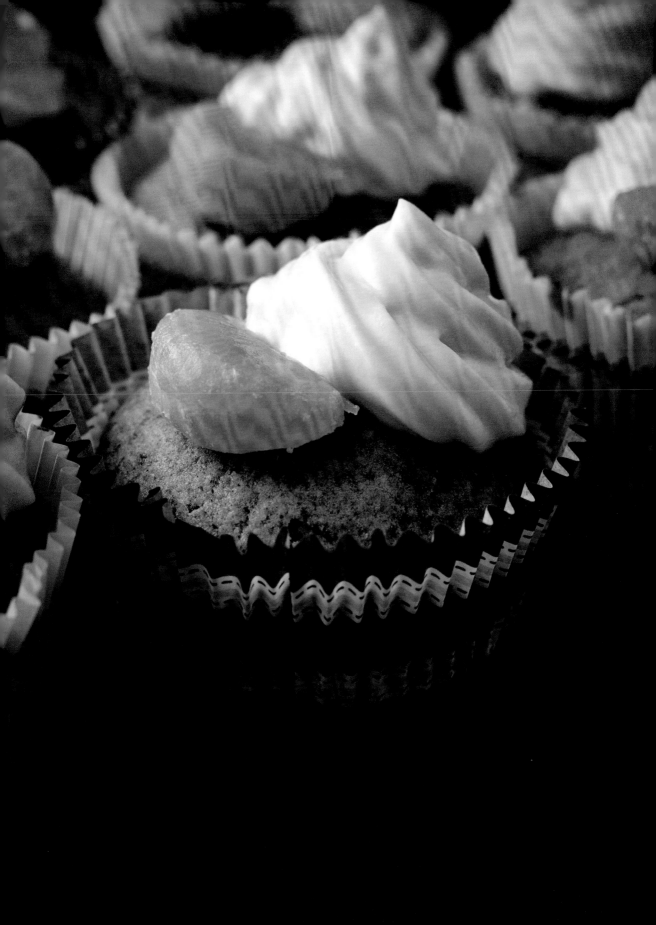

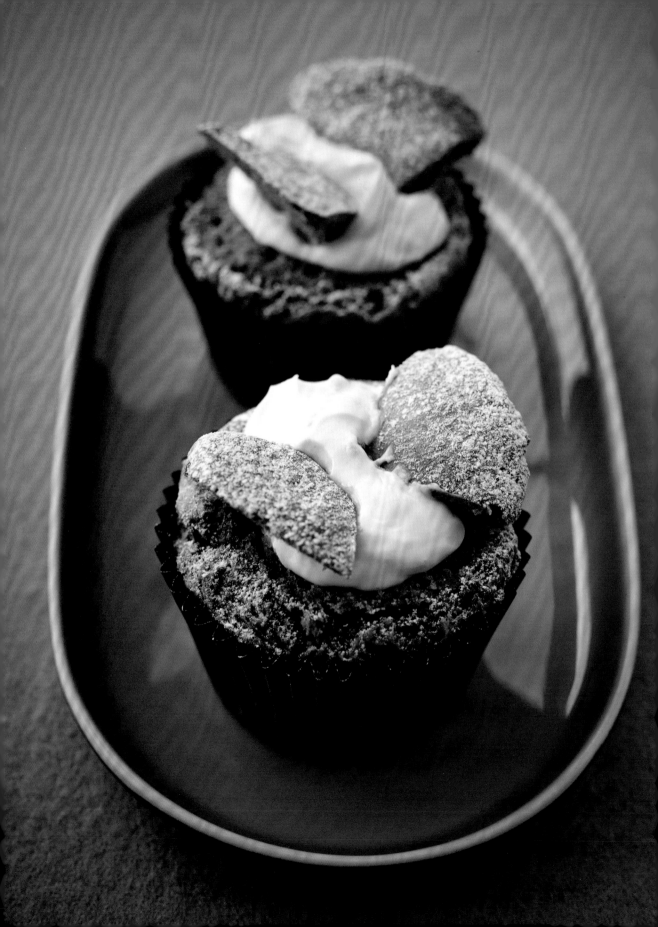

SKINNY CAFFE LATTE BUTTERFLY CAKES

Who said eating lighter means that you cannot eat cupcakes? Feast your eyes on these deliciously, delectable morsels.

Makes

12 cakes

Equipment

12-hole muffin tin, muffin cases, food mixer fitted with the beater attachment or a large bowl

Sponge

75g unsalted butter, softened
100g caster sugar
2 eggs
1 egg white
2 tbsp low-fat Greek yogurt
150g self-raising flour
1 tsp baking powder
Seeds of 1 vanilla pod or 1 tsp vanilla extract
2 tbsp instant coffee granules
Icing sugar, for dusting

Frosting

200g low-fat crème fraîche
50g icing sugar, sifted
1 tbsp Baileys Irish cream liqueur

Preheat the oven to 180°C, (Fan 160°C), 350°F, Gas Mark 4. Line a 12-hole muffin tin with 12 paper muffin cases.

Beat the butter and sugar in a large bowl (or food mixer set with a beater) until well combined. Then beat in the eggs, egg white and Greek yogurt. The mixture will start to look, well a bit curdled, but keep on beating it for a moment or two, and then add the flour, baking powder and vanilla extract or seeds. Blend the coffee granules with 1 tablespoon of hot water and add to the mix. Stir everything together until it is all combined. Pouring the mixture into a jug or using two spoons (or I like to use a mechanical ice-cream scoop), divide the mixture among the 12 cases.

Bake in the oven for 20–25 minutes or until a skewer inserted into the centre of a cupcake comes out clean and the cakes feel springy to the touch. Once the cupcakes are cooked, remove them from the oven and leave to cool in the tray.

Meanwhile, make the frosting. Simply mix together the crème fraîche, icing sugar and Irish cream liqueur in a medium bowl, using as few stirs as possible. Cover and set aside in the fridge until ready to use.

Once the cupcakes are cool, slice the top off each cake and cut the pieces in half down the centre to give two 'wings'. Put a dollop of the frosting on top of each cake, then stick the two 'wings' into the frosting of each one, with the centre cut downwards and the underneath cut outwards. Arrange on a platter or cake stand, dust with icing sugar and serve.

(PER BUTTERFLY CAKE)	ENERGY	FAT	SAT FAT	SUGAR	PROTEIN	SALT
LORRAINE'S RECIPE	185 Kcal	9g	5.4g	14.2g	3.4g	0.29g
COMPARISON RECIPE	207 Kcal	11.5g	6.8g	13.4g	2.9g	0.36g

APPLE, CALVADOS & MAPLE SYRUP UPSIDE-DOWN CUPCAKES

It is well documented in my cookbooks that I like to mini-size things and my favourite classic English pud was not going to get away with not being shrunk. The trick to this dish is to be bold and daring with the apples. Get the butter and maple syrup really hot and quickly caramelize the apples. The butter and the maple may get really dark, but the liquid from the apples will make sure that it does not burn. Once the apples are a dark golden brown, you've nailed it.

Makes
12 cupcakes

Equipment
12-hole muffin tin, muffin cases, food mixer fitted with the whisk attachment

Caramel apples
50g maple syrup
50g butter
5 Granny Smith apples, peeled, cored and cut into 1cm cubes
2 tbsp Calvados or brandy

Sponge
125g caster sugar
100g unsalted butter, softened
100g full-fat Greek yogurt
2 eggs, lightly beaten
250g self-raising flour
4 egg whites
2 tsp baking powder
½ tsp vanilla extract

Preheat the oven to 180°C, (Fan 160°C), 350°F, Gas Mark 4. Line a muffin tin with 12 paper muffin cases.

Put the maple syrup and butter in a wide, shallow pan over a high heat and allow the butter to melt. Leave to bubble away for 1 minute until thickened and syrupy. Then, reduce the heat a little, add the apples and cook them for about 2–3 minutes, stirring occasionally, until the liquid has reduced and the apples have become sticky and golden. Increase the heat and add the Calvados (or brandy), being careful of any splashing. Cook for 30 seconds and then remove from the heat. Spoon the mixture evenly among the muffin cases and set aside.

Put the sugar, butter and yogurt into a large bowl and beat like mad with a whisk until well combined. A food mixer would be great for this job, otherwise get your whisk, roll up your sleeves and just go for it. Now, this mix is not going to go all light and fluffy and pretty like its full-fat cousin, but you are just looking for some semblance of uniformity (it will have quite a few little lumps in, but that is okay).

Next, add the whole eggs and half of the flour and beat for a good few minutes, until the mixture is well blended and starts to look a little smoother. Then, whisk the egg whites until they are light and frothy and fold them into the mixture with the remaining flour, the baking powder and vanilla extract and beat until you have a smooth, pale batter.

Pouring the mixture into a jug or using two spoons (or I like to use a mechanical ice-cream scoop), divide it among the 12 cases, spooning it on top of the apple mixture. Bake in the oven for 20 minutes or until a skewer inserted in the centre of a cupcake comes out clean.

Once cooked, remove from the oven and leave in the tin until cool enough to handle. Then, remove from the tin and leave to cool completely on a wire rack. These are most delicious when eaten warm. Simply peel the paper off and turn them upside down to reveal the caramelized apple.

(PER CUPCAKE)	ENERGY	FAT	SAT FAT	SUGAR	PROTEIN	SALT
LORRAINE'S RECIPE	270 Kcal	12.5g	7.4g	19.8g	4.9g	0.5g
COMPARISON RECIPE	331 Kcal	12.3g	7g	38g	4.1g	0.62g

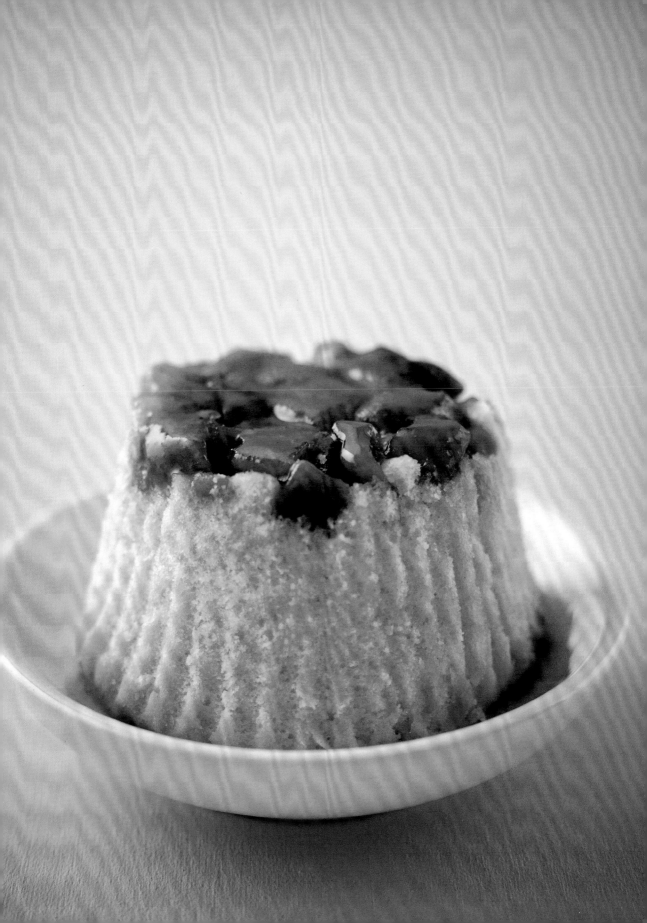

ALMOND, BLACKBERRY & PEACH FRIANDS

So, I made these on a freezing May afternoon trying to recreate a feeling of summer in the UK rain. My daughter came bowling in from school looking for things to eat and spotted these little plump blackberry sponges sitting on the work surface. She took a few and then came back an hour later after a long phone call with a friend and advised me that they were nice, but needed a little something more. So I went back to the drawing board and added a bit of spice and another fruity friend. These are not friands in the traditional sense as they require lorry loads of butter; instead this is my slightly more guilt-free friand.

Makes
12 friands

Equipment
Friand tin or 12-hole muffin tin

Spray oil
100g icing sugar, sifted
75g ground almonds
75g wholemeal flour
50g self-raising flour
1 tsp baking powder
1 tsp ground cinnamon
Pinch of salt
6 egg whites
Seeds of 1 vanilla pod or 1 tsp
    vanilla extract
50g unsalted butter, melted
25ml vegetable oil
3 tinned peach halves (or 15
    tinned peach slices), drained
    and chopped into 1cm cubes
12 blackberries
2 tbsp honey

Preheat the oven to 180°C, (Fan 160°C), 350°F, Gas Mark 4. Spray a friand tin with oil (or if you don't have one of these, use a 12-hole muffin tin either lined with muffin cases or, again, sprayed with a little oil instead) and set aside.

Toss the icing sugar, ground almonds, flours, baking powder, cinnamon and salt together in a large bowl and make a well in the centre. In another bowl, whisk up the egg whites and vanilla seeds or extract until they just start to become frothy (not super white and frothy like meringue, but just like bubble bath before it starts to disappear because of the soap!) Pour this into the centre of the dry ingredients along with the butter and oil and mix everything together using as few stirs as possible. Gently fold the peach pieces through and divide the mixture evenly among the friand tin holes (or muffin cases or holes).

Gently push a blackberry onto the top of each friand and then pop the cakes into the oven to bake for 15–20 minutes until golden on top and a skewer inserted into the centre of one cake comes out clean. As soon as they come out of the oven, mix the honey in a small bowl with 1 tablespoon boiling water and brush this all over the tops of the friands evenly. Then leave to cool. Like so many cakes, these are SO good served warm.

(PER FRIAND)	ENERGY	FAT	SAT FAT	SUGAR	PROTEIN	SALT
LORRAINE'S RECIPE	179 Kcal	9.1g	2.6g	13.8g	4.4g	0.26g
COMPARISON RECIPE	270 Kcal	18.9g	9.1g	18.2g	4.3g	0.36g

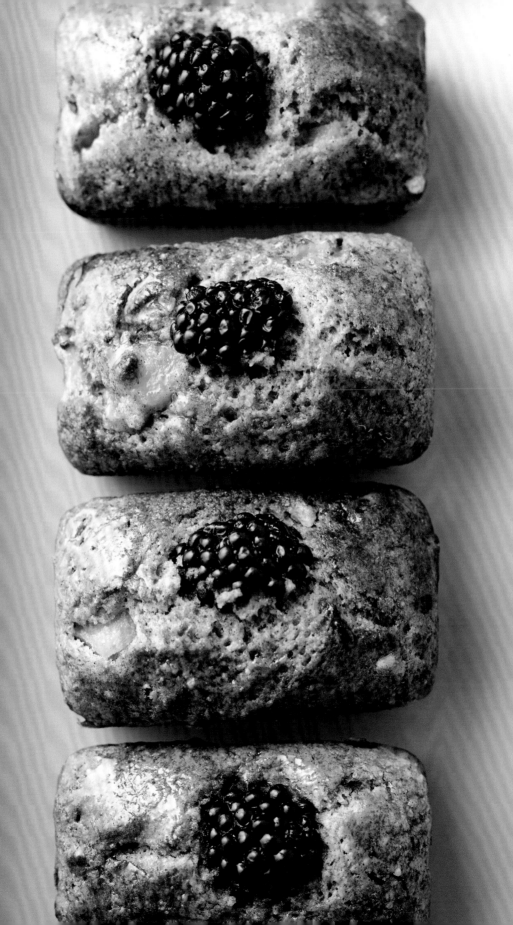

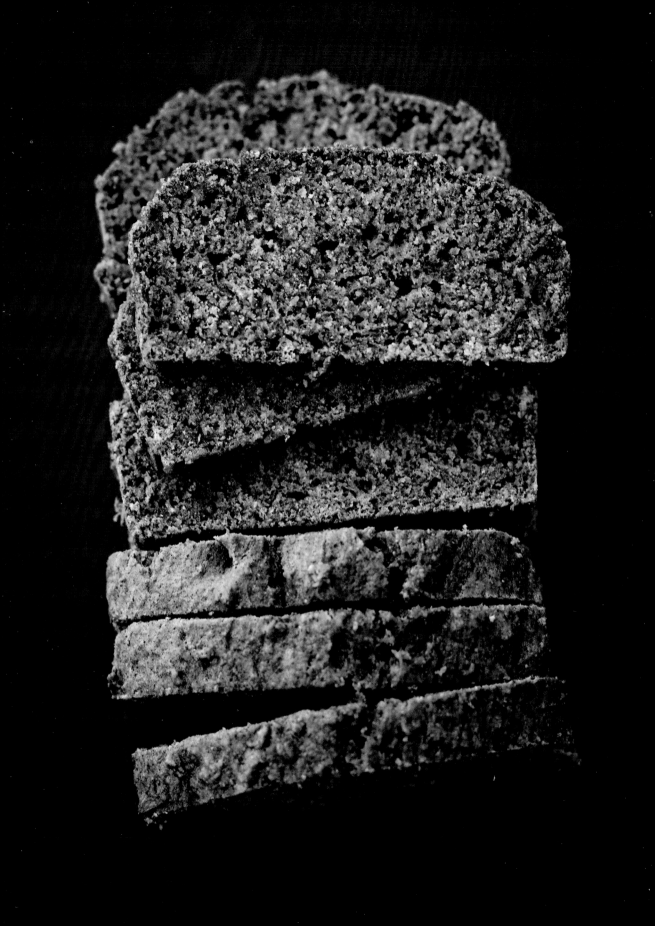

MOIST, MOREISH SPICED PUMPKIN TEA CAKE

This was inspired by a trip to Starbucks stateside where, nestled between the banana bread and the lemon loaf, was this dark orange slice. Pumpkin is not really something I use very often in my cooking, but recently the shops have started to stock pumpkin purée in a jar, which makes things loads easier and faster. There is a whole teaspoon of ground cloves in this recipe, which may prove too much for some, if so, then half a teaspoon will do the trick.

Makes
1 loaf with 12 slices

Equipment
22 x 10cm loaf tin

Spray oil
175g pumpkin purée
75g soft light brown sugar
75g self-raising flour
75g wholemeal flour
50ml rapeseed or sunflower oil
1 egg white
1 tsp ground ginger
1 tsp ground cinnamon
1 tsp ground allspice
1 tsp ground cloves
1 tsp baking powder
Pinch of salt

Preheat the oven to 180°C, (Fan 160°C), 350°F, Gas Mark 4. Grease a 22 x 10cm loaf tin with a light spray of oil and then line with baking parchment. I just cut a long strip of paper to cover the bottom and come up either side of the tin with the excess hanging over a little. This makes it easier to lift the baked loaf out of the tin.

Put all of the ingredients in a bowl and mix them together to give a soft, sticky mixture. Spoon the mixture into the prepared tin and level the top off evenly with the back of a spoon. Then bake for 30–35 minutes or until a skewer inserted into the centre comes out clean.

Once baked, remove the loaf from the oven and allow it to cool a little in the tin. Then lift it out, peel the paper off, cut into 12 slices and serve.

(PER SLICE)	ENERGY	FAT	SAT FAT	SUGAR	PROTEIN	SALT
LORRAINE'S RECIPE	104 Kcal	4.1g	0.3g	7.1g	1.9g	0.21g
COMPARISON RECIPE	143 Kcal	8.4g	0.8g	10.9g	1.6g	0.25g

CHEWY COCONUT MACAROONS WITH A CHEEKY TOUCH OF LIME

No, not those macaroons — the smooth-topped French ones, resplendent in their brightly coloured glory. These macaroons are the little pyramids of coconut wonderment. I absolutely adore these, but make no mistake, desiccated coconut is not to be played around with when it comes to the calorie and fat stakes. I was very surprised to see just how laden with naughties these macaroons usually are. So, in short, this recipe is not going to be an incredible difference to other varieties, but there is a little wholemeal flour to make things a teeny bit better.

Makes

15 macaroons

5 egg whites (about 175ml in total)
50g caster sugar
150g desiccated coconut
2 tbsp wholemeal flour
Finely grated zest of 1 lime
   (optional)

Preheat the oven to 180°C, (Fan 160°C), 350°F, Gas Mark 4 and line a baking sheet with baking parchment.

Put the egg whites in a large bowl and lightly whisk them until they become frothy (like a bubble bath). Then add the sugar, coconut and flour and mix it all together to give a sticky mixture.

Using damp hands, divide the mixture into 15 even-sized pieces. The mixture will be sticky but crumbly, but don't worry too much for now. Then squidge each piece into a pyramid shape, with a flat bottom and pointy top. This will take a bit of time and patience to get a good shape. Rinse your hands as you shape them, leaving them damp, which helps avoid the mixture sticking too much to you. Place them upright on the baking sheet as you go.

Bake for 15–20 minutes or until the macaroons are going golden brown all over. The sharp edges and top will be a bit darker golden. When they are ready, remove them from the oven and set aside to cool. Once cool, arrange them on a serving plate, scatter the lime zest over (if using) and serve.

(PER MACAROON)	ENERGY	FAT	SAT FAT	SUGAR	PROTEIN	SALT
LORRAINE'S RECIPE	87 Kcal	6.3g	5.3g	4g	2.1g	0.1g
COMPARISON RECIPE	127 Kcal	10.1g	7.9g	6.9g	1.9g	0.1g

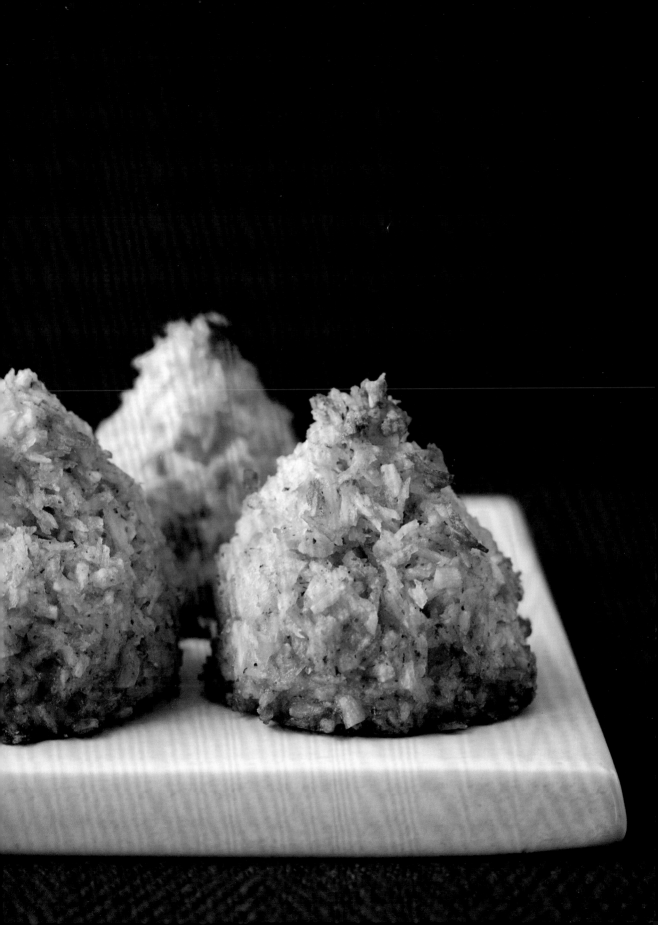

PEACHES & 'CREAM' ÉCLAIRS WITH WHITE CHOCOLATE & RASPBERRIES

I hunted like a crazy woman to find a comparable recipe to this one and came up with nothing exactly the same. I did find, however, a recipe for peaches and cream éclairs with a bourbon caramel sauce on a well-known website and have used their filling and topping for a comparison. And I took one of my old choux recipes from another book as a base to develop the lighter version on page 267.

Makes
12 large or 24 small éclairs

Equipment
Disposable piping bag

Choux pastry
475g Yumsters Wholemeal Choux Paste (see page 267)

Cream cheese 'cream' filling
300g low-fat cream cheese
1 tbsp crème fraîche
3 tbsp icing sugar, sifted
Seeds of 1 vanilla pod or 1 tsp vanilla extract
410g tin of peaches, drained and cut into ½ cm cubes

Topping
100g white chocolate, preferably Milkybar, roughly chopped
12 or 24 raspberries (depending on how many éclairs you are making)

Preheat the oven to 200°C, (Fan 180°C), 400°F, Gas Mark 6 and line two large baking sheets with baking parchment.

Lay a disposable piping bag down flat and cut the tip off with scissors where the width of the bag is 4cm. This gives a nozzle hole of 2½cm, perfect for large éclairs. For small éclairs, cut the tip off the bag where the width is 2½cm, giving a nozzle opening of 1½cm. Spoon the just-made choux paste into a piping bag.

For large éclairs, pipe out 12 sausage shapes each about 16cm long and 4cm wide, spaced apart on the baking sheets. Bake for 30 minutes, without opening the oven door before about 25 minutes or the buns will deflate like a tyre with a slow puncture and they will never really be the same again! For small éclairs, pipe out 24 sausage shapes each about 8cm long and 2cm wide, spaced apart on the baking sheets. Bake for 25 minutes and again, same rule applies, about not opening the door too soon. Once the choux buns have risen, are golden and feel really firm, take them out of the oven and cut them completely in half across their equator. Then, return them to the oven on the baking sheets, cut side up, for about 5 minutes to dry the middles out. Remove them from the oven and leave to cool.

Meanwhile, make the filling. Beat the cream cheese and crème fraîche together in a medium bowl until smooth. Add the icing sugar and vanilla seeds or extract and mix together well. Cover the filling and pop it into the fridge to firm up a little until ready to use.

Once the buns are cool, lay the choux bun halves out, cut side up, on a large serving platter and reserve the tops. Using a knife, dollop and spread the cream cheese filling on each piece of éclair. Then divide the peach pieces among the bottom halves only, spooning them on top. Pick the éclair tops up and sit them, cream cheese side down, on top of the peaches and set them aside.

Break the chocolate into a medium heatproof bowl. I like to melt chocolate in a microwave in 30 second blasts, stirring between each blast. Alternatively, melt the chocolate by sitting the bowl on a medium pan filled with about 3cm deep of boiling water. Make sure the bowl doesn't touch the water as this could make the chocolate grainy. Leave the chocolate sitting until it melts.

Spoon the melted chocolate over the top of each éclair, spreading it out evenly with the back of the spoon. Pop a raspberry on the top at the end of the éclair to stick to the chocolate and serve.

(PER ÉCLAIR (INCLUDING PASTRY) - 12 ÉCLAIRS)	ENERGY	FAT	SAT FAT	SUGAR	PROTEIN	SALT
LORRAINE'S RECIPE	186 Kcal	10.6g	6.3g	10.3g	6g	0.37g
COMPARISON RECIPE	236 Kcal	16g	9.3g	13.9g	3.4g	0.21g

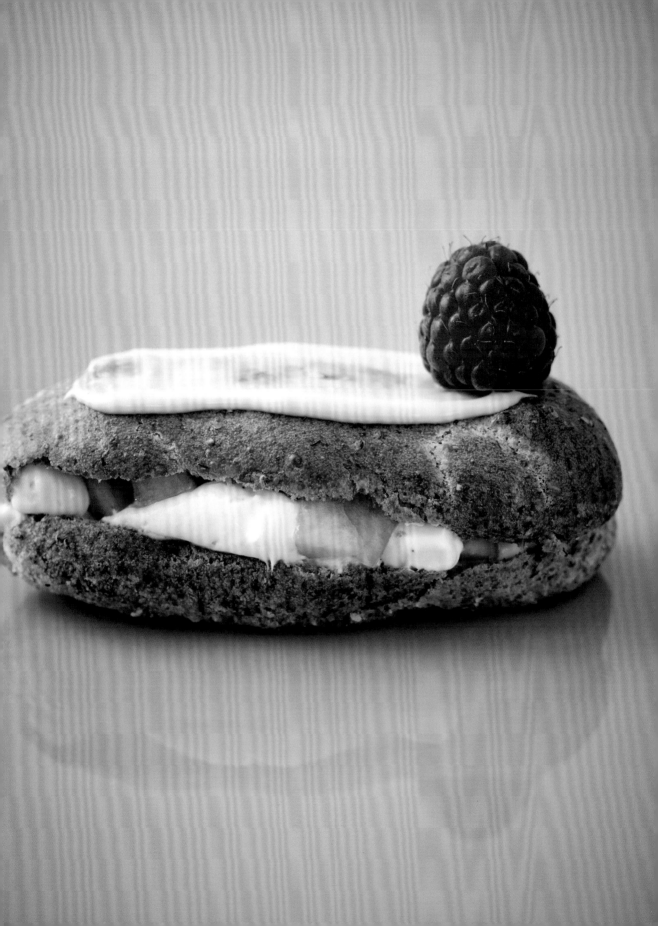

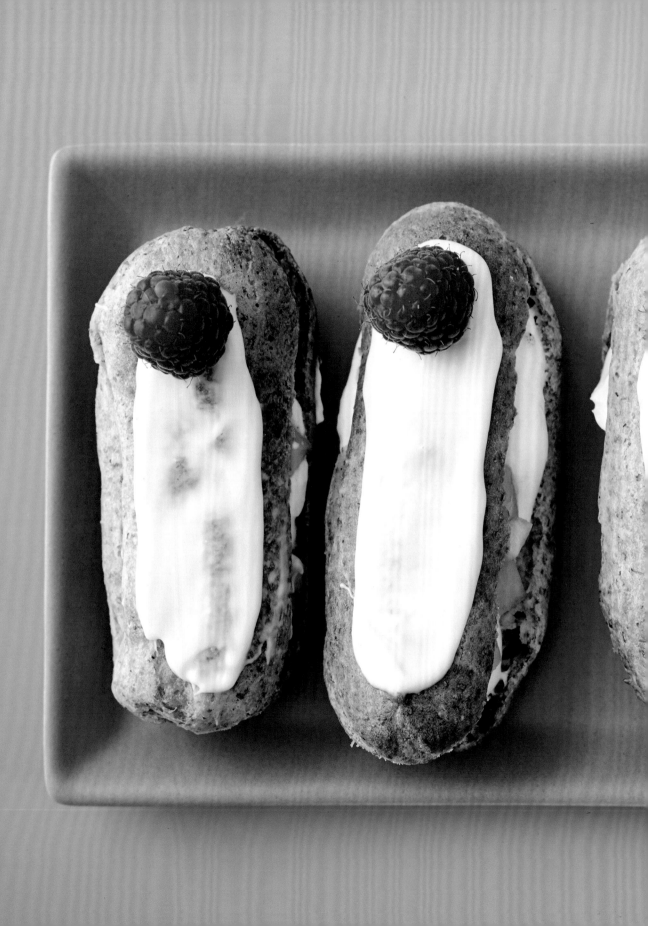

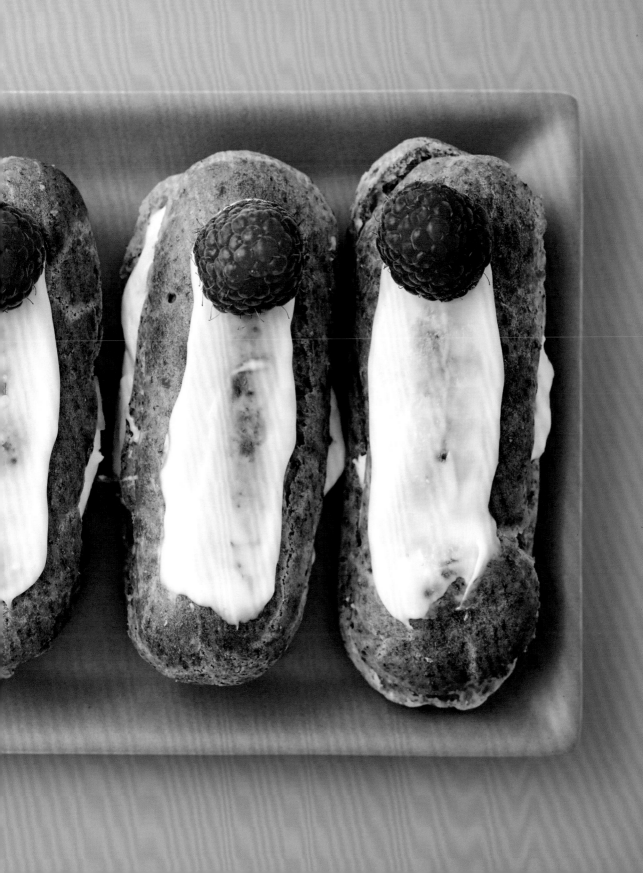

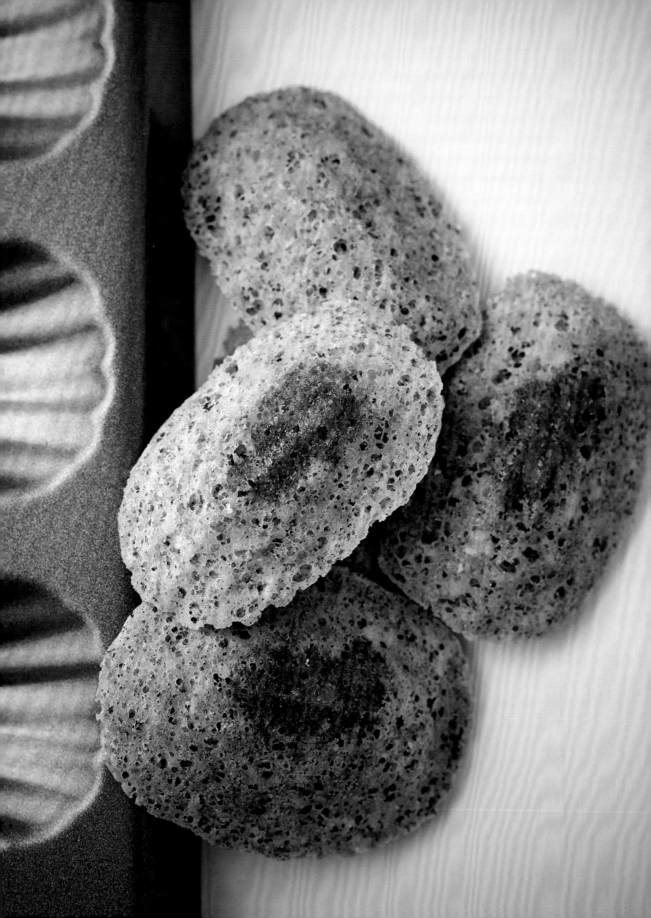

STICKY PEAR, AMARETTO & ALMOND MADELEINES

I made these at home first with a madeleine tin made out of metal: I got into all sorts of trouble, but eventually convinced the madeleines not to stick. Try a flexible mould for these buttery pillows of air if you can find one so you don't have the same problem!

Makes
12 madeleines

Equipment
12-hole madeleine mould

Spray oil

Glazed pears
1 tbsp honey
½ a pear, peeled, cored and very finely diced (to give about 50g)

Madeleines
1 egg
2 egg whites
Seeds of ½ a vanilla pod or ½ tsp vanilla extract
2 tbsp soft light brown sugar
50g plain flour
25g wholemeal flour
3 tbsp ground almonds
¾ tsp baking powder
Pinch of bicarbonate of soda
Pinch of salt
25g unsalted butter, melted
1 tbsp Amaretto (optional)

Preheat the oven to 180°C, (Fan 160°C), 350°F, Gas Mark 4, with the middle shelf at the ready. Spray a 12-hole flexible madeleine mould (see intro above) with oil and set it aside.

Put the honey in a small pan over a medium heat and bring it to a gentle bubble. Then add the pears and cook them for about 2–3 minutes, keeping them moving so nothing burns. The honey should reduce, start to go a darker brown and glaze the pears, which should be just softened without breaking up. Tip the glazed pears out into a bowl and leave to cool.

Put the egg, egg whites and vanilla seeds or extract into a large bowl and whisk them up until they double in size and become glossy. Then add the sugar and continue to whisk to dissolve. This whole process should take a good 2–3 minutes. The eggs won't go really mousse-like due to the proportion of egg white to whole egg, but they will froth up a little. Once the eggs are ready, gently scatter the flours, ground almonds, baking powder, bicarb and salt over them. Pour the melted butter around the side of the whisked eggs so you don't knock out any of the air. Then gently fold everything together really carefully until nicely combined.

I find the easiest way to fill the moulds is to gently pour the mixture into a large jug and then pour from this into the mould holes to come just to the top. Then, carefully place a teaspoon of the glazed pears in the centre of the top of each one. Bake for 12–14 minutes, or until they are golden brown and firm but springy to the touch. Once cooked, remove from the oven and brush the Amaretto over, if using, and serve.

(PER MADELEINE)	ENERGY	FAT	SAT FAT	SUGAR	PROTEIN	SALT
LORRAINE'S RECIPE	78 Kcal	3.7g	1.4g	4.5g	2.4g	0.17g
COMPARISON RECIPE	95 Kcal	5.5g	3.2g	6.3g	1.5g	0.03g

BROWN SUGAR ESPRESSO CHOCOLATE-DIPPED MERINGUE KISSES

I have done lots of meringues in my time and I realize that if there is less sugar in them, they simply do not work. So rather than omit meringues from the book entirely, I have made teeny-tiny ones, which can be put in a dry place and eaten as a 29-calorie snackette when the munchies take hold.

Makes

About 50

Equipment

Large bowl and hand whisk or hand-held electric whisk or freestanding electric mixer set with the whisk attachment, piping bag fitted with a 2cm plain nozzle

150g caster sugar
50g soft light brown sugar
4 medium egg whites
2 tsp instant coffee granules
150g dark chocolate (minimum 70% cocoa solids), roughly chopped

Preheat the oven to 110°C, (Fan 90°C), 225°F, Gas Mark ¼. Line two large baking sheets with baking parchment and set aside.

You can do this by hand, but as that would take a very, very, long time, you are best off using a food mixer fitted with a whisk or electric hand whisk. Put both sugars and one of the egg whites into a large bowl (or food mixer bowl) and whisk together on high for about 30 seconds until well blended. Then add another egg white and whisk for another couple of minutes until the mixture begins to become a bit stiffer. Continue to add the next two egg whites separately until the meringue mix is stiff and shiny. If you stick a fork into the meringue and make a peak with some of the mixture, it should literally hold its shape and not fall back down. That is a nice stiff peak. It will take longer doing it this way with the sugar in first, but it will give you a really stiff and shiny meringue and it is impossible to over whisk it.

Dissolve the coffee granules in 1 teaspoon hot water. Drizzle it around the edge of the meringue mixture and then gently fold it in.

Spoon the mixture into a piping bag fitted with a 2cm plain nozzle (or snip a disposable piping bag to give a hole of this size). Pipe about 50 blobs spaced apart on the baking sheets. Each one should be about 3–4cm wide on the sheets and with a little peak at the top. This is the classic shape for kisses. Bake in the oven for about 2 hours or until the meringue kisses are crisp on the outside, but still mallowy and soft inside.

Once the kisses are baked, remove them from the oven and set aside to cool. Once cool, melt the chocolate in a microwave in 30 second blasts, stirring between each blast. Or put about 3cm depth of water in the bottom of a pan and bring it to the boil. Turn the water down so its starts to simmer. Then put a bowl over the pan, making sure that the bottom of the bowl does not touch the water. Put the chocolate into the bowl and leave it to melt for a few minutes.

Holding a kiss gently at the top without crushing, dip its bottom into the chocolate to come up about 3mm and shake off the excess. Then sit it back onto the baking sheet and repeat until all of the kisses are done. Leave for about 30 minutes until the chocolate has set, and then arrange on a platter and serve.

(PER MERINGUE KISS)	ENERGY	FAT	SAT FAT	SUGAR	PROTEIN	SALT
LORRAINE'S RECIPE	29 Kcal	0.7g	0.4g	5.7g	0.4g	0.02g
COMPARISON RECIPE	30 Kcal	0.8g	0.5g	5.6g	0.4g	0.01g

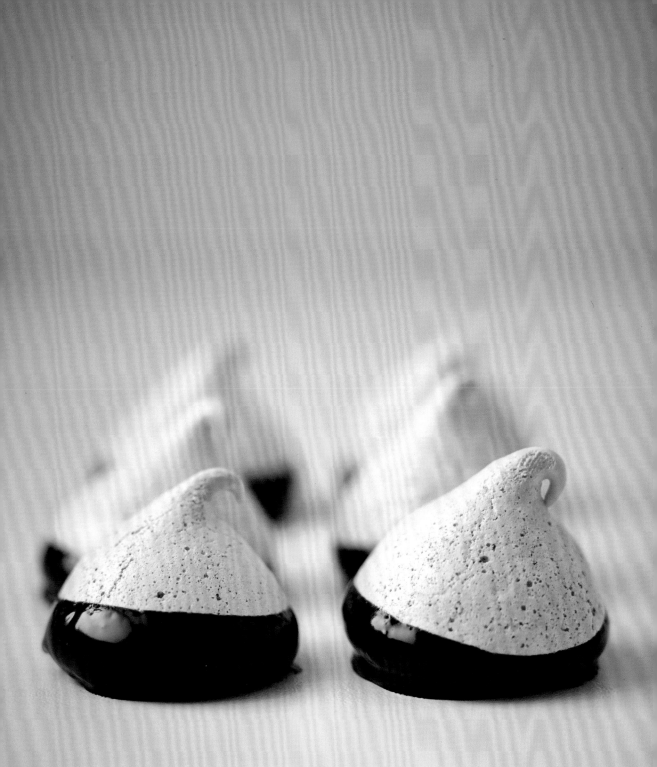

TOASTED COCONUT & ALMOND PASTRY (THINS)

This pastry is an unusual and welcome treat. Toasting desiccated coconut is not an obligatory step but it does take away the sometimes over-chewiness of the coconut and rounds off the flavours, making them more nuttier. This technique definitely gets my vote and it only takes a few minutes. Just chuck the coconut into a frying pan with no oil in and cook it on a medium to high heat until the coconut starts to go a bit golden brown and crispy around the edges. Then take it off the heat, allow it to cool a bit and continue with the recipe.

Makes
22 thins

Equipment
Food processor or large bowl, 6cm round, straight-sided cookie cutter

150g wholemeal flour, plus extra for dusting
50g unsalted butter, diced
Pinch of salt
50g ground almonds
25g desiccated coconut, toasted (see recipe intro)
3 tbsp soft light brown sugar
2 egg yolks
2 tbsp water

Put all of the ingredients in a food processor and blitz until the mixture starts to form lumps. Scrape down the sides of the bowl to get any wet patches that may have bceome stuck and blitz again.

Alternatively, to make by hand, put the flour, butter and salt into a large bowl. Pick up bits of the mixture with the tips of your fingers and rub your thumb into your fingers to blend the ingredients together, allowing it to fall back into the bowl. Keep doing this until the mixture resembles fine breadcrumbs. Stir in the ground almonds, coconut and sugar, and then add the egg yolks and water. Stir everything together really well with a small knife until it starts to form lumps. Scrape the side of the bowl down in case some of the egg or the water has stuck there.

Dust a clean surface with a little flour. Tip the dough onto the surface and squidge the mixture with your hands so it comes together in a ball. Knead lightly for a few seconds until smooth and then wrap with cling film. Refrigerate for 20 minutes to relax and firm up.

Use this pastry as you wish. It is perfect to use as a tart case, for example, or another idea is to simply use it to make my pastry thins.

Preheat the oven to 180°C, (Fan 160°C), 350°F, Gas Mark 4. Line two large baking sheets with baking parchment.

Roll the pastry out to about 4mm thin on a lightly floured surface. Stamp out 22 discs using a 6cm round, straight-sided cookie cutter. Arrange the discs on the baking sheets and bake for 15 minutes until crisp and lightly golden. These thins are lovely served with a cup of tea.

(PER THIN)	ENERGY	FAT	SAT FAT	SUGAR	PROTEIN	SALT
LORRAINE'S RECIPE	77 Kcal	4.6g	2.1g	3.2g	1.8g	0.01g
COMPARISON RECIPE	95 Kcal	7.3g	4.2g	1.2g	1.2g	0.13g

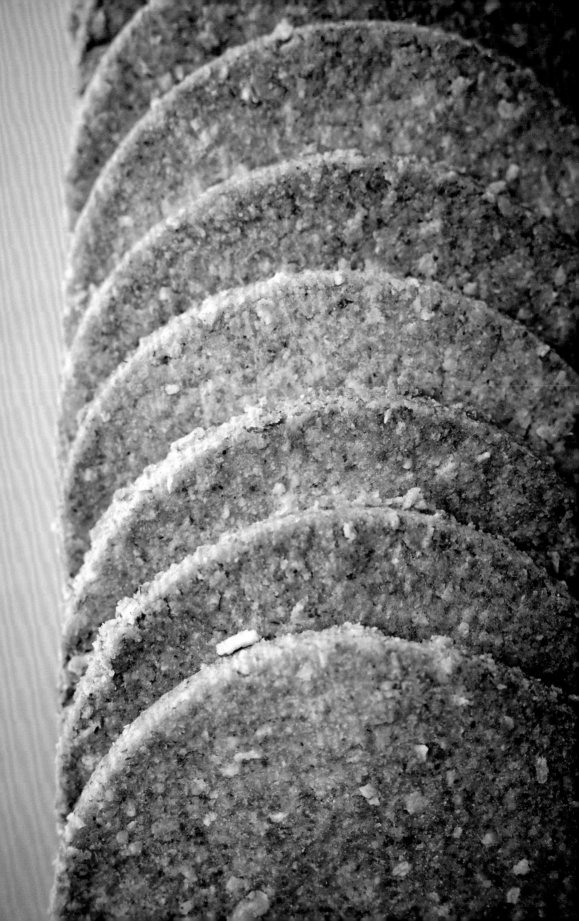

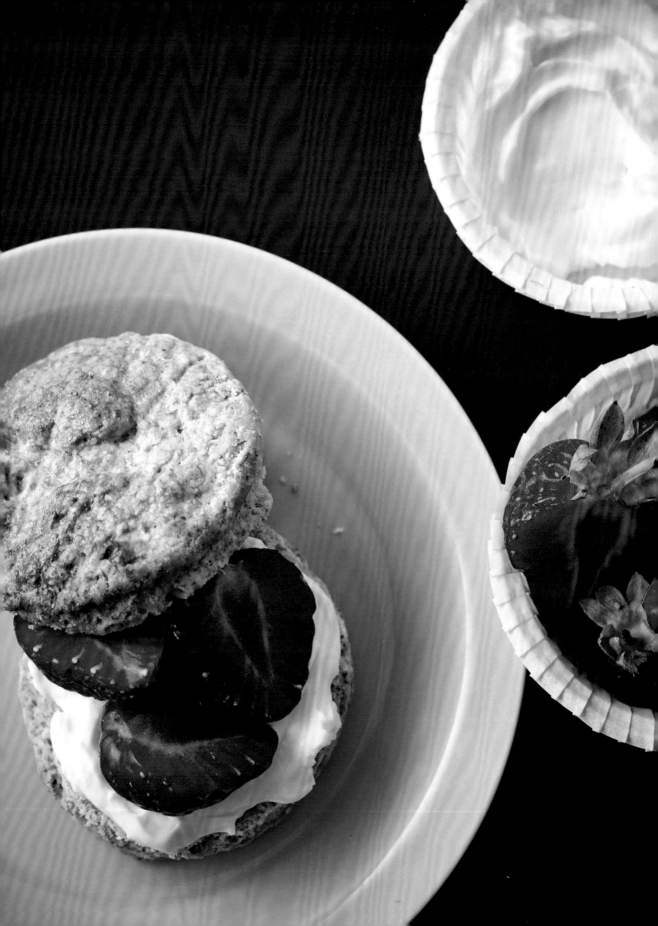

HEAVENLY HONEY SCONES

I remember being driven down to visit an aunt in Bath many, many moons ago. As a young child of less than eight, the schlep from Witney seemed epic. When we finally arrived, my mother parked her mustard Ford Capri outside a little tea room. Aunt was met, greetings were made, and then from the shadows a blue-rinsed, bespectacled lady came out carrying a plate of carbohydrate wholemeal heaven. I could never find that tea shop again, no doubt it has been turned in to a mini supermarket, but my goodness those scones were good. Scones are by their very nature low in fat and sugar, so these have similar nutritional content to typical scone recipes, but are just a teeny bit more angelic.

Makes

8 scones

Equipment

6cm straight-sided round cutter

225g self-raising flour, plus extra for dusting
100g wholemeal flour
1½ tsp baking powder
Pinch of salt
50g cold unsalted butter, diced
2 tbsp honey
1 tsp vanilla extract
150ml semi-skimmed milk
1 small egg, lightly beaten
Light cream cheese, to serve (optional)
Fresh strawberries, halved, to serve (optional)

Preheat the oven to 220°C, (Fan 200°C), 425°F, Gas Mark 7. Line a large baking sheet with baking parchment.

Put the self-raising and wholemeal flour, baking powder, salt and butter into a large bowl. Using your fingertips, pick up bits of the flour with the butter and rub them between your thumb and fingertips. Continue in this way until everything is well mixed together. It should look like flour with no lumps of butter.

Make a well in the centre and add the honey, vanilla extract and milk, then, using a knife, mix everything together. It will become several large lumps, but just get your hands in and squeeze the mixture into one piece of soft, smooth dough.

Dust a clean work surface with a little flour and tip the dough out onto it. Use a rolling pin to roll the dough out to about 2cm thick. Using a 6cm straight-sided round cutter, stamp out scones, arranging them spaced apart on the baking sheet as you go. When cutting the scones out, just push the cutter straight down, rather than twisting it down. This will help avoid them from rising up wonky and twisted. You will need to re-scrunch up the mixture and re-roll it out until all of the dough is used up and you have eight scones in total.

Brush the top of the scones with the egg, making sure it does not drip down the sides. If it does, it may stop the scones from rising up so much. Bake in the oven for 10–12 minutes or until the scones are well risen and golden brown.

Remove and leave until cool enough to handle. These are best served warm, fresh from the oven, and are delightful halved across the middle, slathered with cream cheese and topped with strawberry halves.

(PER SCONE)	ENERGY	FAT	SAT FAT	SUGAR	PROTEIN	SALT
LORRAINE'S RECIPE	213 Kcal	6.3g	3.6g	6.2g	5.1g	0.56g
COMPARISON RECIPE	213 Kcal	7.4g	4g	7g	6g	0.69g

BITE-SIZED PINWHEEL SNACKS

I have made these super-small on purpose, so you can have a little almost guilt-free snack when you want a very tiny treat.

Makes
20 pinwheels

75g butter, softened
35g caster sugar
Pinch of salt
Seeds of 1 vanilla pod or 1 tsp
  vanilla extract
100g plain flour

After splitting mixtures
10g cocoa powder
10g plain flour

Cream the butter and sugar, salt and vanilla seeds or extract together in a medium bowl. Add the flour and smoosh the mixture against the sides of the bowl to really mix it in and create a really soft dough, then split the mixture in half between two bowls. I like to weigh the whole amount and then divide it out evenly. Knead the cocoa powder through one dough piece and the extra flour through the other until well blended. Then, wrap the dough balls in cling film and put them into the fridge for a good 30 minutes to 1 hour to firm up.

When you are ready to cook the pinwheels, preheat the oven to 180°C, (Fan 160°C), 350°F, Gas Mark 4. Line a large baking sheet with baking parchment and set aside.

Once firm, roll each dough ball out on a piece of baking parchment to a 20 x 12cm rectangle. The dough can be tricky to handle, as it can break up and become soft very easily, but just work slowly and carefully to get the right shape and size. I like to straighten and neaten the sides by tapping a ruler or palette knife against them. Once done, pop the chocolate rectangle directly on top of the plain one. The easiest thing to do is to pick it up on the baking parchment and flip it over on top of the plain rectangle before peeling the paper away.

Then, with the longest side facing you, roll the layers up together away from you, like a Swiss roll. Use the bottom sheet of baking parchment to help you lift and roll. Wrap the roll in the baking parchment and refrigerate once again for a good 30 minutes or so until really firm.

Once set, use a sharp knife to cut the roll into 20 x 1cm-thick slices to reveal the swirl shape, and arrange them (lying down) on the prepared baking sheet. Bake in the oven for 15–20 minutes until just firm to the touch but starting to take on some colour. Once cooked, remove from the oven and leave to cool completely and firm up on the tray. I keep these in a little airtight jar for when I fancy a teeny bit of chocolate as a small, naughty snack.

(PER PINWHEEL)	ENERGY	FAT	SAT FAT	SUGAR	PROTEIN	SALT
LORRAINE'S RECIPE	56 Kcal	3.3g	2g	2g	0.6g	0.03g
COMPARISON RECIPE	62 Kcal	4.3g	2.7g	1.4g	0.6g	0.09g

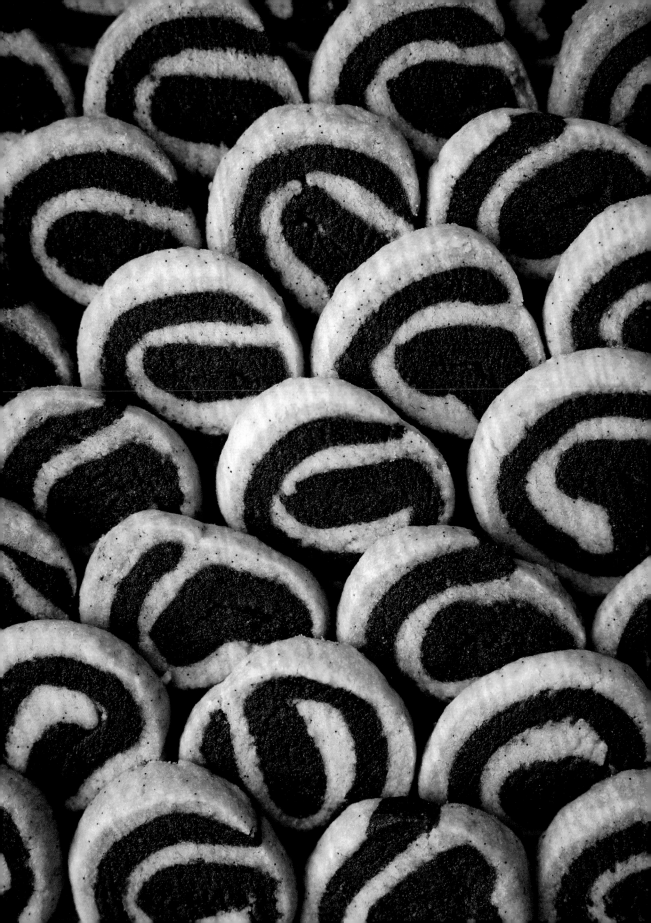

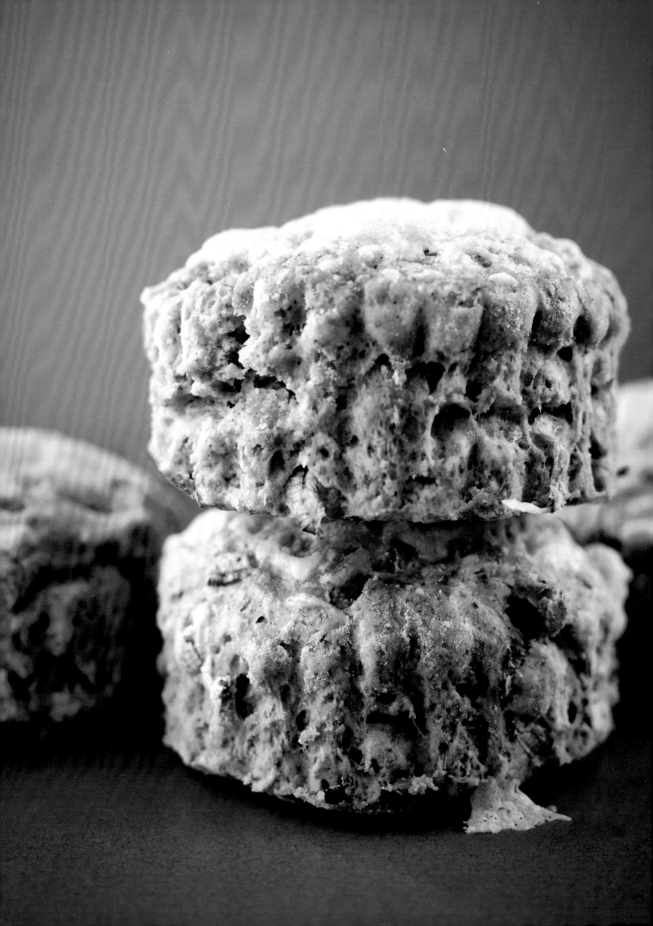

CHEDDAR CHEESE SCONES WITH SPRING ONIONS & PAPRIKA

The brown sugar scones with mascarpone from *Baking Made Easy* were rich and sumptuous to the extreme and something I still make often, however I have had repeated requests by way of tweets, Facebooks and yells from passing cars, to make some of my dishes a little bit lighter (so that people can have a choice of which one they want to make). I was challenged a little with these savoury scones due to my desire to get the cheese flavour strong enough, but I got there in the end. The wholemeal flour is naturally better for us and, funnily enough, the flour that I prefer. I implore you to eat these fresh from the oven with the teeniest bit of butter to moisten. Utterly delicious.

Makes
8 scones

Equipment
Food processor or large bowl, 6cm fluted cutter, pastry brush

Spray oil
5 spring onions, finely chopped
200g self-raising flour, plus extra for dusting
100g wholemeal flour
50g unsalted butter
50g low-fat cream cheese
1 tsp baking powder
2 tsp paprika
Big pinch of salt
100ml skimmed milk
1 small egg, lightly beaten or 1 egg yolk, mixed with 1 tbsp cold water
25g Cheddar cheese, finely grated

Preheat the oven to 200°C, (Fan 180°C), 400°F, Gas Mark 6. Line a large baking sheet with baking parchment and set aside.

Heat a medium frying pan over a medium heat and spray in a little oil. Gently fry the spring onions for 4–5 minutes until softened, but not coloured.

Put both flours, the butter, cream cheese, baking powder, paprika and salt into a food processor and pulse until they form fine crumbs. Add the milk and the cooked spring onions and pulse again briefly until they come together into a soft dough ball.

If you don't have a food processor, then put the ingredients into a large bowl and use your thumb and forefingers to pick up bits of the butter and cream cheese along with the flour mixture and rub them all together. Keep doing this until the mixture resembles fine breadcrumbs, then add the milk and cooked spring onions. Mix everything together quickly with a table knife before getting your hands in and squidging it all together to form a smooth, soft dough. Make sure you get all the dry bits in the bottom of the bowl and really squidge them into the dough.

Dust a clean surface with a little flour and roll the dough out to about 2cm in thickness. Use a 6cm fluted cutter to stamp out rounds and arrange them on the baking sheet as you go. Make sure that when you cut them out, you don't twist the cutter as this will result in the scones not rising straight up. Re-squidge the leftover dough pieces together and re-roll out to give eight scones in total. Brush the tops with the egg, avoiding letting any drip down the sides, which could prevent a good rise. Finally, sprinkle a little cheese over the top of each.

Bake for about 10–12 minutes or until the scones are cooked through, nicely risen and are golden brown. These are delicious served warm.

(PER SCONE)	ENERGY	FAT	SAT FAT	SUGAR	PROTEIN	SALT
LORRAINE'S RECIPE	206 Kcal	7.9g	4.6g	1.6g	6.2g	0.54g
COMPARISON RECIPE	262 Kcal	12.8g	7.7g	5.8g	5.1g	0.68g

THERE IS ONLY ONE WAY TO AVOID CRITICISM:
DO NOTHING, SAY NOTHING, AND BE NOTHING.
ARISTOTLE

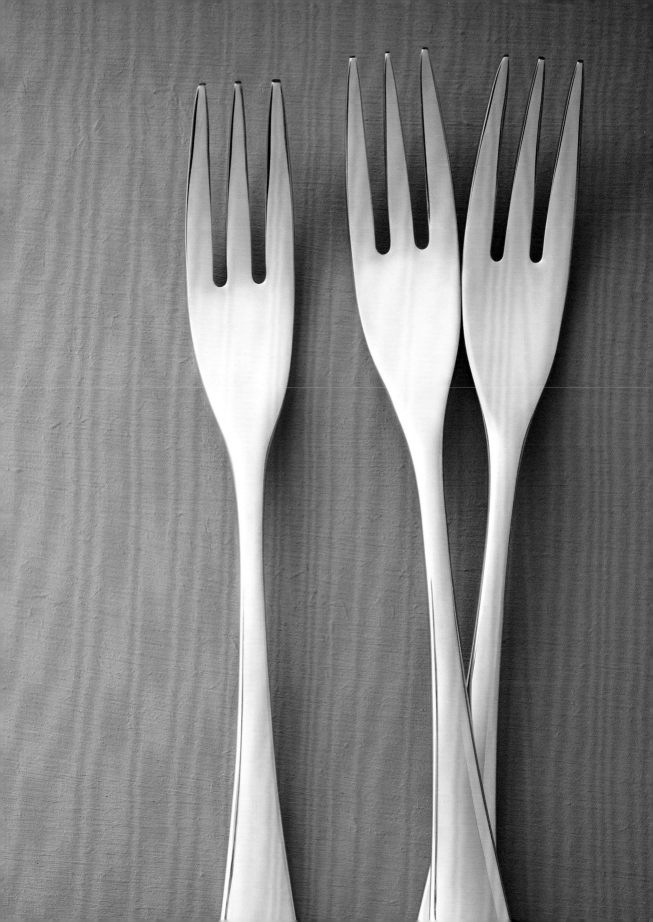

SPECIAL OCCASIONS & ENTERTAINING

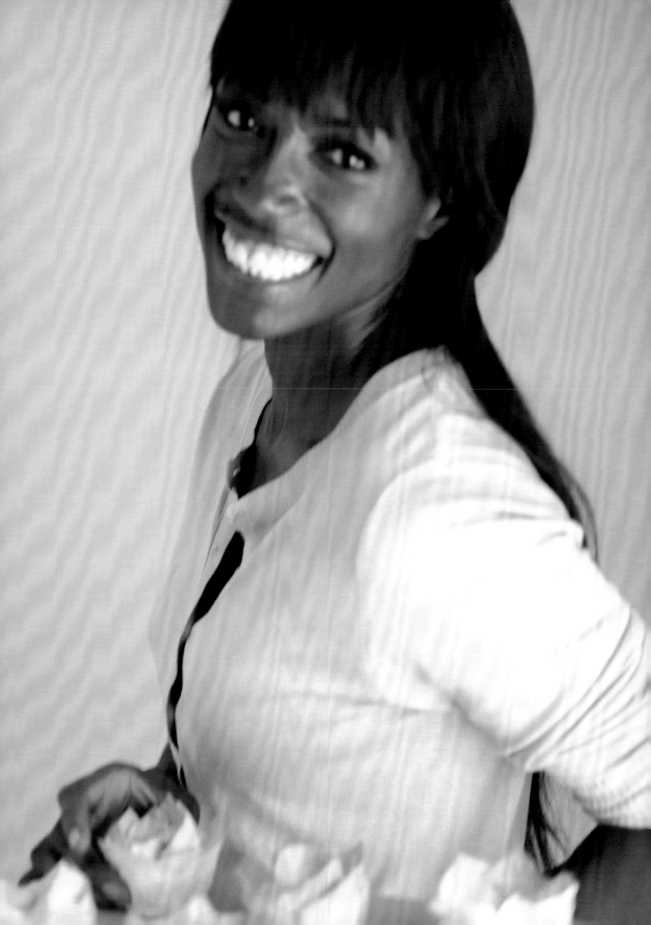

PETITE FILO QUICHE LORRAINE (PASCALE) WITH RED ONION, BACON & THYME

I first made a quiche at catering school, a large one with a sprinkling of bacon and veg. *Baking Made Easy* saw me take quiche to a whole new level with full fat crème fraîche, cream and a whole host of other naughties. This trimmed-down version makes use of lower-fat alternatives and egg whites, and a little bit of mustard on the pastry boosts the flavour and gives a subtle and gentle hint of heat. They are lovely to eat warm and great for your picnic hamper or lunchbox.

Makes
12 quiches

Equipment
12-hole muffin tin

Spray oil
1 red onion, finely sliced
150g back bacon, trimmed of any fat and diced
Leaves from 3 sprigs of fresh thyme
200g half-fat crème fraîche
75ml semi-skimmed milk
25g Parmesan, finely grated
2 eggs
2 egg whites
Pinch of freshly grated nutmeg
4½ sheets of filo pastry, defrosted
1 tbsp yellow mustard
Sprinkle of chopped fresh chives, to garnish
Salt and freshly ground black pepper

To serve
Crisp green salad

Preheat the oven to 180°C, (Fan 160°C), 350°F, Gas Mark 4. Place a baking sheet into the oven to heat up. This will give extra bottom heat to the quiches so that the bases cook through and are not soggy. Grease a 12-hole muffin tin with spray oil and set aside.

Spray a little oil into a large frying pan and gently cook the onion for 6–8 minutes until it just begins to soften, but not colour. Add the bacon and thyme and continue to cook gently for 3–4 minutes until the bacon is cooked through. Remove from the heat and leave to cool.

Next, whisk the crème fraîche, milk, Parmesan, whole eggs, egg whites, nutmeg and a little salt and pepper together well in a large jug and set aside.

Lay the four whole sheets of filo pastry out on top of each other and cut them in half across the width. Then, sit the extra half of filo on top of one of these stacks and cut each stack into quarters. I find scissors really handy to cut these out, but a sharp knife will do. You should now have lots of smaller filo pieces measuring about 12cm square.

Line each hole of the muffin tin with three filo squares. I like to take a square at a time and press it into the hole, each one slightly staggered from the previous so the resulting pastry case edge looks like a kind of star. Make sure to push the pastry down so it is in the 'corners' of each muffin hole. Keep any filo not being worked on under a lightly dampened tea towel so that it doesn't dry out.

Next, brush the base of each mini quiche with a little of the mustard (which adds great flavour and kick!). Divide the onion and bacon mixture among the cases and then carefully pour the creamy egg mixture over to as full as you can get it. Spray the exposed pastry with a little oil.

Place in the oven on the heated baking sheet to bake for 30 minutes or until the egg mixture is just set and the pastry is crisp and golden brown. Sprinkle with the chopped chives and serve at once with a crisp green salad.

(PER QUICHE)	ENERGY	FAT	SAT FAT	SUGAR	PROTEIN	SALT
LORRAINE'S RECIPE	141 Kcal	6g	2.9g	1.6g	7.4g	0.74g
COMPARISON RECIPE	191 Kcal	10.4g	4.7g	1g	7.8g	0.59g

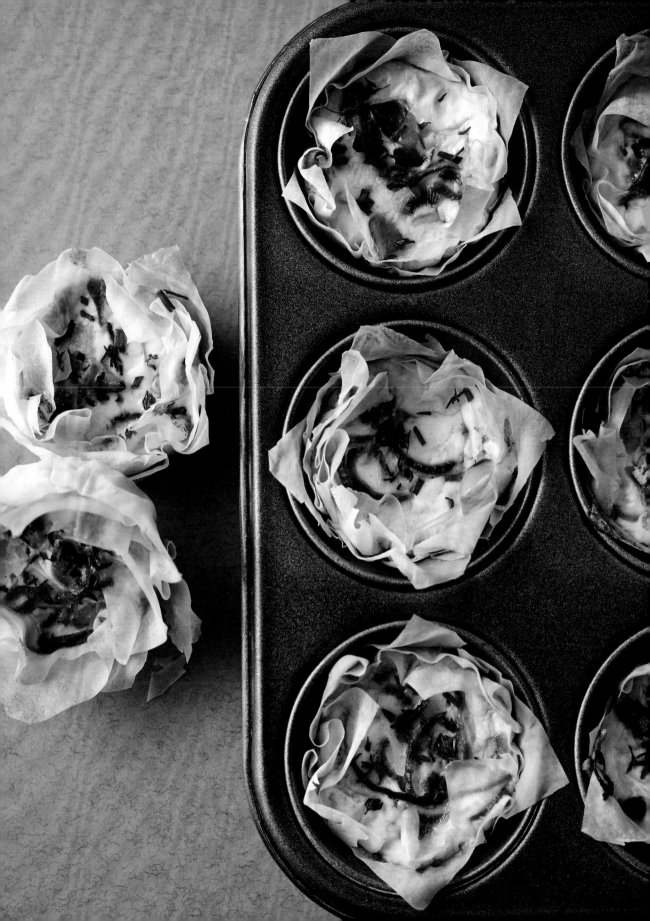

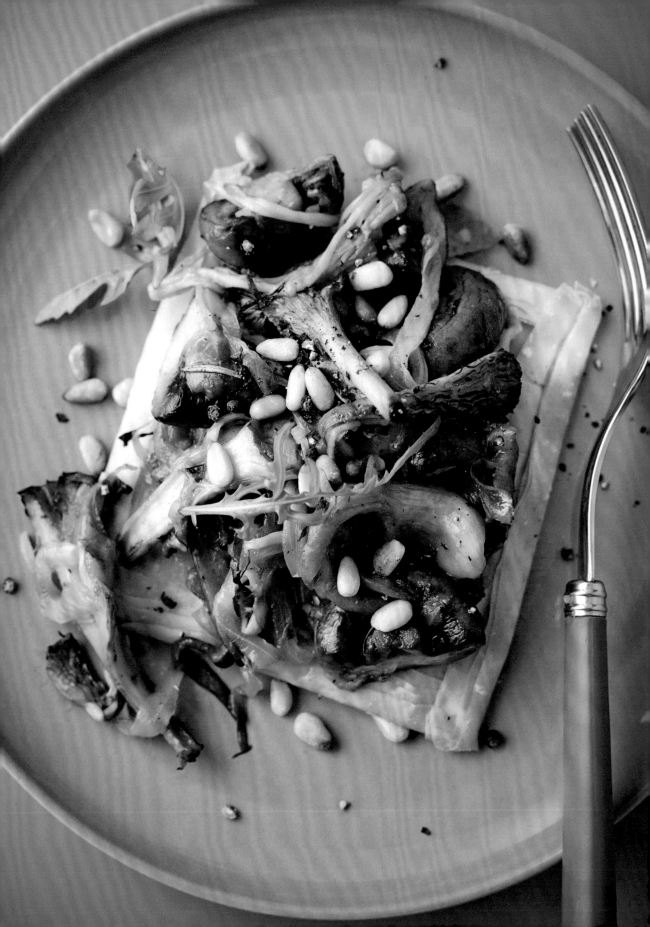

WILD MUSHROOM TART WITH SHERRY & ONIONS

I think in every one of my books I have included a recipe which somehow contains mushrooms and sherry. I simply love the combination of flavours. This tart is good eaten both hot and cold and is great for a picnic if transportation distance is limited – or if you can secure it better than I did when I took it to the park one summer!

Serves

8 as a starter or 4 as a main

4 sheets of filo pastry, defrosted
Spray oil
2 onions, finely sliced
200g chestnut mushrooms, halved or quartered
100g oyster mushrooms, sliced
100g mixed exotic or wild mushrooms, sliced, halved or quartered depending on their size and shape
25g unsalted butter
1 garlic clove, finely chopped
Leaves from 4 sprigs of fresh rosemary, roughly chopped
100ml sherry
50g pine nuts, toasted
50g wild rocket
Salt and freshly ground black pepper

Preheat the oven to 180°C, (Fan 160°C), 350°F, Gas Mark 4. Line a large baking sheet with baking parchment and set aside.

Lay the four sheets of filo out on top of each other and cut the stack in half down the length and then divide it into quarters across the width. This will give you eight stacks of about 12cm squares.

Fold an edge of about 1cm wide inwards all the way around each of the stacks to create a small border. Arrange each one on the baking sheet as you go, and then spritz with a little oil and bake in the oven for 20 minutes until crisp and golden brown.

Meanwhile, spritz a little spray oil into a large frying pan set over a medium heat and gently fry the onions for about 6 minutes or until they are just going soft and a little golden brown. Then, add the mushrooms and cook for a further minute, before adding the butter, garlic, rosemary and seasoning, stirring around to coat the mushrooms. Continue to cook this for 8–10 minutes until everything is really soft. Then turn the heat up to high, pour in the sherry and allow to bubble down for 2–3 minutes. Be careful, as the sherry may flame up a bit, in which case the flames will go as soon as the alcohol burns off. Taste the mushroom mixture, season if you feel it needs more and remove from the heat.

Remove the pastry squares from the oven once they are cool enough to handle and arrange on serving plates. Divide the mushroom mixture between each square, scatter the pine nuts and rocket over, and serve.

(PER SERVING – BASED ON 8 STARTER SERVINGS)	ENERGY	FAT	SAT FAT	SUGAR	PROTEIN	SALT
LORRAINE'S RECIPE	183 Kcal	8g	2g	3.8g	4.6g	0.17g
COMPARISON RECIPE	320 Kcal	21.5g	10.7g	1.1g	7.9g	0.7g

GRUYÈRE & THYME SOUFFLÉ

These are a little higher in sat fat than I would have liked (like pretty much all cheese soufflés), but I played around with them a bit and have got it right down as low as I can. To make them healthier, I have done things like omitted the breadcrumbs on the side of the dish as I find the soufflés rise without them and replaced some of the butter with olive oil to lower the saturated fat. These are as light as air and collapse so, so quickly, so get them to the table as soon as you can!

Makes

6 soufflés

Equipment

6 x 175ml ramekins, bowl and hand whisk or hand-held electric whisk or freestanding electric mixer set with the whisk attachment

Spray oil
25g unsalted butter
1 tbsp olive oil
50g plain flour, plus extra for dusting
1 tsp English mustard powder
300ml semi-skimmed milk
75g Gruyère cheese, roughly grated
4 eggs, separated
2 tsp finely chopped fresh chives
Leaves from 3 sprigs of fresh thyme
Salt and freshly ground black pepper

To serve

Crisp green salad

Preheat the oven to 200°C, (Fan 180°C), 400°F, Gas Mark 6. Put a baking sheet into the oven to get nice and hot. This will ensure that the soufflés have some bottom heat, which will help them shoot up (and also, putting all the ramekins on a sheet makes it much easier to take them in and out of the oven). Spray the insides of six 175ml ramekins with oil, dust lightly with flour and set aside.

Put the butter and olive oil into a medium pan on a medium heat and allow the butter to melt. Then add the flour and mustard powder and mix well to form a thick paste before removing from the heat. Add the milk gradually, stirring all the time until well blended. If you add it slowly while stirring, then you will avoid any lumps forming in the mixture. Once all of the milk is added, return the pan to the heat and bring it to the boil, stirring continuously. Reduce the heat to simmer for 5–6 minutes, continuing to stir all the time now until it begins to get nice and thick. Add the cheese, mixing well until fully melted, and then remove from the heat. Beat in the egg yolks, chives, thyme and seasoning until it is all combined and uniform. Scoop it out into a mixing bowl and set aside.

Next, put the egg whites into a bowl and whisk them up until they are nice and frothy, almost meringue-like. Be careful not to over-whisk them or they will go like bubble bath and not mix into the sauce well at all (and I have been there many times! The soufflé still tastes good and will rise, but the texture is a bit different and not quite as good). Stir a third of the egg whites into the reserved sauce. Don't worry about folding it in this time, just mix it in really quickly and well so that it loosens the sauce. Then, add the remaining egg whites to the sauce in two batches, folding it in more gently this time to keep the air in. Everything should now be well combined.

Next, divide the mixture equally among the six ramekins. Bang the ramekins on the work surface to make sure the mixture has fallen in to all the 'corners'. Then run your thumb down into the edge of the soufflé and along the inside of the ramekin, going all the way around. This will help to prevent the soufflé from sticking to the sides and therefore rise more easily.

Carefully remove the hot baking sheet from the oven and place the ramekins on it. Bake the soufflés in the oven for 12–15 minutes or until golden on the top and well risen. Don't open the oven before the soufflés are cooked as they will collapse. Having said that, once they are back in the oven they will rise up somewhat, but not to the heights of their pre-oven opening former glory!

Once ready, remove the baking sheet from the oven, take it straight to the table and serve asap.

(PER SOUFFLÉ)	ENERGY	FAT	SAT FAT	SUGAR	PROTEIN	SALT
LORRAINE'S RECIPE	213 Kcal	15.1g	6.9g	2.6g	11g	0.45g
COMPARISON RECIPE	245 Kcal	17.2g	9.3g	1.6g	13.6g	1.14g

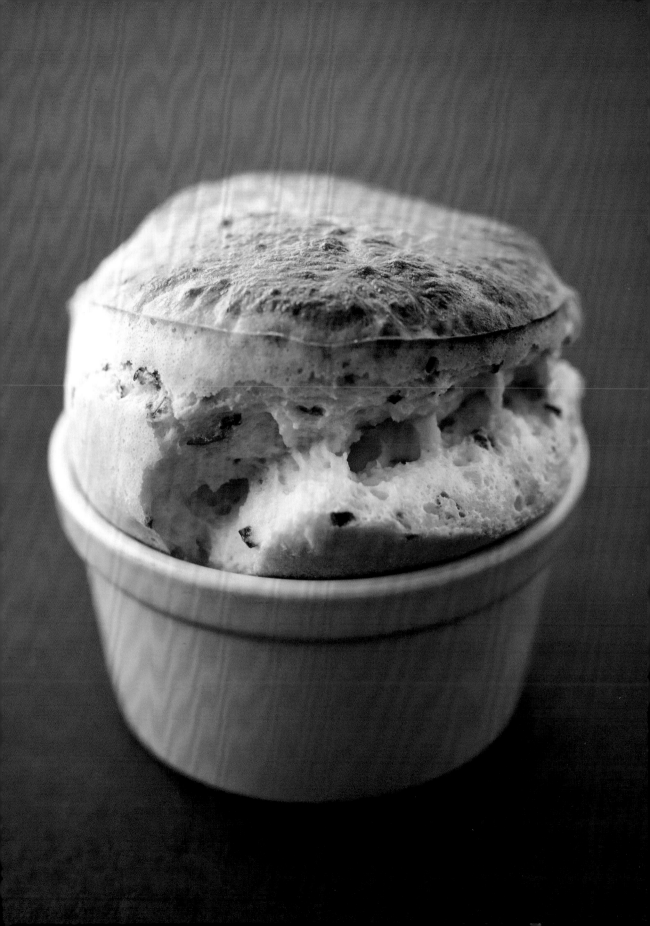

BEEF, GUINNESS & PORCINI PUFF PIE

I had a request from my family to include a puff pie. 'A puff pie,' I yelled, 'in a lighter baking book?' 'Yes,' they yelled back, with equal force, 'and don't go putting that filo on the top of it either!' So I attempted my idea of a lower-fat puff. I tried, I tried and I cried, and I kept pulling flat pieces of dry stiff pastry out of the oven. Then, during one of my loiters in the chilled aisle of the supermarket, I noticed that a little miracle tightly wrapped in plastic lay right there between the croissant dough and the shortcrust. Light ready-rolled puff pastry! There you go, my family, here is your puff pie – with bells on!

Serves
6

Filling
Spray oil
1kg lean beef (stewing steak pieces)
4 tbsp plain flour
2 medium onions, quartered, with root left intact
500ml beef stock
330ml Guinness
2 tbsp Worcestershire sauce
2 garlic cloves, finely chopped
Leaves from 4 sprigs of fresh rosemary, finely chopped
2 bay leaves
2 large carrots, cut into chunks
25g dried porcini mushrooms
Salt and freshly ground black pepper

Pastry
320g sheet of light ready-rolled puff pastry, defrosted
1 egg yolk
1 tbsp semi-skimmed milk

To serve
Garden peas

Preheat the oven to 170°C, (Fan 150°C), 325°F, Gas Mark 3. Line a large baking sheet with baking parchment and set aside.

Spritz a large non-stick casserole pot with spray oil and set over a high heat. Toss the beef in a large bowl with the flour and season. Then, working in three batches, brown the meat well in the pan to get some good colour on it. This will add lots of extra flavour to the finished stew. Scoop the meat out into a bowl as you go and spray a little more oil between batches if necessary.

Once all the beef has been browned and removed, fry the onion wedges over a medium heat for 4–5 minutes, stirring occasionally, until just turning golden. Return the meat to the casserole pot, add the stock, Guinness, Worcestershire sauce, garlic, rosemary, bay leaves and season. Bring to the boil, then pop the lid on and place in the oven for 3 hours.

Meanwhile, unroll the puff pastry sheet onto the prepared baking sheet. Cut it in half down the length and then across the width in thirds to give six evenly sized squares (approximately 12cm square). Separate out the squares a little, cover with cling film and place in the fridge to firm up until you are ready to cook.

Stir the carrots and porcini mushrooms into the casserole for the last half-hour. At this point don't put the lid back on, and also turn the heat up to 180°C, (Fan 160°C), 350°F, Gas Mark 4.

As soon as you have put the casserole back into the oven, mix the egg yolk and milk together in a small bowl and brush this over the puff pastry pieces. Then, bake the pastry in the oven with the casserole for the final 30 minutes of cooking.

Once cooked, the pastry should be puffed and golden. To check that the meat is tender, you should be able to literally cut it with a spoon. Check seasoning and adjust if necessary. To serve, remove the bay leaves from the casserole then divide it between six plates or wide bowls. Put a puff pastry square on top and serve with some peas.

(PER SERVING)	ENERGY	FAT	SAT FAT	SUGAR	PROTEIN	SALT
LORRAINE'S RECIPE	487 Kcal	15.7g	6.9g	6.9g	47.1g	1.8g
COMPARISON RECIPE	580 Kcal	30.1g	14.1g	8.2g	49.6g	1.1g

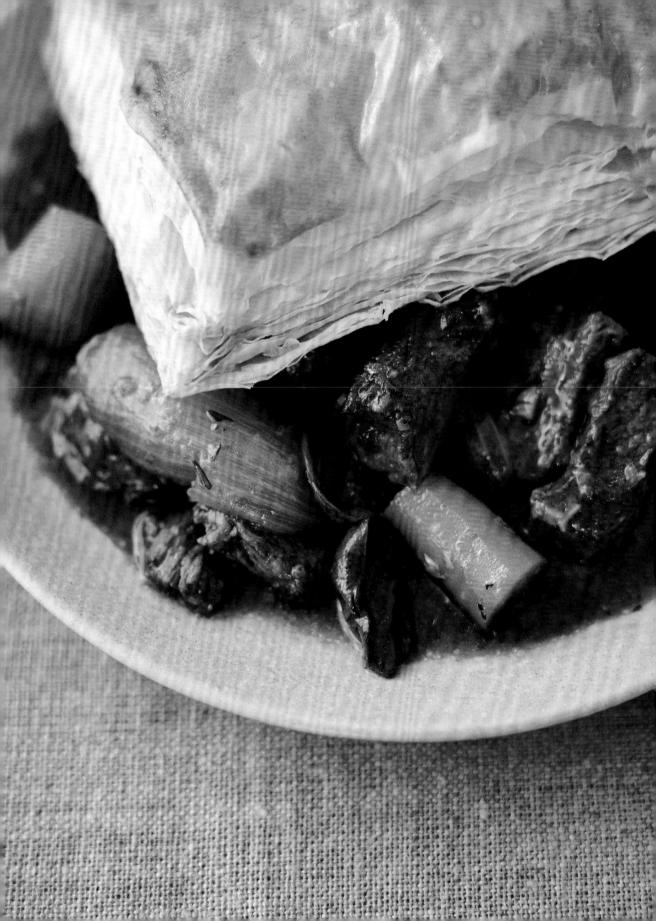

RASPBERRY, VANILLA & WHITE CHOCOLATE CAKE WITH ALMOND FLOWERS

You can use blackberries for this cake and, of course, redcurrants, blueberries or sneak in some chocolate chips.

Serves
10

Equipment
2 x 20cm sandwich tins, food
    processor

Sponge
Spray oil
125g soft light brown sugar
100g unsalted butter, softened
100g low-fat crème fraîche
2 eggs, lightly beaten
250g self-raising flour
1 egg white
2 tsp baking powder
Seeds of 1 vanilla pod or 1 tsp
    vanilla extract
Finely grated zest of 1 unwaxed
    lemon

Icing
75g white chocolate
300g low-fat cream cheese, at
    room temperature
2 tbsp icing sugar, sifted
Seeds of 1 vanilla pod or 1 tsp
    vanilla extract

Sugar syrup
2 tbsp caster sugar

Decoration
250g raspberries
About 50g flaked almonds
    (unbroken flakes, preferably),
    toasted (you will need about
    210 flakes in total)

Preheat the oven to 180°C, (Fan 160°C), 350°F, Gas Mark 4 with the middle shelf at the ready. Grease two 20cm sandwich tins with spray oil, line the base of each with baking parchment and set aside on a baking sheet.

To make the cake, beat the sugar, butter and crème fraîche in a large bowl until smooth and uniform. Then add two-thirds of the beaten egg and half of the flour and beat together again. Add the remaining egg and flour, the egg white (whisked until light and frothy), baking powder, vanilla seeds or extract and lemon zest and stir everything together well. Divide the mixture evenly between the two tins, levelling the tops with the back of a spoon. Bake in the oven for 20 minutes or until the cakes feels spongy to the touch and a skewer inserted in the centre comes out clean.

Meanwhile, prepare the icing. Tip the chocolate into a small heatproof bowl. I like to melt chocolate in a microwave in 30-second blasts, stirring between each blast. Alternatively, melt the chocolate in a bowl that just sits on top of a medium pan with a little bit of boiling water. Just make sure the bowl doesn't touch the water as this could make the chocolate grainy. Leave the chocolate to sit until it melts, then put aside to cool to room temperature but not set.

Meanwhile, beat the cream cheese, icing sugar and vanilla seeds or extract in a large bowl until smooth. Add a little bit of the cream cheese mixture to the cool melted chocolate and stir together gently. Then fold this white chocolate mixture into the cream cheese mix. I do it this way so that the white chocolate mix does not seize or go all grainy and firm. Cover and refrigerate until ready to use.

Prepare the sugar syrup about 5 minutes before the cake is ready. Simply put the sugar into a mug, add 2 tablespoons of boiling water and stir until dissolved. As soon as the two halves of the cake are out of the oven, brush them liberally with the sugar syrup and then leave them to cool in the tin. This will keep them nice and moist. Once cool, remove them from the tin and put one half on a serving plate.

Dollop about a quarter of the filling on the cake half and spread the icing evenly over it. Pick out about 30 of the smallest raspberries and reserve them for the flower decorations. Then scatter the remaining raspberries over the icing and pop the other cake half on top. Spread the remaining icing all over the cake sides and top to give a smoothish finish. Spread it around so that the edges are kind of straight and flat.

To decorate, put one of the reserved raspberries on the cake and place about seven flaked almonds around it so that the flakes stick up and out like 'petals' (rather than flat on the cake) and as if you have put an actual flower on the cake. Repeat this with the fruit and almonds to make flowers all over the cake, spaced apart on the top and sides. Then serve! Keep this in the fridge if not serving straight away.

(PER SERVING)	ENERGY	FAT	SAT FAT	SUGAR	PROTEIN	SALT
LORRAINE'S RECIPE	268 Kcal	13.9g	7.3g	18.3g	6.2g	0.39g
COMPARISON RECIPE	401 Kcal	22.3g	13.4g	32.3g	5g	0.64g

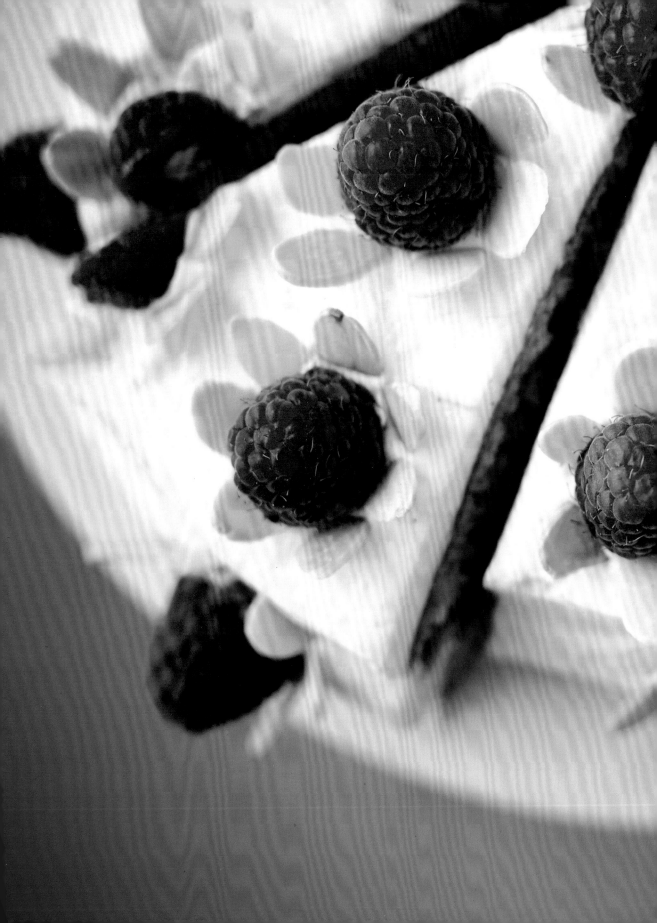

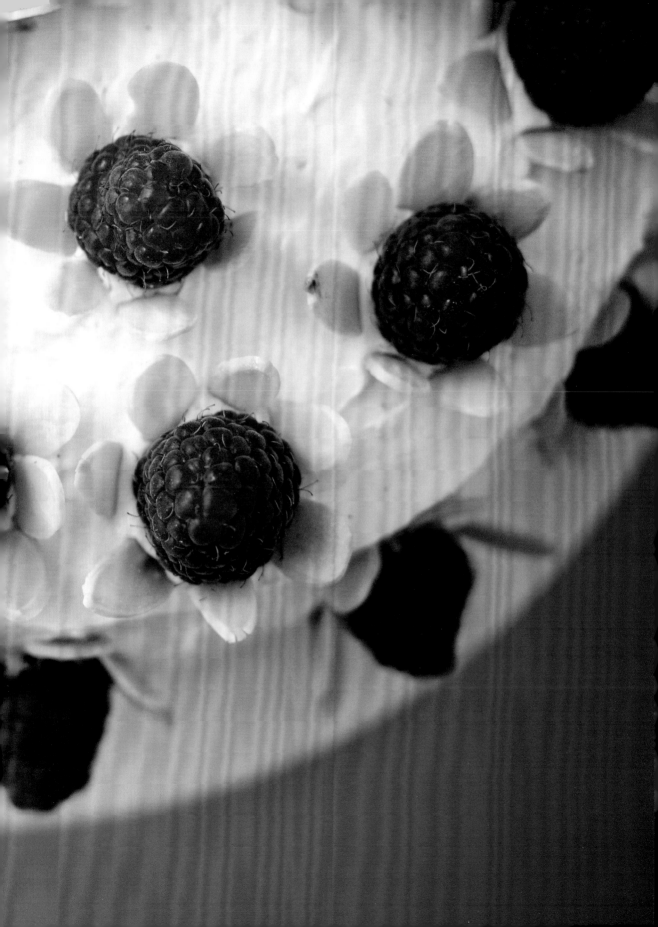

CHOCOLATE, GUINNESS & BLACKCURRANT CAKE

To the slightly older folk reading this book: ever been a young 20-something drinking Guinness and blackcurrant in your local pub? If you enjoyed the drink in the glass, then you will like it even more in this cake.

Serves
12

Equipment
4 x 20cm sandwich tins, food processor

Sponge
Spray oil
100ml Guinness
175g unsalted butter
1 tsp instant coffee granules
200g soft light brown sugar
75g cocoa powder, sifted
200g low-fat crème fraîche
5 eggs
Seeds of 1 vanilla pod or 1 tsp vanilla extract
300g self-raising flour
150g wholemeal flour
2 tsp baking powder

100g reduced-sugar blackcurrant jam

Filling
400g low-fat cream cheese
100g light sour cream
3 tbsp icing sugar, sifted
Seeds of 1 vanilla pod or 1 tsp vanilla extract

To serve
100g blackberries

Preheat the oven to 180°C, (Fan 160°C), 350°F, Gas Mark 4. Grease four 20cm sandwich tins with a little spray oil, line the base with baking parchment and set aside on two baking sheets. If you only have two sandwich tins you can just cook this in two batches.

Heat the Guinness, butter and coffee together in a large pan over a medium heat until the butter has melted. Then, remove from the heat, and stir through the sugar and cocoa followed by the crème fraîche, eggs and vanilla seeds or extract to give a smooth and glossy, chocolaty liquid. Finally, add the flours and baking powder and give it a good mix until well blended.

Divide the mixture evenly between the four tins, levelling the top with the back of a spoon (or just use half the mixture to fill two for now if you are working in two batches). Bake for 15–18 minutes or until the sponge is springy to the touch and a knife comes out clean when inserted into the centre. Swap the trays around on the shelves halfway through cooking to ensure an even cook and rise.

Meanwhile, mix the jam in a small bowl with 3 tablespoons of boiling water until well blended, and set aside. (You can sieve out the seeds if you want to at this stage, but I usually leave them in.)

Next, prepare the filling. Beat the cream cheese, sour cream, icing sugar and vanilla seeds or extract in a large bowl until well blended. Cover and refrigerate until ready to use.

Once the sponges are baked, remove them from the oven and spread a quarter of the jam mixture over each one. Then, if you have four cake tins, leave them to cool in the tin. If you have two cake tins, just leave the cakes until cool enough to handle before carefully removing them from the tin. Grease and re-line the tins with fresh baking parchment, pour in the remaining batter and cook as before. Again, spread them with the jam mixture once they are cooked.

Once all your cakes are cool, lay them out on a clean surface. Spoon a quarter of the cream cheese filling on top of each one and spread it out evenly with a palette knife. Keeping the prettiest one for the top, stack the four cakes on top of each other on a serving plate or cake stand, then scatter the top with the blackberries. This is a simple but stunning cake which will look just as amazing when it is cut into, showing off all those layers.

(PER SERVING)	ENERGY	FAT	SAT FAT	SUGAR	PROTEIN	SALT
LORRAINE'S RECIPE	456 Kcal	23.6g	13.7g	25.2g	11.9g	1.07g
COMPARISON RECIPE	663 Kcal	41.4g	25.3g	51.7g	6.6g	1.04g

RASPBERRY PISTACHIO NAPOLEONS WITH VANILLA CRÈME FRAÎCHE CHANTILLY

I interchange the words 'Napoleon' and 'Mille-feuille', although I am sure a food historian would prove me wrong on this somehow. But despite the hole in my French patisserie knowledge, I know these Napoleons are very much a lighter way to bake. Traditionally made with puff pastry, filo has taken over in this version – not so much a thousand layers (which is what *Mille-feuille* means) but more like a dozen crispy crunchy layers with all the taste and (almost half) the fat.

Makes
8

Pastry
4½ sheets of filo pastry, defrosted
1 tbsp icing sugar, plus a little extra for serving

Edible glue
4 tbsp rapeseed oil
2 tbsp honey

Crème fraîche Chantilly
350g low-fat crème fraîche
50g icing sugar, sifted
Seeds of 1 vanilla pod or 1 tsp vanilla extract

Filling
600g raspberries
75g shelled pistachios, roughly chopped (you can buy them green – don't use the white ones in the shells)

Preheat the oven to 200°C, (Fan 180°C), 400°F, Gas Mark 6. You will need two large, heavy baking sheets and two sheets of baking parchment cut to fit.

Lay the four full sheets of filo on top of each other in a stack and cut them in half across the width. Including the other half of the filo you should now have nine pieces. Lay three pieces of the filo out individually. Mix the oil and honey together in a small bowl and brush a thin layer of it evenly over each piece. Put another sheet of filo directly on top and brush with a little more honey mix. Place the remaining filo sheet on top of this and lightly dust icing sugar evenly over it. You should now have three stacks of three. Using a sharp knife, cut each stack into eight even-sized rectangles of about 12 x 6cm to give 24 in total.

Lay them out on one of the prepared baking sheets. Then, take the other piece of baking parchment and lay this on top of the filo, followed by the second baking sheet on top of this. This will keep the filo flat. Bake in the oven for 20–25 minutes, or until the filo is crisp and golden brown. The filo rectangles near the edges of the baking sheet may start to catch and burn, so remove them ahead of the others if necessary. Handle them carefully, as they can be very brittle. Once cooked, remove from the oven, remove the top tray and paper and leave until completely cool.

Meanwhile, mix the crème fraîche Chantilly ingredients together in a small bowl, using as few stirs as possible so the mixture does not get too thin. Cover with cling film and place in the fridge until ready to use.

When ready to assemble, put a small splodge of the cream on a serving plate and put a filo rectangle down on it. This helps stick it down and secure it in place. Spoon a teaspoon of the cream onto the pastry and spread it out with the back of the spoon. Arrange eight raspberries in two rows on top, pointing upwards, then scatter over a few of the pistachios. Take another filo rectangle, put a small blob of the cream underneath and place this, cream side down, on top of the fruit. Layer that rectangle again with the cream, raspberries and pistachios. Top it off with another rectangle with a blob of cream underneath to stick it down. Sprinkle the top with a little icing sugar and a small scattering of pistachios. Repeat with the remaining ingredients to make eight stacks in total, and serve at once.

(PER SERVING)	ENERGY	FAT	SAT FAT	SUGAR	PROTEIN	SALT
LORRAINE'S RECIPE	328 Kcal	17.3g	5.5g	17.4g	6.6g	0.18g
COMPARISON RECIPE	466 Kcal	35.3g	19.7g	11.7g	5.1g	0.52g

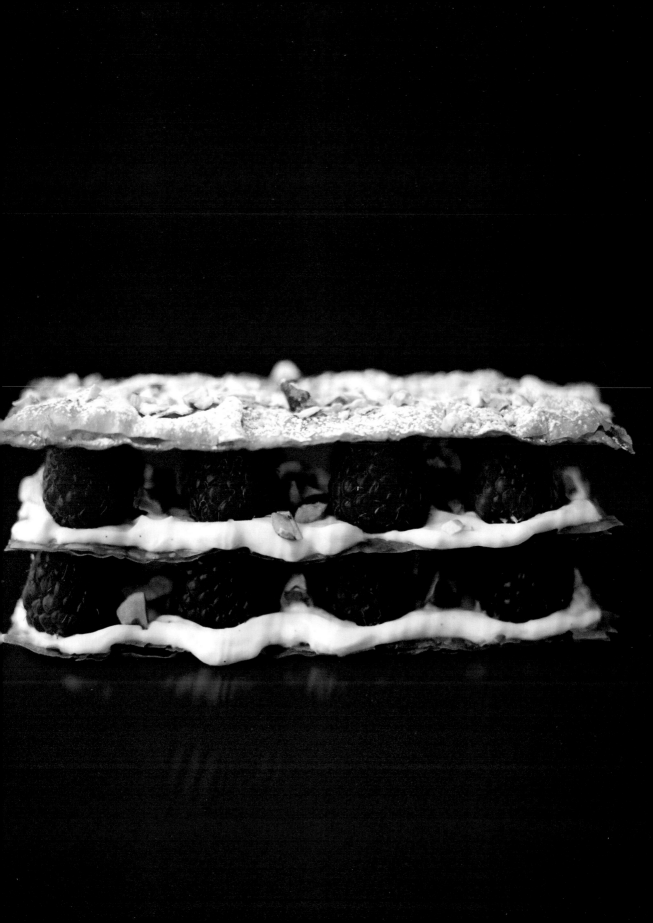

'LET THEM EAT
MORE CAKE',
CAKE WITH
BLUEBERRIES &
WHITE CHOCOLATE
ICING

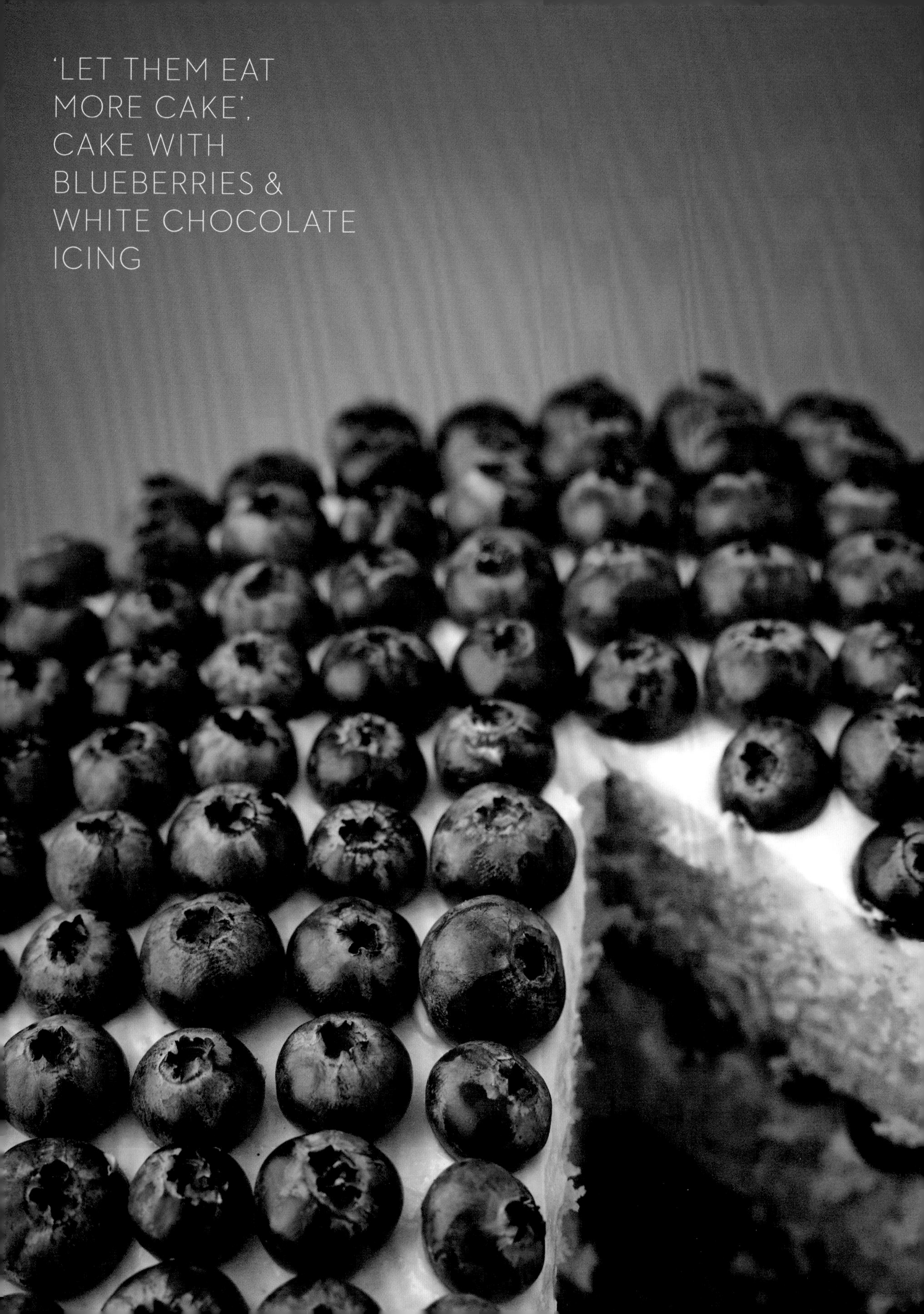

This cake has oodles of wow factor, making it perfect for a celebration.

Serves

10

Equipment

2 x 20cm loose-bottomed sandwich tins

Sponge

Spray oil
125g caster sugar
100g unsalted butter, softened
100g full-fat Greek yogurt
2 eggs, lightly beaten
250g self-raising flour
1 egg white
2 tsp baking powder
Seeds of ½ a vanilla pod or ½ tsp vanilla extract

Icing

75g white chocolate, roughly chopped
300g light cream cheese, at room temperature
2 tbsp icing sugar, sifted
Seeds of ½ a vanilla pod or ½ tsp vanilla extract

Sugar syrup

2 tbsp caster sugar

Topping

600g blueberries

Preheat the oven to 180°C, (Fan 160°C), 350°F, Gas Mark 4, with the middle shelf at the ready. Lightly grease two 20cm loose-bottomed sandwich tins with spray oil and line the base of each with a circle of baking parchment. Set them aside on a baking sheet.

Put the sugar, butter and yogurt into a large bowl and beat like mad. This will not go the way of a usual sponge cake and get light and creamy, but after a couple of minutes it should start to look a little more uniform. Then, add half of the beaten egg and half of the flour and beat it again until smooth. Add the remaining egg and flour, the egg white (whisk it until it is light and frothy before adding to the mix), the baking powder and the vanilla seeds or extract and beat to combine. Divide the cake batter evenly between the two tins, levelling the tops with the back of a spoon. Then place them into the oven to bake for about 20 minutes until the sponge is golden brown and feels springy to the touch.

Meanwhile, prepare the white chocolate icing. Tip the chocolate into a small heatproof bowl. I like to melt chocolate in a microwave in 30-second blasts, stirring between each blast. Alternatively, melt the chocolate in a bowl that just sits on top of a medium pan with a little bit of boiling water. Just make sure the bowl doesn't touch the water as this could make the chocolate grainy. Leave the chocolate to sit until it melts, then set the chocolate aside to cool to room temperature but not set.

Meanwhile, beat the cream cheese, icing sugar and vanilla seeds or extract in a large bowl until smooth. Add a little bit of the cream cheese mixture to the cool melted chocolate and stir together gently. Then fold this white chocolate mixture into the cream cheese mix. I do it this way so that the white chocolate mix does not seize or go all grainy and firm. Cover and refrigerate until ready to use.

Prepare the sugar syrup about 5 minutes before the cake is ready. Simply put the sugar into a mug, add 2 tablespoons of boiling water and stir until dissolved. As soon as the cakes are out of the oven, brush them liberally with the sugar syrup and then leave the cakes to cool in the tin. Once cool, remove them from the tin, peel the paper off and sit one half on the serving plate or cake stand.

Using a palette knife, spread this cake half with a quarter of the icing and then scatter about 100g of the blueberries over. Pop the second cake half on top and spread the remaining icing all over the cake sides and top to give a smoothish finish. Then stick the remaining blueberries all over the cake. Those who have tried my 'Let them eat cake', cake will know that I do like my berries to be nice and straight in a row. Once the cake is completely covered (and admittedly this does take a little time, but I find it very relaxing), serve the cake exultantly… and eat with purpose! If not serving straight away then keep this in the fridge to keep the icing as firm as possible.

(PER SERVING)	ENERGY	FAT	SAT FAT	SUGAR	PROTEIN	SALT
LORRAINE'S RECIPE	373 Kcal	16.7g	9.9g	29.6g	8.2g	0.88g
COMPARISON RECIPE	571 Kcal	39.1g	23.3g	35g	7.4g	0.37g

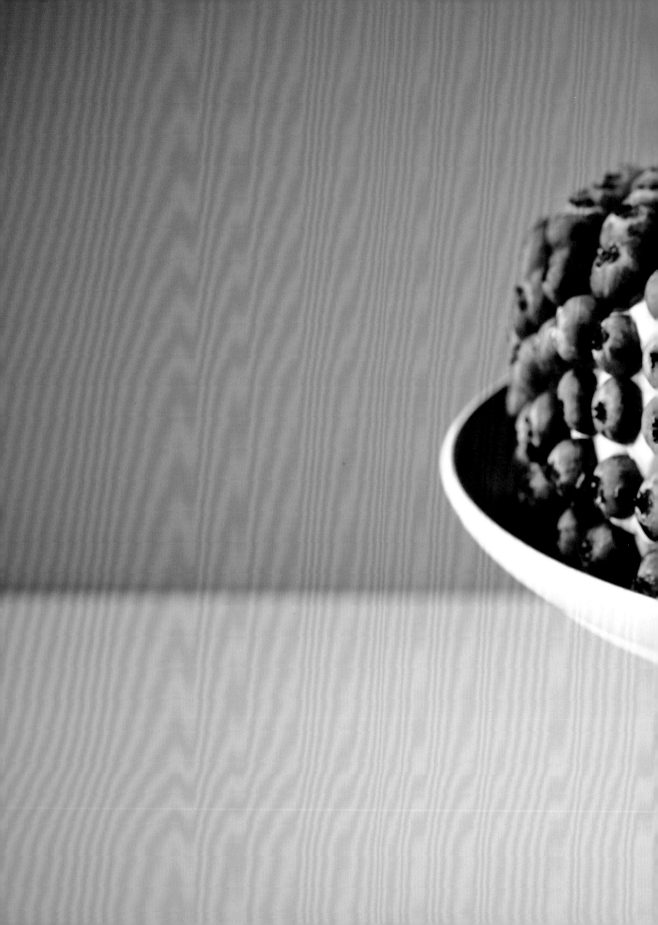

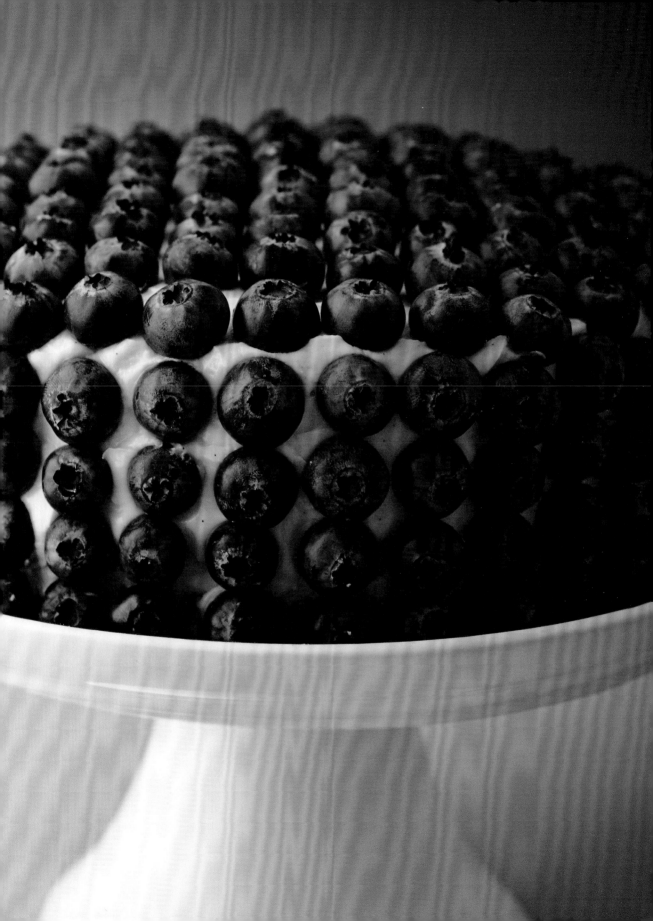

CRISPY FILO MINCE PIES WITH PEAR & APPLE MINCEMEAT

These light bites are made from filo pastry and the mincemeat filling has fresh fruit to replace some of the dried fruit (fresh fruit has a lot less sugar than dried). If you are really craving regular pastry, then just use one of the pastry recipes, such as the one on page 258, to give you a shortcrust pastry crunch. If you do this, the nutritional value on the calories, fat and protein will obviously increase.

Makes
12 mince pies

Equipment
12-hole muffin tin

Spray oil
12 sheets of filo pastry, defrosted
1 egg, lightly beaten
Icing sugar for dusting (optional)

Filling
3 Granny Smith apples, peeled, cored and cut into 1cm chunks
1 perfectly ripe pear, peeled, cored and cut into 1cm chunks
100g raisins
100ml apple juice
75g dried cranberries
50g pecan nuts, finely chopped
2 tsp ground ginger
2 tsp ground cinnamon
Big pinch of ground cloves
Big pinch of freshly grated nutmeg
Seeds of 1 vanilla pod
Finely grated zest of 1 orange
1cm piece of fresh ginger, peeled and very finely chopped
A few twists of cracked black pepper
3 tbsp cider, Calvados, rum or brandy (optional)

To serve (optional)
200g low-fat Greek yogurt
50g icing sugar, sifted
Seeds of 1 vanilla pod or 1 tsp vanilla extract

Preheat the oven to 180°C, (Fan 160°C), 350°F, Gas Mark 4. Place a baking sheet into the oven to heat up. This will give extra bottom heat to the pies so that the bases cook through and are not soggy. Grease a 12-hole muffin tin with a little spray oil and set aside.

Put all of the filling ingredients and the alcohol (if using) into a medium pan over a medium heat. Allow to cook gently, stirring occasionally, for about 10 minutes or until the apples begin to soften. Then remove from the heat and leave the mixture to sit and infuse while you make the pastry cases.

Lay the sheets of filo pastry out on top of each other and cut them in half across the width. Then cut each half into quarters to give eight stacks of about 12cm squares of filo. I find scissors really handy to cut these out, but a sharp knife will do.

Line each hole of the muffin tin with three squares of filo. I like to take a square at a time and press it into the hole, each one slightly staggered from the previous so the resulting pastry case edge looks like a kind of star. Make sure to push the pastry down so it is in the 'corners' of each muffin hole. Keep any filo not being worked on under a lightly dampened tea towel so that it doesn't dry out. After lining the tin, you should still be left with 12 squares of filo, which you can reserve under the damp tea towel for now.

Spray each stack in the tin with a little oil and bake in the oven for 6–8 minutes until crisp and pale golden. Then, divide the filling evenly among the cases. Next, take the remaining squares of filo, scrunch each one up lightly and place one on top of each pie so that it looks like a scrunched-up tissue. Brush them lightly with the beaten egg.

Pop in the oven on the heated baking sheet for 10–12 minutes or until the pies are crisp and golden. While they are baking, prepare the yogurt for serving, if using: gently mix together the yogurt, icing sugar and vanilla in a bowl. Cover and set aside in the fridge until ready to use.

Once ready, remove the pies from the oven, dust with a little icing sugar (if using) and serve with a dollop of the yogurt, if you like.

(PER MINCE PIE)	ENERGY	FAT	SAT FAT	SUGAR	PROTEIN	SALT
LORRAINE'S RECIPE	162 Kcal	4.1g	0.4g	12g	3.2g	0.14g
COMPARISON RECIPE	328 Kcal	16.4g	9.5g	23.2g	3.1g	0.3g

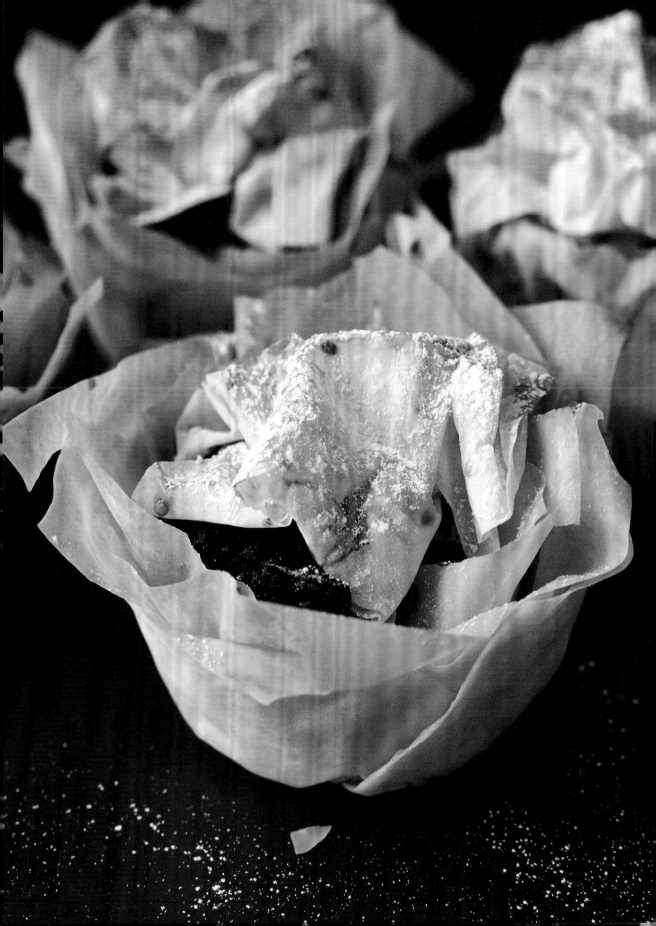

PECAN & MAPLE CHRISTMAS CAKE WITH A CHEEKY DASH OF PORT

This totally tasty Christmas cake will keep for about a week if you put it in a cake tin and then wrap up the cake tin with cling film. Leave it out of the fridge and keep it in a cool dry place.

Serves
20

Equipment
23cm round cake tin, food mixer fitted with the beater attachment, 25cm cake board

Sponge
2 eating apples, peeled, cored and diced into 1cm cubes (to give about 300g)

1 ripe pear, peeled, cored and diced into 1cm cubes (to give about 100g)

75g cranberries

200g raisins

200ml golden rum, port, sherry, brandy or your fave Christmas tipple

Spray oil

100g unsalted butter, softened

150g soft dark brown sugar

2 eggs

1 egg white

200g wholemeal or plain flour

75g pecan nuts, roughly chopped

50g ground almonds

4 tbsp maple syrup

2 knobs of stem ginger, roughly chopped (optional)

2 tsp baking powder

3 tsp mixed spice

Pop the apples, pear, cranberries and raisins into a large bowl. Pour your chosen alcohol over and toss everything together well. If you have time, do this the night before so the fruit can steep while you sleep. But, if you, like me, are a bit of a last-minute Larry then just prepare the fruit at least 30 minutes or so before you are going to bake the cake. The cake will still taste fabulous.

When you are ready to cook, preheat the oven to 150°C, (Fan 130°C), 300°F, Gas Mark 2. Grease a 23cm round cake tin with a little spray oil and then line the bottom and insides with two layers of baking parchment. This prevents the outside of the cake burning while it cooks.

Beat (by hand or machine) the butter and sugar in a large bowl until well mixed together. Then, add the eggs and egg white, one at a time, beating well between each addition. The mix may not look its best at this stage but it will soon come good! Add three-quarters of the wholemeal flour (reserving the remainder for a minute), the pecan nuts, ground almonds, maple syrup, stem ginger (if using), baking powder and mixed spice. Mix everything together really well and set aside.

Drain and reserve the alcohol from your mixed fruit in a small jug. You can use this to 'feed' your cake once it is baked. Toss the remaining flour through the fruit to evenly coat and then stir this through the cake mixture. Coating the fruit in flour will stop it from sinking to the bottom during cooking. Spoon the cake mixture into the prepared tin and smooth the surface with the back of a spoon. Bake the cake in the top of the oven for around 2½ hours or until a skewer inserted into the centre of the cake comes out clean.

As soon as you remove the cake from the oven, use a skewer to poke about 10 holes on the top of it (about a couple of centimetres deep). Then drizzle half of the reserved alcohol over slowly, allowing it to sink down inside. Leave the cake to cool completely in the tin, before removing it and peeling the baking parchment off. Wrap the cake up really well with a layer of cling film followed by tin foil. Then store in an airtight container in a cool, dark place (but not in the fridge, as this will dry it out). Feed the cake with the remaining alcohol a day or two later and wrap up well again until ready to decorate (leave up to a maximum of two weeks).

contd...

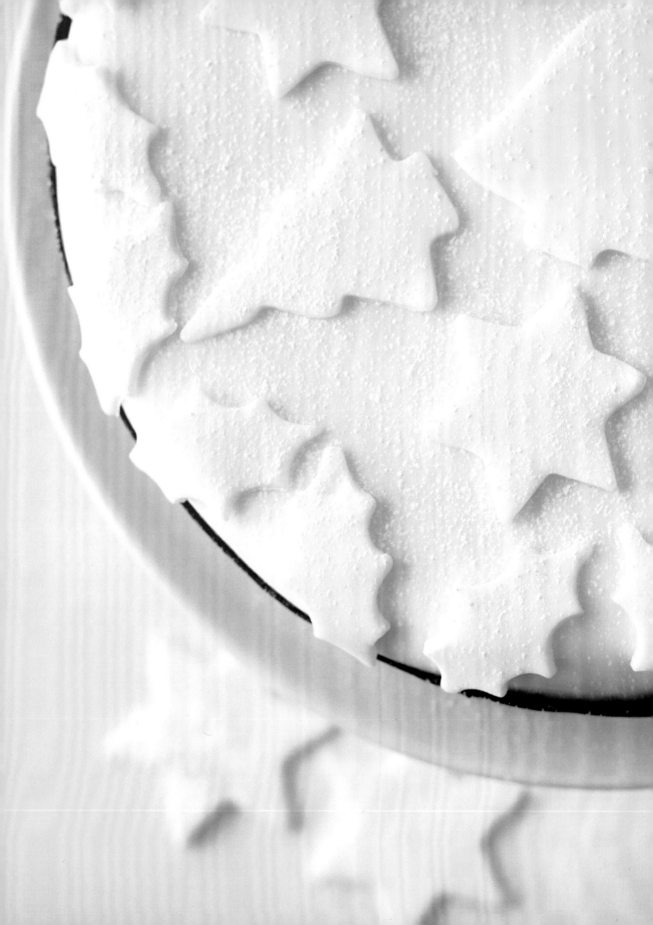

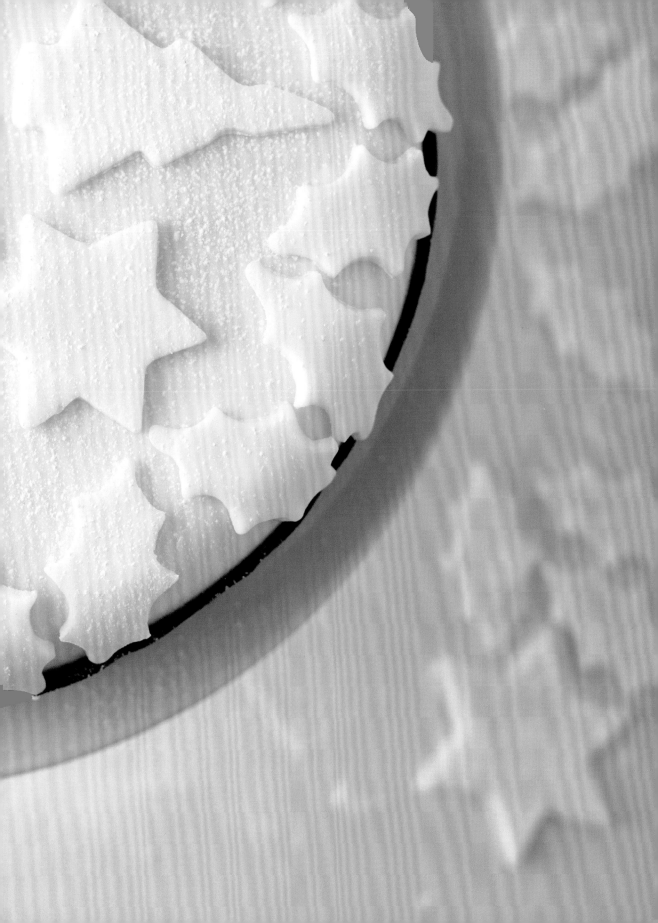

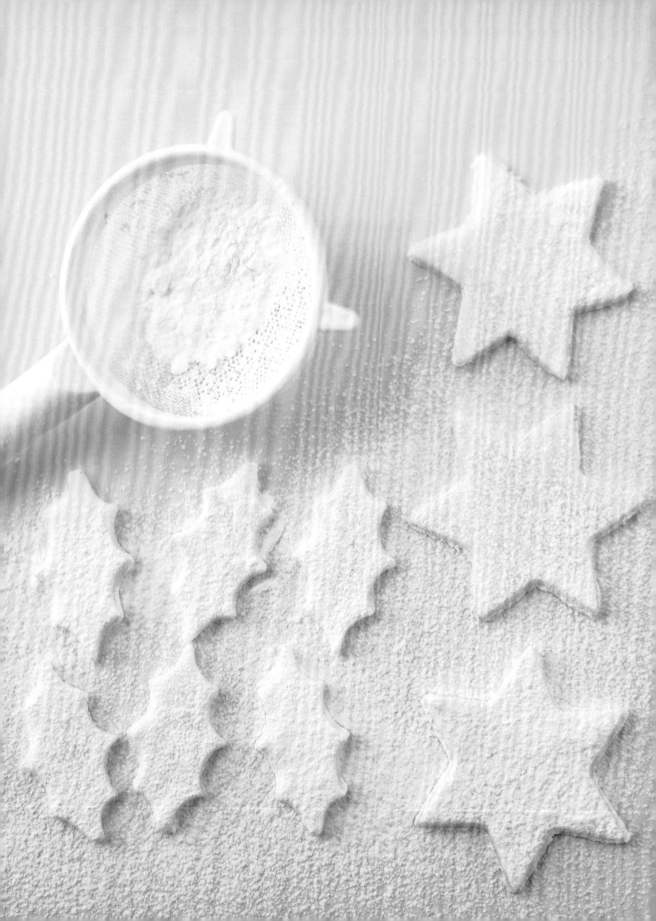

DECORATION FOR THE CHRISTMAS CAKE

Decoration

750g white Regalice/ready-to-roll icing (in the baking section of the supermarket)
2 tbsp maple syrup
Icing sugar for rolling out
500g natural or white marzipan

Brush a 25cm cake board all over with a little maple syrup. Roll out a small handful of the Regalice/ready-to-roll icing on a sheet of baking parchment to a fairly thin 25cm circle, and stick this onto the board. Trim the edges to neaten and brush a little more maple syrup in the centre.

Next, unwrap your cake and sit it, flat side down, on a large flat plate or board. Brush it evenly all over with a little more of the maple syrup.

Then, onto the marzipan. Dust a good amount of icing sugar on a clean work surface. If the marzipan is a bit stiff, knead it for a moment or two to soften it and then roll it out into about a 40cm round, the thickness of a £1 coin. Carefully lift the icing up, draping it over the rolling pin, and then drape it over the cake. Use your hands to smooth the marzipan over the cake, so it is nice and flat. Cut away any excess from around the bottom where it meets the board. Then, brush the marzipan all over with the maple syrup once again and set the cake aside.

If the remaining Regalice/ready-to-roll icing is in more than one block, knead them together on a surface dusted with icing sugar to give one smooth ball. Roll it out in the same way as the marzipan to a 40cm round, again about the thickness of a £1 coin. Drape the icing over the rolling pin, pick it up and then drape it over the cake, smooth well with your hands and then trim off the excess around the bottom to give a good neat finish.

Now, the slightly tricky bit of transferring the iced cake onto the cake board. Without too much fuss, simply slide a wide fish slice underneath and with your other hand supporting one side, quickly pop it onto the centre of the cake board. Or, sometimes I get brave and simply grab it gently from both sides with the palms of my hands and lift it on that way. Either way, any damage to the icing can be easily smoothed out by rubbing the palms of your hands over it.

Then, the final fun bit. Use festive-shaped cookie cutters to cut shapes out of any remaining icing and stick them onto the cake with a little maple syrup brushed onto the back of them.

Tie a ribbon around the cake to finish and then store in an airtight container until you are ready to serve. As this cake is not as rich as your usual Christmas cake it will probably only keep for a week or so.

(PER SERVING)	ENERGY	FAT	SAT FAT	SUGAR	PROTEIN	SALT
LORRAINE'S RECIPE	455 Kcal	12.3g	3.4g	75.9g	5.2g	0.23g
COMPARISON RECIPE	512 Kcal	17.5g	9.6g	76.7g	4.5g	0.40g

LIGHTER CHRISTMAS PUDDING WITH GROUND ALMONDS & SPICE

This is the ultimate Christmas showstopper – I remember many a Christmas with the pud being brought from the kitchen with its dancing blue flame on top. I loved and still love the drama of it all, but always found that puddings can just be so rich and heavy. This is easier to make lighter than many recipes – just limit the amount of dried fruit, which is rich in sugar, and in its place put fresh fruit (and carrots, which are quite sweet). Fresh fruit still has lots of sugar in but a whole lot less than dried, so the carb content and calorie content have been greatly reduced. I am hoping you and the family will enjoy this at your leisure! If you choose to flame the pudding with booze for serving, then it's best to set the pudding on a deep plate to catch the alcohol as it pours off. That way the flames stay there too! Please be careful when doing this. Due to its lightness the cake will be a little crumbly on the inside, and will only last for around a week once cooked.

Serves
8

Equipment
1.2 litre pudding basin, food mixer fitted with the beater attachment

Pudding
Spray oil
100g unsalted butter
100g soft dark brown sugar
225g wholemeal flour
2 eggs
1 egg white
1 large carrot, peeled and roughly grated (to give about 100g)
1 large eating apple, peeled, cored and roughly grated (to give about 100g)
100g raisins
50g ground almonds
3 tsp baking powder
3 tsp mixed spice
1cm piece of fresh ginger, peeled and finely grated
Finely grated zest of 1 orange
Seeds of 1 vanilla pod or 1 tsp vanilla extract
Pinch of salt

Preheat the oven to 170°C, (Fan 150°C), 325°F, Gas Mark 3. Use a little spray oil to grease a 1.2 litre pudding basin and set aside.

Beat (by hand or machine) the butter and sugar in a large bowl until well mixed together. Add half of the flour and the whole eggs and mix well. Then, add the remaining flour, the egg white, carrot, apple, raisins, ground almonds, baking powder, mixed spice, ginger, orange zest, vanilla seeds or extract and salt. Stir everything together until well combined. Dollop the mixture into the pudding basin and level the top with the back of a spoon.

Put a kettle full of water on to boil. Sit a trivet or upturned heatproof small plate in the bottom of a large, deep pan (wide and deep enough to take the pudding basin comfortably). Pour a few centimetres of the boiled water into the bottom of the pan, pop a tight fitting lid on and set it over a medium to high heat.

Cover the top of the pudding basin with foil, making sure that the covering is airtight but leaves a little bit of room for the pudding to grow. Tie the tin foil down with string by running it all the way around the rim of the basin. Leave one of the ends of string long enough to go across the top of the pudding to form a handle, tying it down on the opposite side. This will be handy for lifting the pudding out of the pan of water. Carefully lower the pudding basin into the pan. Make sure the water comes halfway up the sides of the basin, adding a little more water from the kettle if necessary. Allow it to come back to the boil before reducing the heat to a simmer. Pop the lid back on and leave to cook for 1 hour 45 minutes or until a skewer inserted into a centre part of the pudding comes out clean. Carefully remove the pudding from the pan when checking and wrap it back up well if returning. It's also important to remember to top the water up regularly during cooking to avoid it drying out and burning.

Brandy cream

150g low-fat cream cheese
3 tbsp brandy
1 squidge (about 25ml) honey or
  maple syrup

Topping

100ml brandy, rum or whisky

Meanwhile to make the brandy cream, simply mix all of the ingredients together in a small bowl until well blended. Cover and set aside in the fridge until ready to use.

Once the pudding is cooked, leave it to cool for a few moments in the basin. Then, run a small sharp knife all around the edge of the pudding to loosen it. Put your deep serving plate (see intro) upside down over the top of the basin and then, holding onto both (using oven gloves if the pudding basin is still too hot), flip the whole thing over so that the plate is on the bottom and the pudding basin is upside down. Then carefully remove the basin to reveal the lovely pudding.

When you are ready to serve the pudding, slowly pour your chosen alcohol over the top. Carefully light it with a match and then go and show off your Christmas centrepiece showstopper!

(PER SERVING - PUDDING ONLY)	ENERGY	FAT	SAT FAT	SUGAR	PROTEIN	SALT
LORRAINE'S RECIPE	337 Kcal	16.3g	7.4g	24.7g	7.8g	0.62g
COMPARISON RECIPE	375 Kcal	13.4g	4.6g	50g	6.1g	0.45g

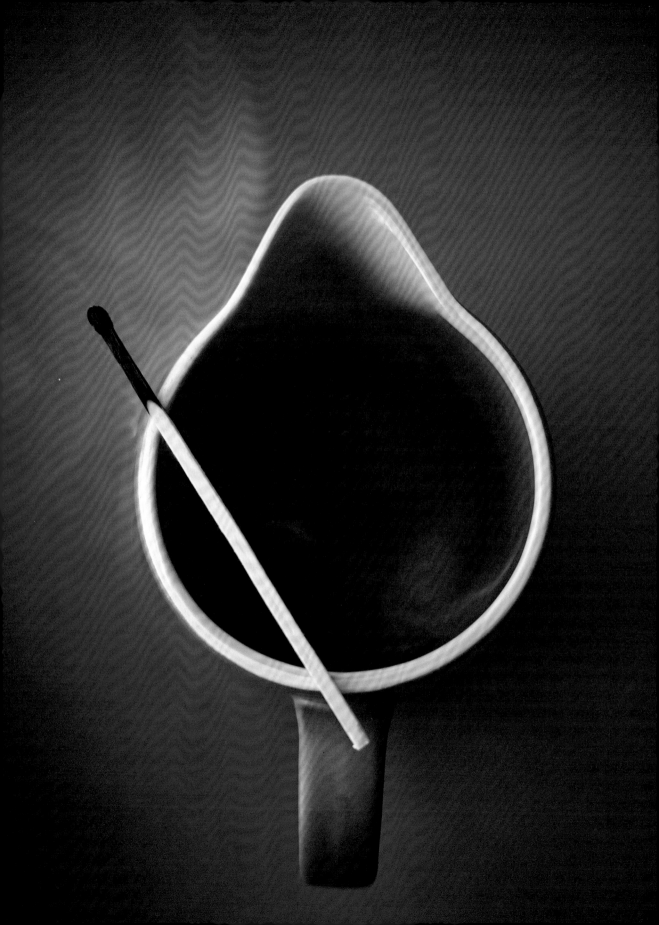

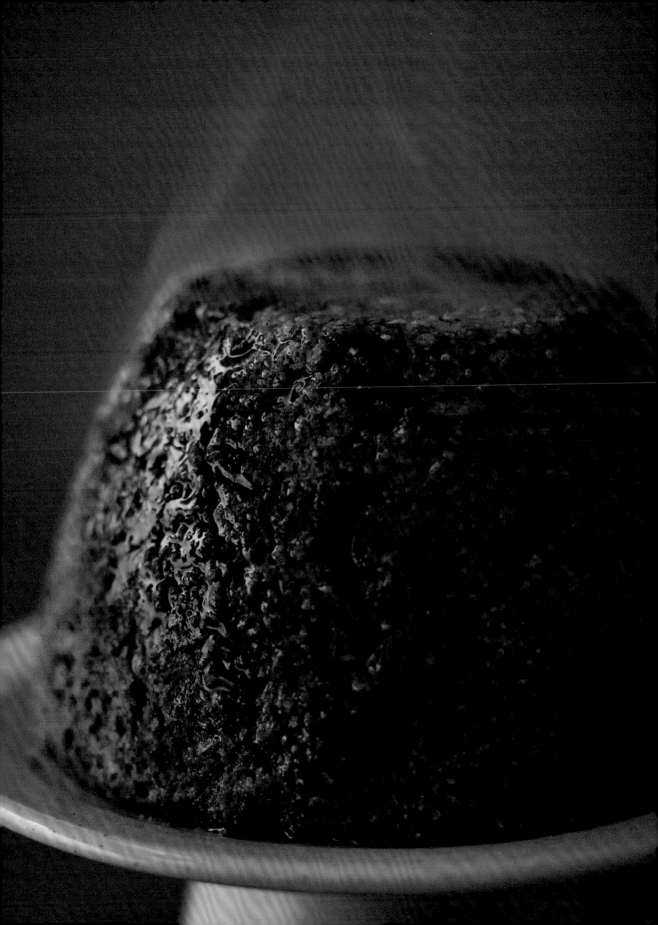

CHRISTMAS CHOCKY YULE LOG

Christmas pudding, Christmas cake, mince pies and all the chocolate strewn around the house at Christmas – it is a wonder we can make any more room for something sweet. In our house we usually have a Christmas cake and a yule log. The yule log is mainly for the young ones who do not yet eat the heavy fruit cake. There are a fair amount of 'parts' to this cake – making the sponge and rolling it up, and then making the sugar syrup and filling – but I have tried to make it as simple as possible, so it's a little bit fiddly but still easy. The pomegranate seeds on top provide nice colour and good texture, but dried cranberries can be used in their place if you see fit.

Makes

12 skinny (but very rich) slices

Equipment

20.5 x 31cm Swiss roll tin, food processor

Sponge

Spray oil
50g soft light brown sugar
1 tbsp instant coffee granules
3 eggs
1 egg whites
Seeds of 1 vanilla pod or 1 tsp vanilla extract
25g wholemeal flour
50g self-raising flour
25g cocoa powder, sifted
1 tsp baking powder
Pinch of salt

Ganache

100g dark chocolate (minimum 70% cocoa solids)
50g milk chocolate
200g low-fat cream cheese, at room temperature
75ml semi-skimmed milk, at room temperature
25g icing sugar, sifted

contd...

Preheat the oven to 190°C, (Fan 170°C), 375°F, Gas Mark 5. Lightly grease a 20.5 x 31cm Swiss roll tin with spray oil and line with baking parchment. I just cut a long strip of paper to cover the bottom and come up on opposite sides of the tin and leave the excess hanging over a little – this makes it easier to lift the baked cake out of the tin.

Blitz the sugar and coffee in a food processor for a few seconds to give a finely chopped mixture. This is really worth doing to help bring out the coffee flavour in the cake.

Put the whole eggs, egg whites and vanilla seeds or extract in a large bowl. Whisk for a good 3–4 minutes until the eggs are mousse-like and have increased in size somewhat. Add the coffee-sugar mixture gradually in stages and keep whisking for another 3–4 minutes or so. To test if the eggs are whisked up enough, take a spoonful of the mixture and drop it back into the bowl. The egg mix should sit on the surface for a second before it disappears back into the mixture. This is called 'to the ribbon' and means you will have a lovely fluffy cake.

Lightly scatter the flours, cocoa powder, baking powder and salt over the top and use a spatula to fold everything in very gently, while trying to retain all of that air which has been whisked into it. I like to use a spatula to really get underneath the mixture, as flour often falls to the bottom of the bowl. Gently pour the mixture into the Swiss roll tin from a low height so you don't knock any air out, and level out with a palette knife or the back of a spoon. Bake in the oven for 10 minutes or until the sponge is springy to the touch and has slightly shrunk away from the sides of the tin. Then remove from the oven and leave to cool completely in the tin.

Meanwhile, make the ganache for filling and coating the yule log. Tip the dark and milk chocolate into a small heatproof bowl. I like to melt chocolate in a microwave in 30-second blasts, stirring between each blast. Alternatively, melt the chocolate in a bowl that just sits on top of a medium pan with a little bit of boiling water. Just make sure the bowl doesn't touch the water as this could make the chocolate grainy. Leave the chocolate to sit until it melts, then give it a stir, then set the chocolate aside to cool to room temperature but not set.

contd...

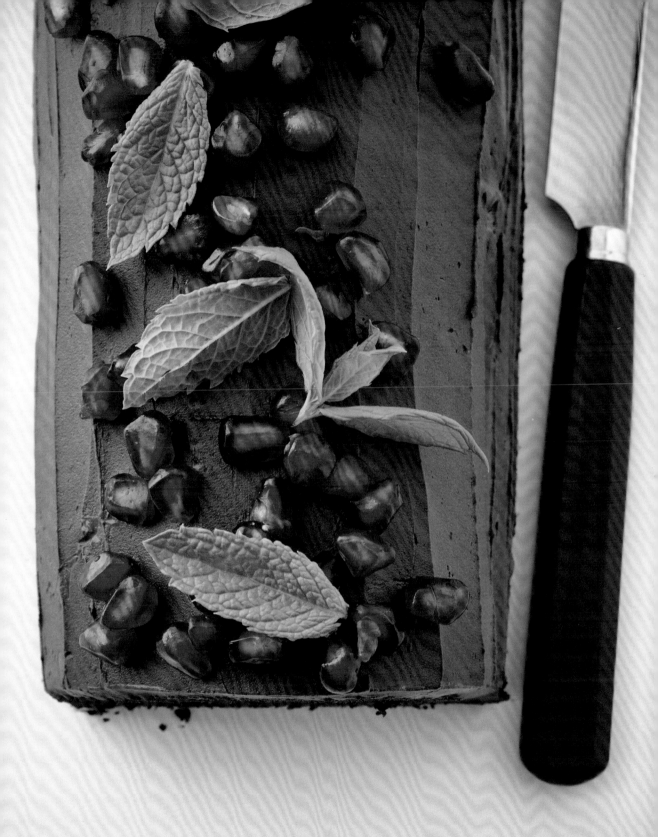

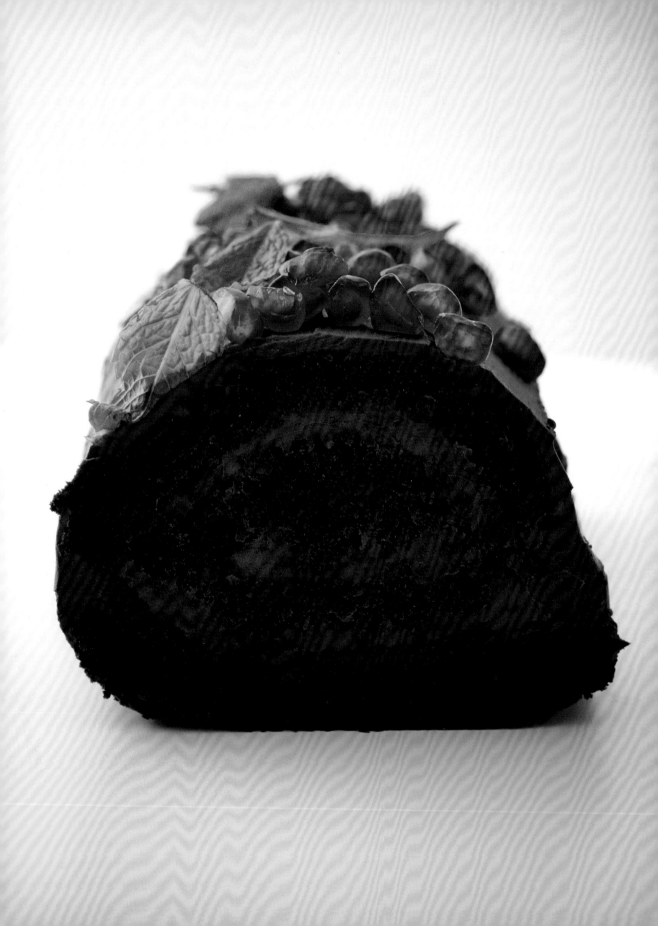

Sugar syrup

2 tbsp caster sugar

Decoration (optional)

2 tbsp pomegranate seeds
Small handful of fresh mint leaves

Once the chocolate has cooled, beat in the cream cheese and milk, mixing well to combine, and then add the icing sugar to taste, mixing until it is uniform. Set aside until ready to use.

When the Swiss roll is almost cool, make the sugar syrup. Put the sugar in a small pan with 2 tablespoons of water over a low heat and stir until the sugar dissolves. Then turn up the heat and let it bubble away for 30–60 seconds until syrupy, before removing from the heat.

Once the Swiss roll is cool, put a piece of baking parchment a little larger than the Swiss roll tin down on the work surface. Lift the cake out of the tin and flip it top side down on the sheet of paper. If the sponge is a bit stuck around the edges of the tin, just carefully run a small sharp knife around the inside edge to release it. Peel the paper off the base of the sponge, which is now facing upwards, and brush the surface all over with the sugar syrup.

Then, with one of the shorter sides facing you, roll the Swiss roll up and away from you. This pre-roll, as I call it, will make the cake more pliable and will help it stay in shape once it is rolled again in a minute. So, unroll it again and then spread the cake with half of the chocolate ganache. Then, again with one of the shorter sides facing you, roll the first bit of the Swiss roll up. It is really good to get the first bit of the roll nice and tight. Roll the whole thing up quite tight and don't worry about anything squidging around the sides.

Dust the plate with some icing sugar and then place the Swiss roll, seam side down, on a serving plate and spread the remaining ganache over the top and sides (but not the twirled ends). Make a tree-bark-type effect on it with a knife or fork. If you are using them, arrange the pomegranate seeds and mint leaves on top. Serve at once, cut into 12 slices.

(PER SLICE)	ENERGY	FAT	SAT FAT	SUGAR	PROTEIN	SALT
LORRAINE'S RECIPE	173 Kcal	7.9g	4.3g	16.3g	5.5g	0.3g
COMPARISON RECIPE	278 Kcal	17.5g	10g	23.3g	4.4g	0.16g

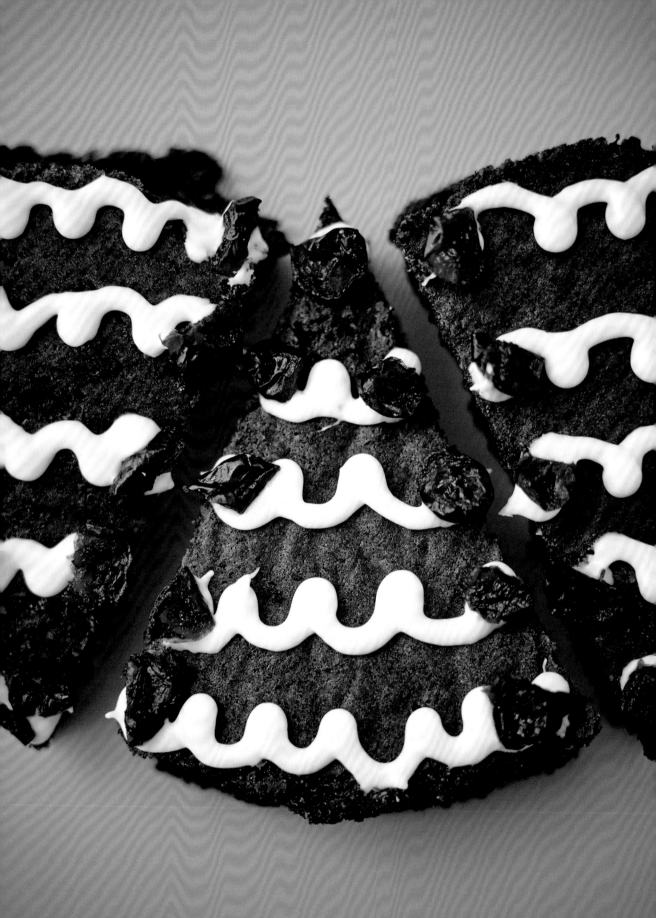

CHOCOLATE & GINGERBREAD CHRISTMAS TREE

Deck the halls with boughs of holly... And make sure there's a good stash of brownies somewhere around too!

Makes

10 Christmas trees

Equipment

20cm round, loose-bottomed cake tin, electric whisk, disposable piping bag

Brownies

Spray oil
100g unsalted butter
75g dark chocolate (minimum 70% cocoa solids), roughly chopped
75g milk chocolate, roughly chopped
3 eggs
2 egg whites
75g soft dark brown sugar
75g wholemeal flour
1 tbsp ground ginger
1 tsp bicarbonate of soda
½ tsp ground cinnamon
Pinch of ground cloves

Decoration

50g white chocolate, roughly chopped
2 tbsp dried cranberries, halved

Preheat the oven to 180°C, (Fan 160°C), 350°F, Gas Mark 4. Grease a 20cm round, loose-bottomed cake tin with a little spray oil, line the base with a disc of baking parchment and set aside on a baking sheet.

Melt the butter in a medium pan over a gentle heat. Then remove from the heat, add the dark and milk chocolate and set aside for the chocolate to melt.

Meanwhile, put the eggs and egg whites into a large bowl and whisk until they go really light, fluffy and foam-like. They will go quite a bit lighter in colour, too. It is best to use an electric whisk for this as it will take a good few minutes. Then, continuing to whisk all the time, add the sugar in three batches. It is important to add the sugar gradually so that it can dissolve before you add the next batch. The mixture should increase in volume a little bit to give a thick, smooth, foamy mixture.

The chocolate should now be melted, so give it a stir to combine the mixture. Pour this chocolate mixture into the eggs around the edges of the bowl rather than the middle so you don't knock out any of the air that you have just whisked into it. Scatter the flour, ginger, bicarb, cinnamon and ground cloves over and carefully fold everything together. The butter and the flour are heavier than the eggs and so they do sink to the bottom sometimes. I use a spatula to scoop everything off the bottom of the bowl and to make sure it is all (well, mostly) combined.

Gently pour the mixture into the prepared tin from a low height and spread it evenly with a palette knife or the back of a spoon to make sure it is level. Bake in the oven for 25–30 minutes, or until the cake is springy to the touch and a skewer inserted into a centre part of the cake comes out clean. Once baked, remove from the oven and leave to cool in the tin.

Once cool, carefully remove from the tin and cut in half across the centre. Cut each half into five equal-sized wedges. Each of these are your Christmas trees. Arrange them on a wire rack sitting on a tray and set aside.

Melt the chocolate for the decoration. I like to melt chocolate in a microwave in 30-second blasts, stirring between each blast. Alternatively, melt it in a bowl that just sits on top of a medium pan with a little bit of boiling water. Just make sure the bowl doesn't touch the water as this could make the chocolate grainy. Leave the chocolate to sit until it melts, then give it a stir.

Spoon the melted chocolate into a small icing bag, snip the end and drizzle over the brownie wedges like tinsel on a Christmas tree. Stick the cranberry pieces onto the chocolate tinsel to look like baubles on the tree and hey presto – Happy Christmas!

(PER TREE)	ENERGY	FAT	SAT FAT	SUGAR	PROTEIN	SALT
LORRAINE'S RECIPE	272 Kcal	16.4g	9.3g	22.4g	5.2g	0.41g
COMPARISON RECIPE	333 Kcal	20.8g	12.3g	30.9g	3.9g	0.43g

CASHEW, CRANBERRY & SPICE BISCOTTI

Cranberries and spice make a classic Christmas combination, but pretty much any other nuts and fruit can be used in place of my suggestions. I do love a cashew, but runners-up in the flavour stakes, and perfect for this recipe, would be pecans or macadamias, although of course the nutritional count will vary. Prettily wrapped, these make a lovely home-made Christmas present.

Makes

30 biscotti

100g wholemeal flour
100g self-raising flour, plus extra for dusting
75g soft light brown sugar
75g dried cranberries
75g cashew nuts (raw and unsalted), roughly chopped
1 tsp bicarbonate of soda
1 tsp baking powder
1 tsp ground cinnamon
1 tsp mixed spice
Pinch of salt
2 eggs
Seeds of 1 vanilla pod or 1 tsp vanilla extract

Preheat the oven to 170°C, (Fan 150°C), 325°F, Gas Mark 3. Line a large baking sheet with baking parchment.

Toss the flours in a large bowl with the sugar, cranberries, cashew nuts, bicarb, baking powder, cinnamon, mixed spice and salt. Then, make a well in the centre and add the eggs and vanilla seeds or extract and mix everything together well. It will start to lump together, but then get your hands in and really squidge it all together to form a dough ball.

On a lightly floured surface, roll the ball out into a sausage shape about 30cm long and 5cm wide. Carefully lift it up and transfer it to the baking sheet. Then, squidge it down gently so it becomes 8cm wide and about 1½ cm high.

Bake in the oven for 30 minutes, until firm and a knife pierced into the centre comes out clean. Remove and leave it until it is cool enough to handle. Then, using a fish slice, carefully lift it from the baking sheet onto a chopping board. Using a sharp serrated-edge knife, cut 30 x 1cm-thick slightly slanted slices. Do this by leaning the blade of the knife back slightly so that it is at an angle. Some bits may crumble off a bit as you cut, but that is okay. I just slice really slowly holding the biscotti 'log' with the other hand. Any bits that fall off are a nice chef's perk! Arrange the biscotti slices lying flat on the baking sheet and return them to the oven to bake for 40 minutes, turning them over halfway through. Once cooked, they should be super-crisp and firm as these are essentially doubled-baked.

When the biscottis are ready, remove from the oven and leave to cool completely. For me these are best served dunked in a cup of something hot.

(PER BISCOTTI)	ENERGY	FAT	SAT FAT	SUGAR	PROTEIN	SALT
LORRAINE'S RECIPE	59 Kcal	1.8g	0.4g	4.4g	1.7g	0.19g
COMPARISON RECIPE	67 Kcal	1.8g	0.2g	6.7g	1.2g	0.40g

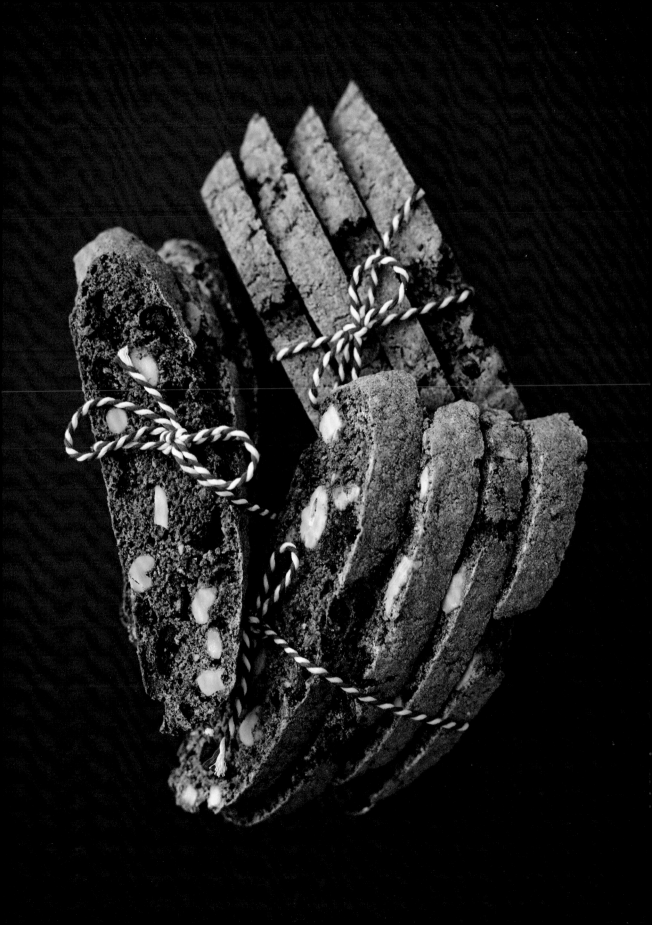

IT DOES NOT MATTER HOW SLOWLY YOU
GO AS LONG AS YOU DO NOT STOP.
CONFUCIUS

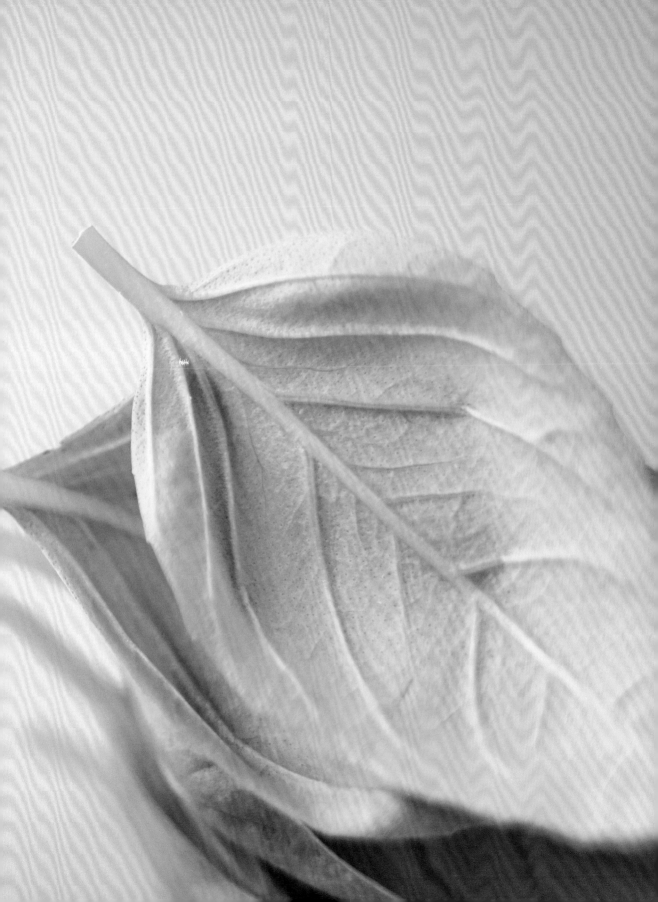

PASTRY
& BASICS

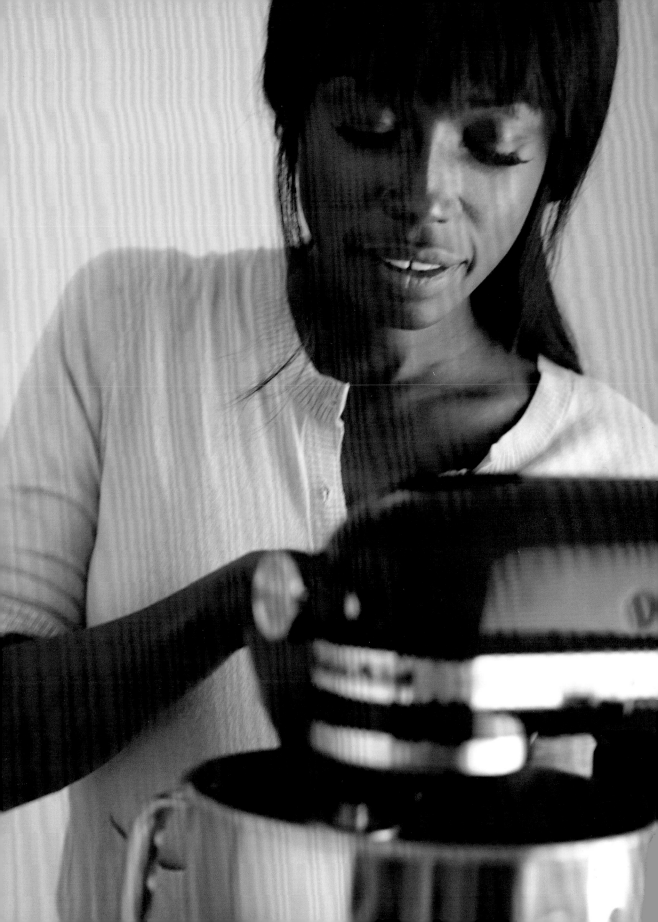

SWEET HONEY SHORTCRUST PASTRY

I have made shortcrust pastry more times than I can count and wanted to develop a recipe with a little something extra. I usually start with the base of one of my other recipes, so in this case the shortcrust, and then try to think of ways to make it different to what I have seen before. Sweetened pastry really is nothing new, but I wondered what else I could sweeten it with to give a different flavour. I started to go through the cupboards for inspiration and then, sitting in a pool of its own stickiness (as honey so often does), it came to me, and I squealed, 'Why did I not think of that before?' So a lovely squidge of honey sweetens the pastry and gives a softer taste than just using regular sugar. Use this as a very tasty base for tarts and sweet flans.

Makes
400g pastry

Equipment
Large bowl or food processor

225g white spelt flour (plain flour will work also), plus extra for dusting
75g unsalted butter
Pinch of salt
1 squidge of honey (about 20g)
1 egg
1–2 tbsp water

Put all of the ingredients in a food processor and blitz them until the mixture begins to clump together.

Alternatively, to make by hand, put the flour and butter into a large bowl. Pick up bits of the mixture with the tips of your fingers and rub your thumbs into your fingers to blend the ingredients together, allowing them to fall back into the bowl. Keep doing this until the mixture resembles fine breadcrumbs. Stir the salt through and add the honey. Lightly beat the egg in a small bowl and stir into the crumbs really well with a small knife until it starts to form lumps. Add 1 tablespoon of the water to bring it together, adding the remaining tablespoon if the dough is still a little dry.

Dust a clean surface with a little flour. Tip the dough onto the surface and squidge the mixture with your hands so it comes together in a ball. Knead lightly for a few seconds until smooth, flatten into a disc shape and then wrap with cling film. Refrigerate for at least 20 minutes to relax and firm up.

Remove the dough from the fridge and use as needed.

(PER SERVING – 8 PORTIONS)	ENERGY	FAT	SAT FAT	SUGAR	PROTEIN	SALT
LORRAINE'S RECIPE	184 Kcal	8.9g	5.1g	2g	5g	0.07g
COMPARISON RECIPE	214 Kcal	11.3g	6.1g	11.1g	3.4g	0.05g

OATY ALMOND & VANILLA PASTRY

Making a decent pastry with all the taste but a little lighter was not the easiest of tasks. I cut down the butter and added some wholemeal flour, which made a perfectly good pastry. I felt it could do with something extra to add to the wholesome stakes so a good amount of oats gave the pastry added body, added texture and a good nutty flavour. Use this pastry for both sweet and savoury dishes.

Makes
425g pastry

Equipment
Large bowl or food processor

100g wholemeal or wholemeal spelt flour, plus extra for dusting
100g plain flour
50g rolled oats
50g ground almonds
Pinch of salt
50g unsalted butter
Seeds of 1 vanilla pod or 1 tsp vanilla extract
1 egg
3 tbsp cold water

Put all of the ingredients in a food processor and blitz them until the mixture begins to clump together.

Alternatively, to make by hand, put the flours, oats, almonds, salt, butter and vanilla into a large bowl. Pick up bits of the mixture with the tips of your fingers and rub your thumb into your fingers to blend the ingredients together, allowing it to fall back into the bowl. Keep doing this until the mixture resembles fine breadcrumbs. Add the egg and water, stirring really well with a small knife until it starts to form lumps. Scrape the side of the bowl down in case some of the egg or water has stuck there.

Dust a clean surface with a little flour. Tip the dough onto the surface and squidge the mixture with your hands so it comes together in a ball. Knead lightly for a few seconds until smooth and then wrap with cling film. Refrigerate for 20 minutes to relax and firm up.

Remove the dough from the fridge and use as needed.

(PER SERVING – 8 PORTIONS)	ENERGY	FAT	SAT FAT	SUGAR	PROTEIN	SALT
LORRAINE'S RECIPE	205 Kcal	10.4g	3.8g	0.7g	6g	0.01g
COMPARISON RECIPE	237 Kcal	14.2g	7.9g	2.1g	4.3g	0.74g

RICH, SWEET WHOLEMEAL SHORTCRUST PASTRY

Shortcrust, by its very definition, contains lots of butter. I tried with less and less fat, but it just does not work well for a true shortcrust. Using wholemeal flour gives a wholesome alternative. The pastry goes quite dark when cooked, but gives a nice snap!

Makes
400g pastry

Equipment
Large bowl or food processor

225g wholemeal flour, plus extra
  for dusting
100g unsalted butter
1 tbsp caster sugar
1 egg yolk
3–4 tbsp water

Put all of the ingredients (using 3 tablespoons of the water) into a food processor and blitz them up until the mixture starts to form clumps. Use a knife to scrape off any bits of dough which are stuck to the sides and the bottom of the food processor and blitz again. If the dough is still very dry, just add the remaining water. Try not to add too much otherwise the pastry will just shrink when it bakes and be very grey and tasteless.

Alternatively, to make by hand, put the flour and butter into a large bowl. Pick up bits of the mixture with the tips of your fingers and rub your thumb into your fingers to blend the ingredients together, allowing it to fall back into the bowl. Keep doing this until the mixture resembles fine breadcrumbs. Stir in the sugar, then add the egg yolk and 3 tablespoons of the water and stir in really well with a small knife until it starts to form lumps. Add the remaining tablespoon of water, if necessary, to bring it together. Scrape the side of the bowl down in case some of the egg or water has stuck there.

Dust a clean surface with a little flour. Tip the dough onto the surface and squidge the mixture with your hands so it comes together in a ball. Knead lightly for a few seconds until smooth and then wrap with cling film. Refrigerate for 20 minutes to relax and firm up.

Remove the dough from the fridge and use as needed.

(PER SERVING – 8 PORTIONS)	ENERGY	FAT	SAT FAT	SUGAR	PROTEIN	SALT
LORRAINE'S RECIPE	203 Kcal	11.7g	6.8g	3.3g	4.2g	0.01g
COMPARISON RECIPE	227 Kcal	15.4g	9.5g	3.7g	3.4g	0.27g

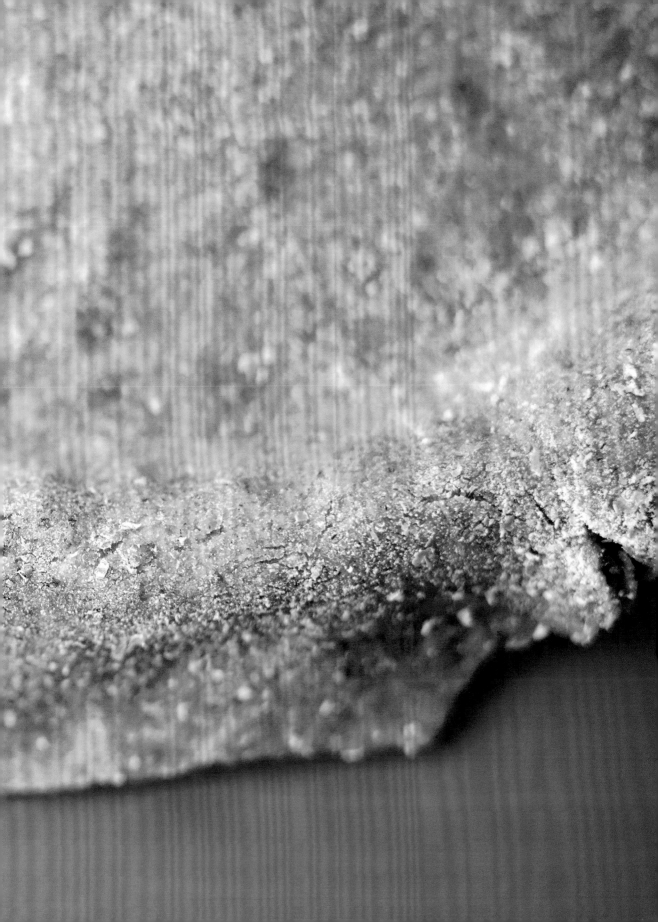

SWEET SHORTCRUST SPELT PASTRY

What is spelt all about, then? It is an ancient grain derived from wheat, and is full of goodness and good stuff. I find it easier to work with than regular flour; it feels softer somehow and I love the nutty taste it has once baked. Give it a whirl, buy a bag and share it with your friends. It might just become your new baking favourite!

Makes
400g pastry

Equipment
Large bowl or food processor

225g white spelt flour (wholemeal or plain flour will also work), plus extra for dusting
75g unsalted butter
1 tbsp caster sugar
1 egg
1 tbsp water

Put all of the ingredients in a food processor and blitz them until the mixture begins to clump together.

Alternatively, to make by hand, put the flour and butter into a large bowl. Pick up bits of the mixture with the tips of your fingers and rub your thumbs into your fingers to blend the ingredients together, allowing them to fall back into the bowl. Keep doing this until the mixture resembles fine breadcrumbs. Stir the sugar through. Lightly beat the egg in a small bowl and stir into the crumbs really well with a small knife until it starts to form lumps. Add the water to bring it together.

Dust a clean surface with a little flour. Tip the dough onto the surface and squidge the mixture with your hands so it comes together in a ball.

This pastry needs to be rolled out straight away, so roll it out to two-thirds of the thickness of a £1 coin and line your flan ring (or whatever you are using) with it. You can then pop it in the fridge for up to 24 hours. Because of the low butter and water content in the pastry and the nature of the flour, if it is left to sit the flour will 'drink' up all of the liquid and then when you come to roll it out, it will just crack and break – this is why it is best to roll it out and use it straight away.

(PER SERVING – 8 PORTIONS)	ENERGY	FAT	SAT FAT	SUGAR	PROTEIN	SALT
LORRAINE'S RECIPE	180 Kcal	9.1g	5.1g	1.9g	4.9g	0.03g
COMPARISON RECIPE	212 Kcal	11g	6g	8.2g	3.5g	0.17g

LOWER-FAT SPREAD WHOLEMEAL 'SHORTCRUST' PASTRY

This recipe gives a pastry that is light and not rich with flavour, but is a great healthy alternative to a butter pastry. I am not usually a fan of using light spreads, but so many people have asked me to do one, so here it is!

Makes
350g pastry

Equipment
Large bowl or food processor

225g wholemeal flour, plus extra
    for dusting
100g light olive oil spread
Pinch of salt
2–3 tbsp water

Put all of the ingredients (using 2 tablespoons of the water) into a food processor and blitz them up until the mixture starts to form clumps. Use a knife to scrape off any bits of dough that are stuck to the sides and the bottom of the food processor and blitz again. If the dough is still very dry, just add the remaining tablespoon of water. Try not to add too much otherwise the pastry will just shrink when it bakes and be very grey and tasteless.

Alternatively, to make by hand, put the flour, olive oil spread and salt into a large bowl. Pick up bits of the mixture with the tips of your fingers and rub your thumb into your fingers to blend the ingredients together, allowing it to fall back into the bowl. Keep doing this until the mixture resembles fine breadcrumbs. Stir 2 tablespoons of the water in really well with a small knife until it starts to form lumps. Add the remaining tablespoon of water, if necessary, to bring it together. Scrape the side of the bowl down in case some of the pastry has stuck there.

Dust a clean surface with a little flour. Tip the dough onto the surface and squidge the mixture with your hands so it comes together in a ball. Knead lightly for a few seconds until smooth and then wrap with cling film. Refrigerate for 20 minutes to relax and firm up.

Remove the dough from the fridge and use as needed.

(PER SERVING – 8 PORTIONS)	ENERGY	FAT	SAT FAT	SUGAR	PROTEIN	SALT
LORRAINE'S RECIPE	135 Kcal	5.4g	1.5g	0.6g	3.7g	0.13g
COMPARISON RECIPE	184 Kcal	11.7g	7.1g	0.65g	3.5g	0.2g

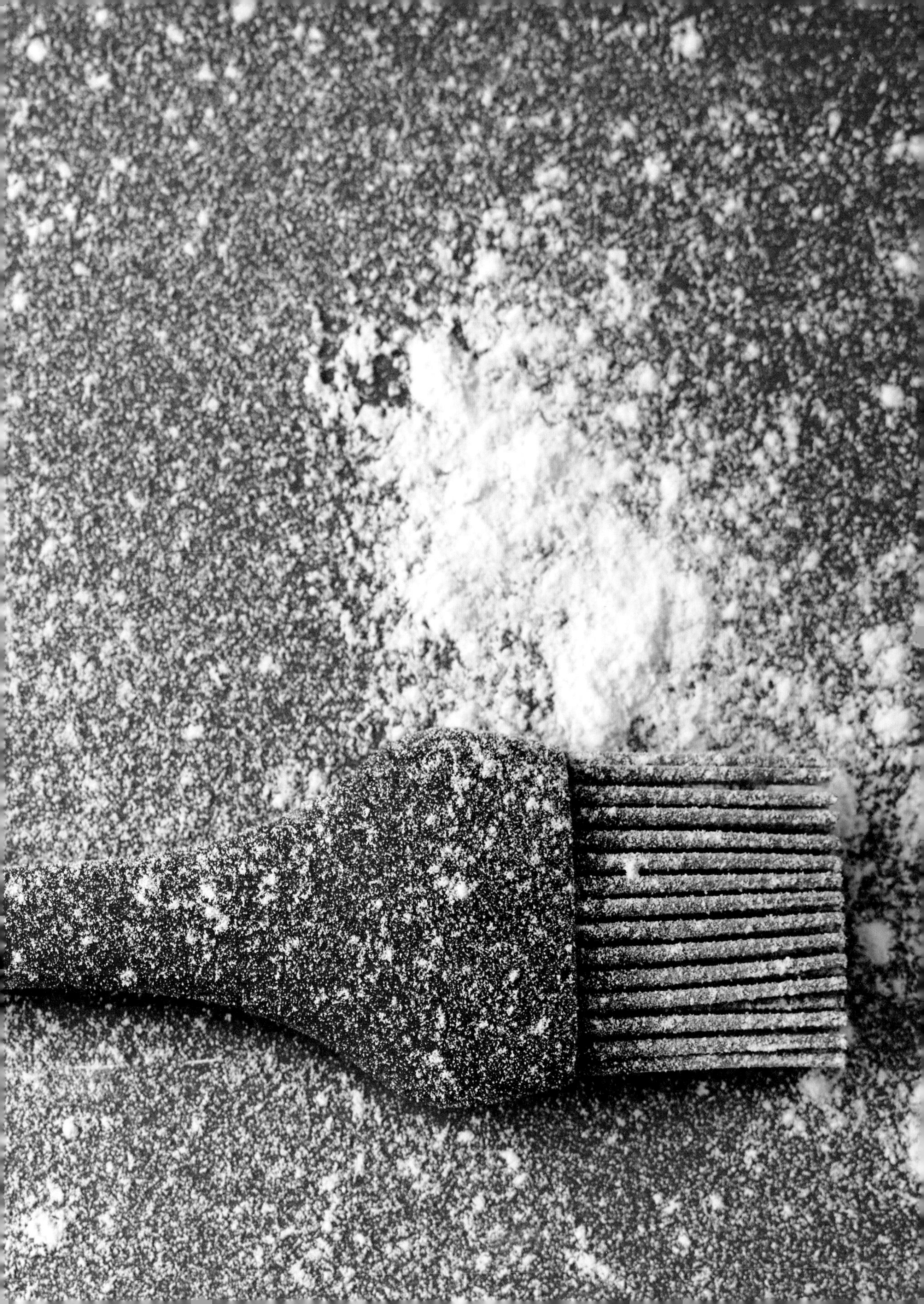

THYME WHOLEMEAL PASTRY

It is lovely to see the flecks of dark green in this pastry when it is baked, but it is hard to get the flavour to come through. It's great to call it thyme pastry, but the flavour has to be there too. So, after a few attempts, I found that 1 tablespoon of dried thyme (I know it sounds a lot, but it does work) or 2 tablespoons of fresh works well for this savoury, nutty, tasty tart pastry.

Makes
350g pastry

Equipment
Large bowl or food processor

225g wholemeal flour, plus extra for dusting
50g unsalted butter
1 tbsp dried thyme or 2 tbsp fresh thyme leaves
1 egg
1 tbsp water

Put all of the ingredients into a food processor and blitz them up until the mixture starts to form clumps.

Alternatively, to make by hand, put the flour and butter into a large bowl. Pick up bits of the mixture with the tips of your fingers and rub your thumb into your fingers to blend the ingredients together, allowing it to fall back into the bowl. Keep doing this until the mixture resembles fine breadcrumbs. Stir the thyme through. Lightly beat the egg in a small bowl and stir into the crumbs really well with a small knife until it starts to form lumps. Add the water to bring it together.

Either way, dust a clean surface with a little flour. Tip the dough onto the surface and squidge the mixture with your hands so it comes together in a ball.

This pastry needs to be rolled out straight away, so roll it out to two-thirds of the thickness of a £1 coin and line your flan ring (or whatever you are using) with it. You can then pop it in the fridge for up to 24 hours. Because of the low butter and water content in the pastry and the nature of the flour, if it is left to sit the flour will 'drink' up all of the liquid and then when you come to roll it out, it will just crack and break – this is why it is best to roll it out and use it straight away.

(PER SERVING - 8 PORTIONS)	ENERGY	FAT	SAT FAT	SUGAR	PROTEIN	SALT
LORRAINE'S RECIPE	342 Kcal	15.1g	8.2g	1.5g	10.8g	0.07g
COMPARISON RECIPE	455 Kcal	27.9g	17.1g	1.4g	7.4g	0.59g

YUMSTERS WHOLEMEAL CHOUX PASTRY

I really, really wanted to make a chocolate choux. I just thought that double chocolate éclairs would be so, so nice. I used cocoa powder in place of some of the flour and the resulting choux was really not a nice thing to eat. Disgruntled, I went back to my pen and paper to think of another way to make these a little healthier. I took one of my choux recipes, threw a bit of wholemeal flour in there, more than halved the butter and replaced two of the eggs with two egg whites. And here it is...

Makes

About 475g choux paste

75g strong wholemeal bread flour
50g plain flour
Pinch of salt
50g unsalted butter
200ml cold water (from the tap)
2 eggs
2 egg whites

Toss the flours and salt together in a small bowl and set aside.

Put the butter into a medium non-stick pan along with the cold water. Heat gently until the butter has melted and then turn the heat up to bring to the boil. As soon as it starts boiling, take it off the heat and add the flour mixture. Beat the mixture like mad, really giving it some elbow grease. It will start to come away from the sides of the pan. Once it has reached this stage, set it aside for a few minutes until it has cooled down to body temperature. If the eggs are added when the choux panade is too hot, the eggs may scramble, giving an eggy taste and texture to the finished product. Not to mention the choux may not rise enough during baking.

Once the choux has cooled a little, add one of the eggs and beat the mixture hard with a wooden spoon to incorporate. At first the mixture will seem quite slippy and that there is not a hope of it ever coming together nicely, but keep going and it will become uniform. This really does take a bit of hard work, but will be worth it for the delicious choux pastry at the end!

Add the next egg and beat well, getting all of the mixture from the 'corners' of the pan mixed in. Next, add one egg white, beating hard again to mix it all in. Then, repeat with the remaining egg white. Take a scoop of mixture up on the spoon and tilt and shake it slightly. The mixture should dollop off in a 'reluctant' dropping consistency.

Use straight away.

(PER SERVING – 12 PORTIONS)	ENERGY	FAT	SAT FAT	SUGAR	PROTEIN	SALT
LORRAINE'S RECIPE	123 Kcal	7g	3.7g	0.3g	4.6g	0.14g
COMPARISON RECIPE	165 Kcal	12.6g	7g	0.25g	4g	0.15g

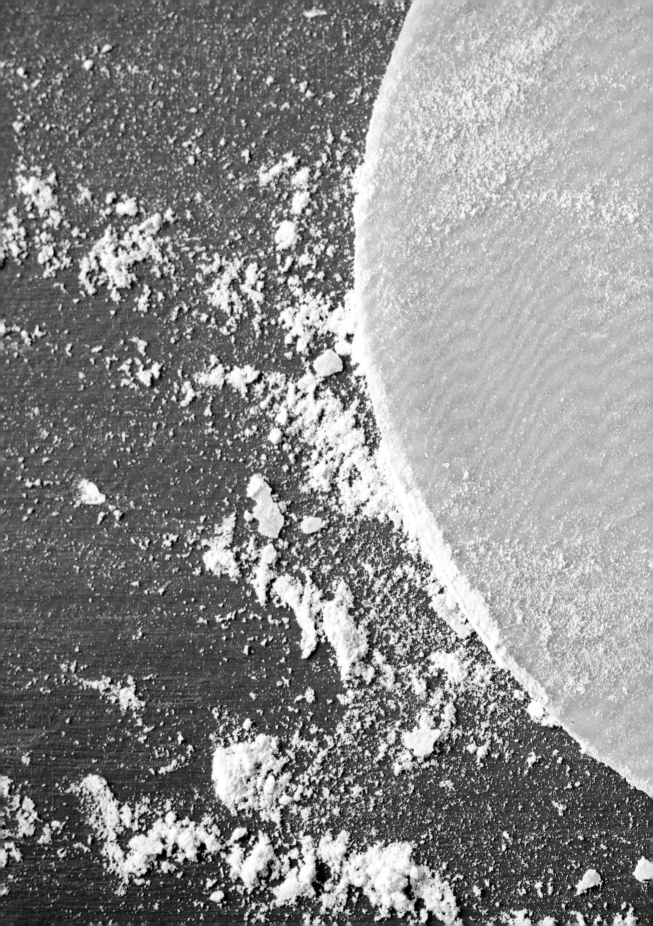

GARLIC & CHIVE MAYONNAISE

I hope you don't mind me slotting in a couple of cheeky non-low-fat recipes. I ended up with so many leftover egg yolks when baking the light cakes and bakes that I felt compelled to pop in a couple of delicious recipes that would use them up (see also Crème Anglaise on page 272). In the past, I have done the shop-bought mayonnaise a disservice. I gave my daughter tuna mayonnaise so many times in her youth that even now when it is mentioned my poor child breaks out in a sweat and feels sick to her stomach. Much as I love the stuff in the jar, this home-made version is a delicious alternative. It takes a bit of patience to get it just right but it is so rewarding served with eggs, or as a dip for some Baked Potato Crispies (see page 87).

Makes

500g

Equipment

Food processor

2 garlic cloves, peeled
4 egg yolks
1 tsp yellow mustard
1 tbsp white wine vinegar
500ml olive oil or vegetable oil
Small bunch of chives,
   very finely chopped
Salt and freshly ground black
   pepper

Take 1 garlic clove and squish it flat. Then add a pinch of sea salt and, using the flat side of a knife, keep pressing the garlic until it forms a paste. It should be nice and smooth. (You can use a garlic press to make this job easier if you want to!)

Pop the garlic in the bowl of a food processor. Add the egg yolks, mustard and vinegar and pulse it a few times. Then, with the blender running, add the oil in a really thin, steady stream. It is important to add it like this so that the yolks and the oil can mix properly. If it is added too quickly, the mixture will not properly combine. Keep adding the oil in this way gradually until the mayonnaise is nice and thick. Then taste it and season as necessary.

Stir through the chopped chives and serve straight away.

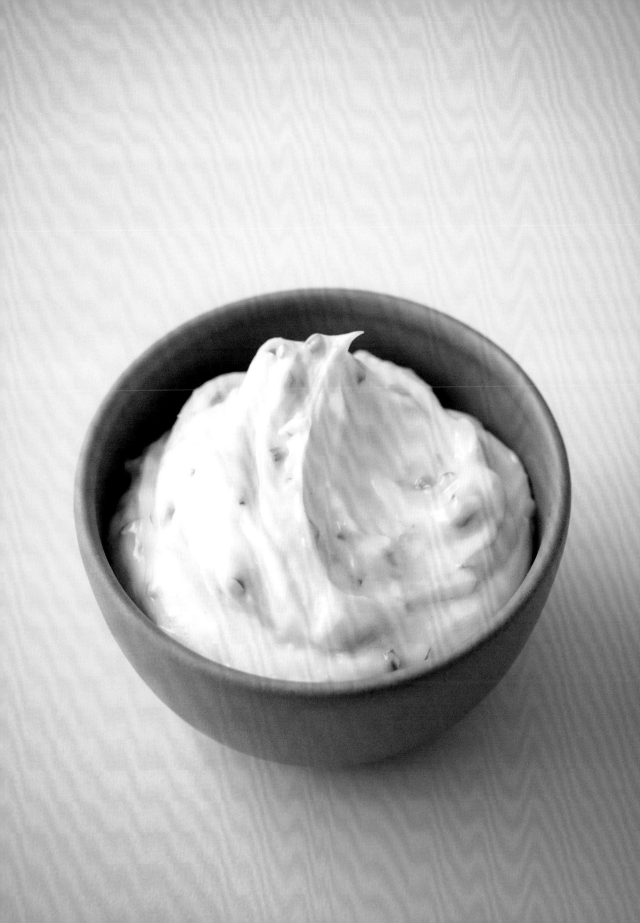

CRÈME ANGLAISE, OR REALLY POSH CUSTARD

Another cheeky non-low-fat recipe, perfect for using up leftover egg yolks if you've been busy baking my lighter cakes! Birds Eye was always in the cupboard during my youth. I say 'in the cupboard', because for the life of me I cannot remember it ever coming out of its place on the shelf just left of the now re-named 'afro-haired jam man in stripy trousers' and right of the unopened jar of Shipman's fish paste. At school custard was a tawdry affair, all pomp and no circumstance and plenty of lumps. It was not until my first trip to my all-time favourite restaurant, Le Gavroche, the Roux brothers' gem nestled in the glamour of Mayfair that I changed my mind about custard. This is a nod to that fine day, when I discovered that custard could indeed be a thing of beauty – silky, smooth and full of delicate, rich flavour.

Serves

4–5 (makes 600ml)

500ml semi-skimmed milk
6 medium egg yolks
Seeds of 1 vanilla pod or a couple
  of drops of vanilla extract
110g caster sugar

Put the milk into a pan and heat gradually until it is just steaming, then take it off the heat. Meanwhile, put the eggs, vanilla and sugar in a bowl and mix together well. Gradually pour the milk over the egg mixture, stirring all the time. As you will be stirring with one hand and pouring with the other, the bowl may slip around a bit. If this happens, just fold up a tea towel and place it underneath the bowl. This will keep the bowl firm.

Put a sieve over a bowl and set aside. (You will need this for later.)

Once the milk is all mixed up with the egg mixture, pour it into a heatproof bowl sitting on top of a pan of simmering water (making sure the bottom of the bowl doesn't touch the water). Cook really gently, stirring all the time with a wooden spoon until the mixture thickens slightly and coats the back of the spoon. The mixture will not go really thick, as crème anglaise is quite a thin custard, but it will start to get slightly thicker. Once it reaches this stage, pour it through the sieve into another bowl. (The key is not to overheat it, otherwise it turns into sweet scrambled eggs!)

Now pour into a jug and serve.

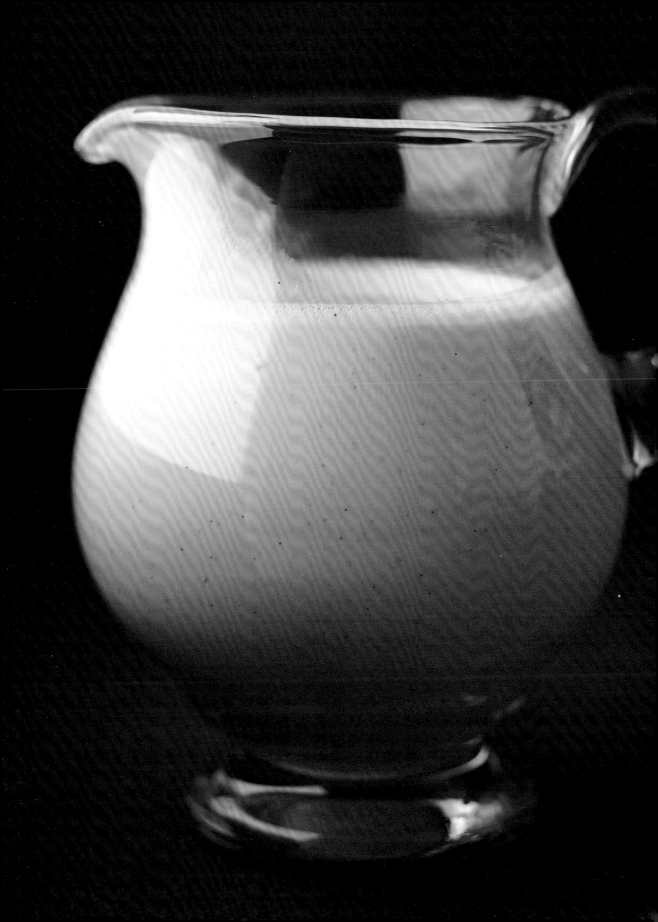

REMEMBER THAT NOT GETTING
WHAT YOU WANT IS SOMETIMES
A WONDERFUL STROKE OF LUCK.
DALAI LAMA

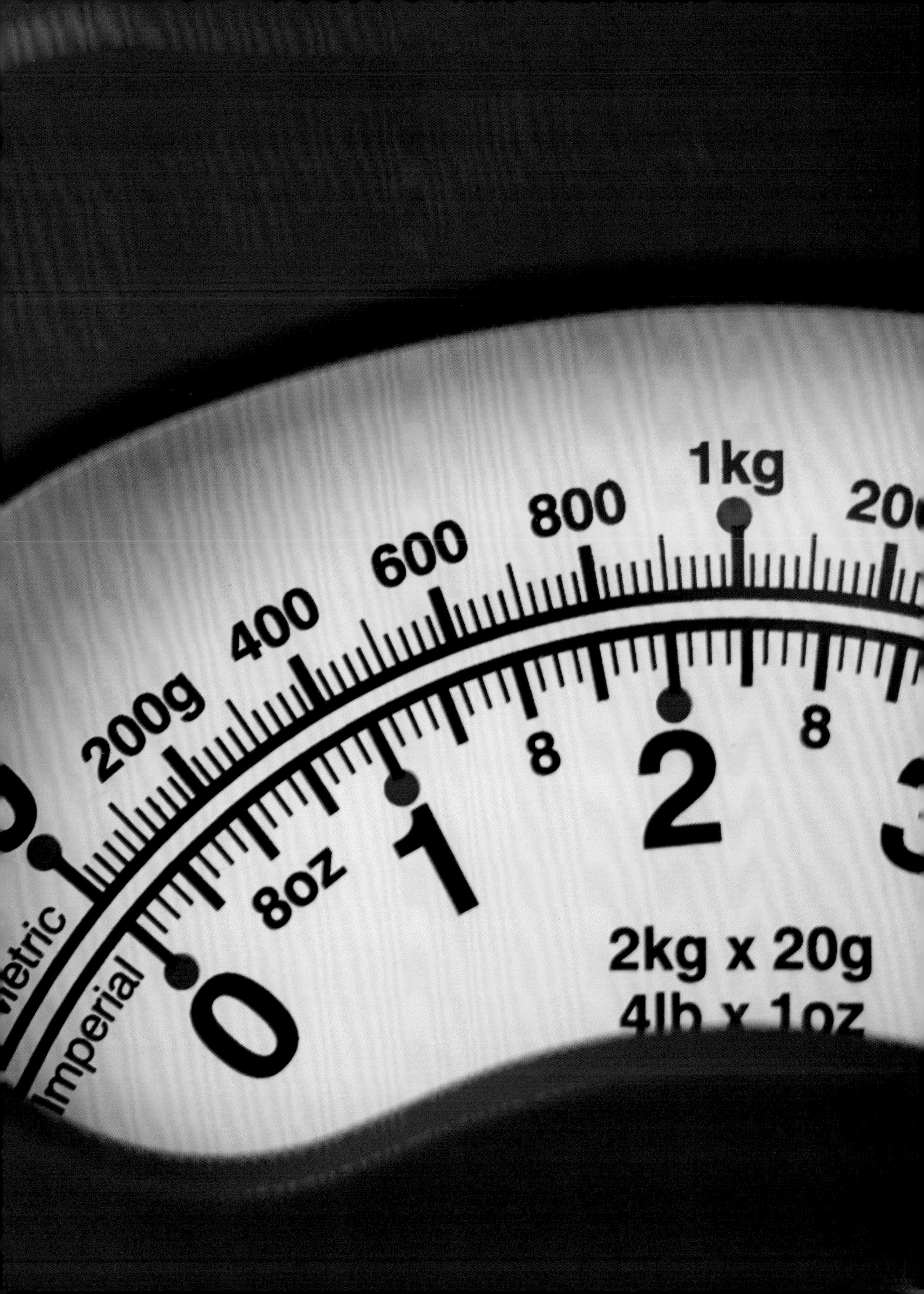

1kg

800

600

400

200g

Metric

Imperial

200

8

8oz

8

0   1   2   3

2kg x 20g
4lb x 1oz

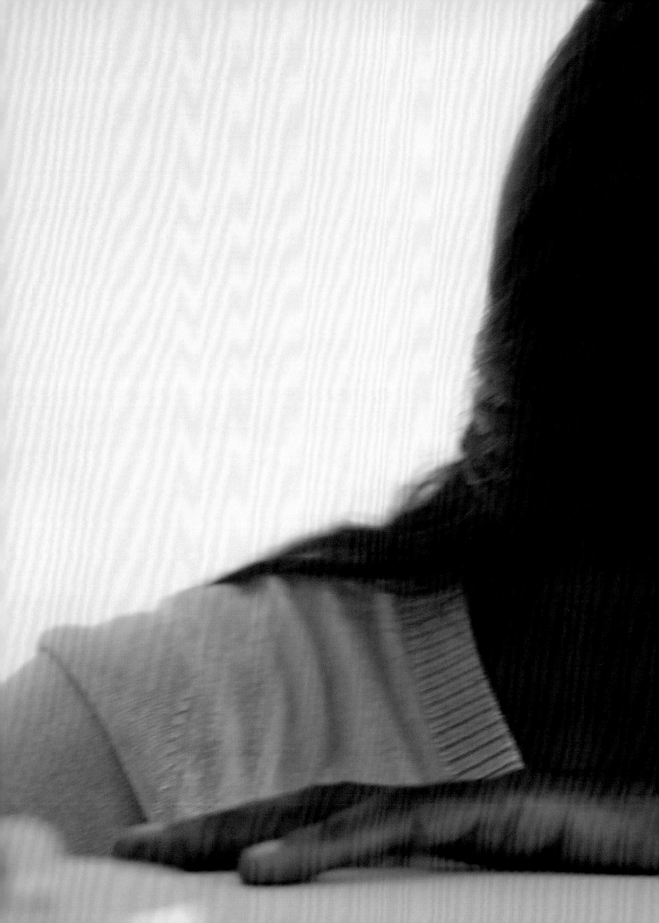

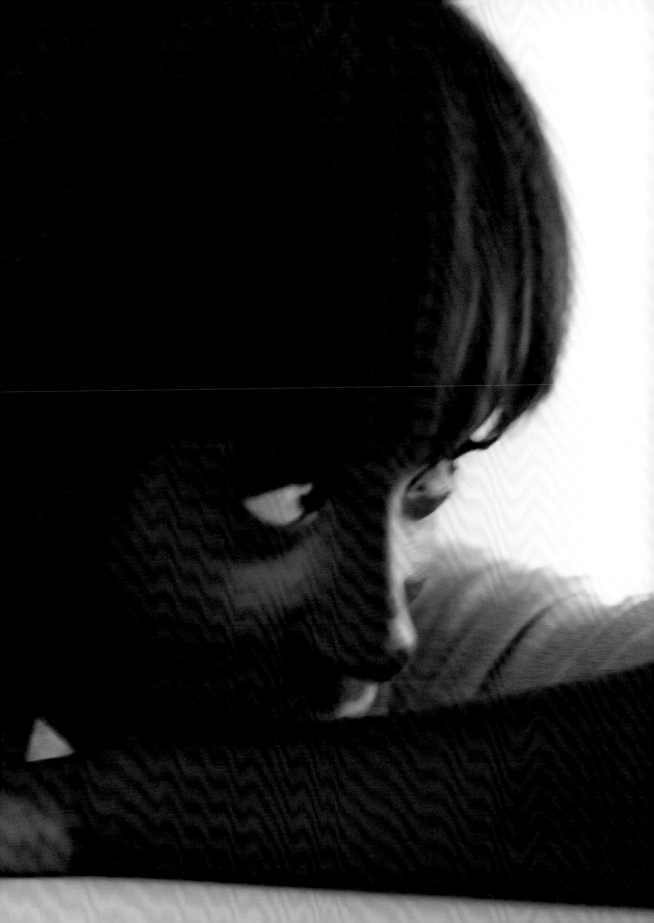

INDEX

ACKNOWLEDGEMENTS

I was sitting at home, faffing about on the internet as you do, looking at all manner of cakes and bakes and then an idea popped into my head. What about cakes that still taste the same but are a little bit lighter? From that moment on I was all systems go, scurrying about speaking to my lovely publishers HarperCollins and a whole host of people in order to see this book come to fruition. I would like to thank those of you who have stood by me and helped me with this book, and my support system that continues to help me day by day as we all try to make it through in this mad, crazy and funny old world.

Thank you so much to the team at James Grant, who continue to help me day in and day out: Nicola Ibison, Mary Bekhait, Eugenie Furniss, Paul Worsley, Darren Worsley, Amy Newman, Karen Mills, Leon Harlow, Georgie White, Isabelle Gill, John Bower, Blaise McGowan and Riz Mansor.

The ever brilliant Sharon Hearne-Smith for her expertise in checking my recipes so efficiently and thoroughly and for propping me up during a slight crisis of confidence when my culinary self-esteem had hit a bit of a low.

The team at HarperCollins and those on the shoot for supporting my lighter way to bake whim and for their inspiration, imagination, tireless hard work and energy: Carole Tonkinson, Georgina Atsiaris, Martin Topping, Myles New, Katie Giovanni, Beatrice Ferrante, Tom Regester, Tony Hutchinson, Laura Nickoll, Kay Halsey, Fiona Hinton, Elsa Robson, Orlando Mowbray and Laura Lees.

Carlos Ferraz for styling me for the book with his magic-like hands for hair and make up.

My fabulous family: mum, dad, Jace, Kate, Fran, Rachel, Auntie Angela, Victoria and James and the very brilliant Ella.

Friends: Satya, Lia, Velma, Rodney, Maggie Draycott, Charlotte Mensah, Diana Waiss and all my friends who are always there for me through thick and thin.

Neil: I just want to say, thank you.

To followers on Twitter, Instagram and Facebook: your humour and information never cease to amaze me, thank you for your support.

And as always I would like to mention the charities that I am involved in and support, amongst them are: TACT Care, Rays of Sunshine, The Princes Trust, Barnardos, Sutton Community Farm, The British Association for Adoption and Fostering and the Tope Foundation. Here is to continued success for you all in 2014 and thanks for letting me be involved.

I have not seen you all enough in 2013, let's hope we can change that in '14.

Thank you so much
Lorraine.

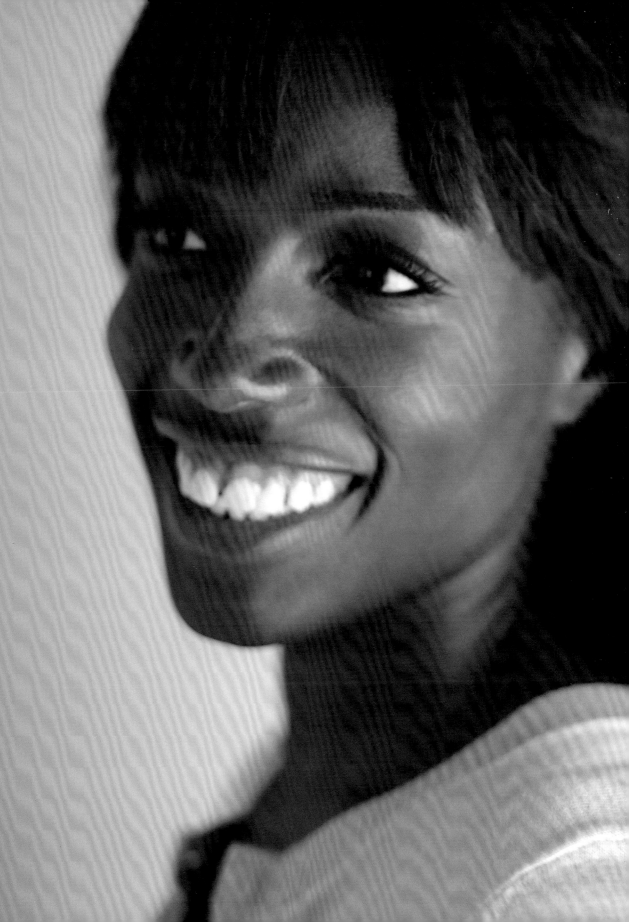